Ranking and Prioritization for Multi-indicator Systems

Environmental and Ecological Statistics

The Springer series **Environmental and Ecological Statistics** is devoted to the cross-disciplinary subject area of environmental and ecological statistics discussing important topics and themes in statistical ecology, environmental statistics, and relevant risk analysis. Emphasis is focused on applied mathematical statistics, statistical methodology, data interpretation and improvement for future use, with a view to advance statistics for environment, ecology, and environmental health, and to advance environmental theory and practice using valid statistics.

Each volume in the **Environmental and Ecological Statistics** series is based on the appropriateness of the statistical methodology to the particular environmental and ecological problem area, within the context of contemporary environmental issues and the associated statistical tools, concepts, and methods.

Previous Volumes in this Series

VOLUME 3
Modeling Demographic Processes In Marked Populations
Edited by David L. Thomson, Evan G. Cooch and Michael J. Conroy

VOLUME 4
Composite Sampling: A Novel Method to Accomplish Observational Economy in Environmental Studies
Ganapati P. Patil, Sharad D. Gore, Charles Taillie

VOLUME 5
Ranking and Prioritization for Multi-indicator Systems: Introduction to Partial Order Applications
Rainer Brüggemann and Ganapati P. Patil

For further volumes:
http://www.springer.com/series/7506

Rainer Brüggemann · Ganapati P. Patil

Ranking and Prioritization for Multi-indicator Systems

Introduction to Partial Order Applications

Springer

Rainer Brüggemann
Department of Ecohydrology
Leibniz Institute of Freshwater Ecology
and Inland Fisheries
Schöneiche, Germany
brg_home@web.de

Ganapati P. Patil
Center for Statistical Ecology
and Environmental Statistics
Pennsylvania State University
University Park, PA, USA
gpp@stat.psu.edu

ISBN 978-1-4614-2968-5 ISBN 978-1-4419-8477-7 (eBook)
DOI 10.1007/978-1-4419-8477-7
Springer New York Dordrecht Heidelberg London

Printed on acid-free paper

Springer is part of Springer Science+Business Media (www.springer.com)

To

Gertraud and Lalit

with love and affection

for your profound understanding

and patience

for this work

Rainer and GP.

Preface

Ranking issues are found everywhere! For example, chemicals can be as harmful to humans and the environment as they are useful. Therefore, it appears rather clear that only those chemicals should be used in the market that do not have an adverse impact on humans and the environment. How do we find out whether they are hazardous? There are many time-consuming and expensive investigations necessary to perform a risk assessment. Hence the question is: With which chemicals should we begin at first? Thus a ranking can be performed to give the more involved investigations a reasonable operating sequence. Once accepted that a ranking is needed, we discover that there is no intrinsic property of a chemical which tells us that it is hazardous. Still worse, one needs to know the hazard of chemicals in different scenarios. Hence, several aspects of a chemical need to be simultaneously considered. And thus the final and central question arises: How to rank chemicals characterized by several attributes.

Child well-being: In a report of UNICEF, a ranking of 21 rich nations was performed with respect to child well-being. For this purpose, six attributes were finally constructed by which the countries were ranked. It is clear that each of these six rankings need not be the same. Therefore, a composite indicator was defined, giving each of the six indicators the same weight. How far is this justified? What influence does this kind of aggregation have on the final result? Italy, for example, could get a better position if the indicator "family" would get more weight on the index. How can we analyze the role of weights?

Integrity of watersheds: Scientists of the Atlantic Slope Consortium (ASC) developed three levels of indicators to describe the health of watersheds. The indicators of the three levels increase in quality and accuracy of the data as well as the amount of cost and efforts needed to obtain the data. An important question is about how well level 1 or level 2 indicators perform compared with level 3 indicators. Partial order can help with this question.

Surface water management strategies: High concentration of nutrients in surface waters is of much concern for environmental protection agencies. What could be done to improve the situation? Clearly one has to study the release paths by which nutrients enter the surface waters. Then one has to develop strategies to control these and limit the emissions into surface waters. How well do such strategies work? In a chapter, we analyze 15 management strategies developed to reduce the concentration of nitrogen in the surface waters of the river. Each strategy is characterized by eight indicators according to the path through which nitrogen enters the surface water. Is there a best strategy? Can we compare, for example, rural and technical strategies? Unfortunately they turn out to be incomparable when partial order is applied. However, we use tools to facilitate the comparison without having to develop weights for all the eight indicators.

In this monograph, we discuss the following main topics of ranking, applying partial order theory:

1. Starting from a data matrix, partial order analysis renders methods to get insights into ranking without crunching the indicators by subjective weights into a composite indicator.
2. Partial order in terms of formal concept analysis renders knowledge about ordinal implication structures inherent in the data matrix.
3. Attributes may serve as proxies for a certain abstract concept. We analyze how well these attributes describe this unknown nevertheless desired concept.
4. Compared with composite indicators, partial order analysis enables comparability knowledge discovery.

These topics need a broad base and this book attempts to provide that. It is not a mathematical textbook about partial order in general but rather discusses how far simple partial order methods can be useful for the ordinal analysis of data matrices. Therefore, this monograph provides in the first 10 chapters axioms of partial order and some basic material, for example, consequences of "crisscrossing" of data profiles, the role of aggregations of the indicators, and the powerful method of formal concept analysis. The interested reader will learn how to apply fuzzy methods in partial order analysis and what "antagonistic indicator" means.

An exclusive chapter dwells on the concepts through some illustrative case studies. For example, we apply fuzzy partial order methods on biomanipulation in lakes. We consider chemicals and compare regions with respect to their pollution. We ask what to do to improve the ecological status of communes. Management strategies are compared to help improve the water quality in a river basin. One illustrative case study is concerned with the quality of information services for drinking water quality and another one with the human environment interface index. The role of a fish species for ranking creeks in a wetland is discussed, and we render how a Hasse diagram "sees" the ecological role of this fish species.

Ranking of complex, multifaceted items is often done by means of composite indicators. So, nowadays and we think in the future, composite indicators will be constructed and used more and more. Composite indicators tend to sit between advocacy (when they are used to draw attention to an issue) and analysis (when they are used to capture complex multidimensional phenomena), to quote Saltelli. Using composite indicators, objects of interest can be compared and an important application is to deduce through the scalar values of the composite indicators a ranking of the objects.

We would like our reader to know of partial order in this connection. Partial order theory is a discipline associated with graph theory and discrete mathematics. Partial order theory is the theory by which objects, characterized by multiple indicators, can be compared and ordered. Partial order as the theory of order is applied to the set of objects and it delivers insights which result in appropriate ranking of objects.

We can derive a measure by which the set of indicators can be checked for its appropriateness and completeness as a proxy for a non-measurable nevertheless important aim. The composite indicator depends on the functional form and especially if a linear combination is selected, it depends on the weights. Independent of whether there is uncertainty about the functional form or the weights, partial order can derive subsets of objects whose relative rankings are invariant with respect to the functional form selected or the weights. In this connection, a key concept in partial order theory is that of a chain. Because of the averaging process in the weighted sum, the individual role of a single indicator cannot be easily traced back. Partial order theory offers some tools to overcome this difficulty. These tools are developed within the context of stepwise aggregation: Start with an indicator, add the next, and see what happens until the composite indicator is finally attained. The averaging process, may affect objects in different ways if weights are uncertain. Uncertainty concerning the weight values results in a rank interval indicative of ambiguity in the ranks of objects. Partial order theory provides an upper limit for the ranges of ranks of objects. We also conduct a Monte Carlo simulation in changing the weights and in observing the corresponding rank frequency distributions for the objects in response to the varied weights. The crucial role and the consequence of weights are well known. Therefore, we offer a method to deduce weights from the data matrix alone, where the rows are defined by the objects and the columns by the indicators. Partial order theory also offers several methods to obtain linear orders of objects (with or without ties). Therefore, one of these partial order methods could be selected if a ranking is desired that does not need to weight the indicators. We may even compare the ranking due to a composite indicator with that obtained from partial order theory, if there are no uncertainties.

Partial order can work even if the data matrix consists of indicators with different scaling levels. This kind of a situation occurs often in scientific fields where quantitative measures are difficult to obtain. Partial order, in its own right, delivers insights to understand the impacts of indicators on the objects in a multi-indicator system. Such results are important, especially when crunching the indicators into a composite indicator is not an option, as it was the case in a study of pollution. There the measurements of single indicators were so expensive that an averaging into a composite indicator was seen to be too disadvantageous.

The Hasse diagram, which is a graph theoretical visualization of a partially ordered object set, is an ideal tool if the number of objects is not too large. Striking feature in Hasse diagrams is the concept of incomparability, which appears if the order of objects due to one indicator contradicts the order of another indicator. Chains can be easily identified from a Hasse diagram. If the Hasse diagram is too messy to get chains by inspection, software tools help find chains. Many concepts can be motivated just by discussing them within a simple Hasse diagram but are still valid, even when the Hasse diagram loses its visual appeal, because it is too complex and messy.

We are thinking of a reader who is concerned with ranking in the broadest sense. So we have in our mind stakeholders, statisticians, scientists, and instructors. We hope to render for them a monograph helpful in the application of tools, insightful with theoretical considerations and motivated by a series of case studies for further applications.

Schöneiche, Germany Rainer Brüggemann
University Park, Pennsylvania Ganapati P. Patil

Acknowledgments

We are thankful to the United States National Science Foundation Project 0307010 for Digital Governance and Hotspot Geoinformatics of Detection and Prioritization for its support of parts of research that have been largely behind the preparation of this monograph.

We are also thankful to the NSF Working Group Project for Surveillance GeoInformatics for its support of the logistics of research and training workshops on topics inclusive of the monograph material.

We greatly appreciate the facilities of the Center for Statistical Ecology and Environmental Statistics in the Department of Statistics at the Pennsylvania State University, where most of the monograph work was carried out.

We thank Paola Annoni, Lars Carlsen, Sharad Joshi, Andrew Lawson, Wayne Myers, Jessica Newlin, and Barry Nussbaum for careful reading of the manuscript and for suggestions to improve its content and usefulness. We thank Shuhua for performing some calculations and Tushar Chaudhari for initial layout control. And Mary McCarty for taking care of it all.

Contents

About the Authors

Dr Rainer Brüggemann has studied chemistry in the Ludwig-Maximilians University, Munich (LMU). He got his PhD working on quantum chemistry. After a post-doc time in the Physikalisch-Chemischen Institut of the LMU, he joined a group performing risk assessment studies with respect to nuclear waste disposal sites in German salt domes (Technical University in Berlin). One of his specific tasks was to apply and to develop geochemical software in order to assess the composition of salt brines. He changed the position to work in the Helmholtz-Center, Munich (formerly, GSF – National Research Center for Environment and Health). There he was one of the authors of the evaluation software code for chemicals "E4CHEM." This code contains simulation models for transport processes of chemicals in the environment, an estimation module for release of chemicals in the technosphere and one for data estimation. To make optimal use of the simulation results, he introduced concepts of partial order theory.

Dr Brüggemann became the commissary leader of a group of scientists concerned with "Hazard Potentials of Environmental Chemicals." He went to the Leibniz-Institute of Freshwater Ecology and Inland Fisheries, Berlin. Since that time, he has been applying concepts of partial order in several fields of environmental sciences and chemistry. He is responsible for the partial order software WHASSE. He is writing the code PyHasse to map actual developments in partial order theory.

Dr Brüggemann has been a lecturer in different universities. His topics are mathematical modeling of chemical's fate and exposure as well as model concepts in ecotoxicology.

He has been a guest scientist in several international institutions.

He has initialized a series of workshops about partial order in environmental sciences and chemistry. He has published several books as author, editor, or co-editor. In total, there are more than 350 scientific publications.

Dr G.P. Patil is a distinguished professor of mathematical and environmental statistics emeritus in the Department of Statistics at the Pennsylvania State University and is a former visiting professor of biostatistics at Harvard University in the Harvard School of Public Health.

He has a PhD in mathematics, D.Sc. in statistics, one honorary degree in biological sciences, and another honorary degree in letters. He is a fellow of American

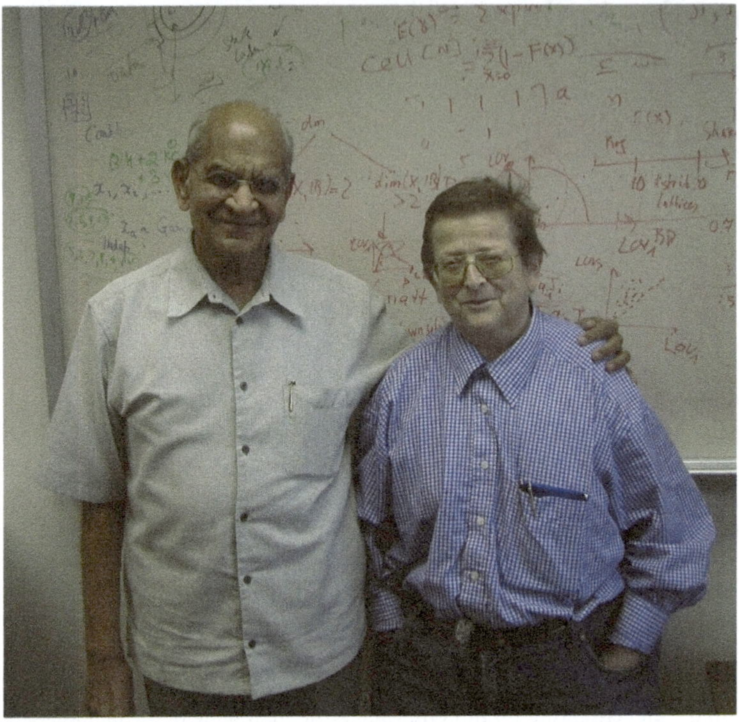

Dr Patil, *left*. Dr Brüggemann, *right*

Statistical Association, fellow of American Association of Advancement of Science, fellow of Institute of Mathematical Statistics, elected member of the International Statistical Institute, and founder fellow of National Institute of Ecology and Indian Society for Medical Statistics.

He has been a founder of Statistical Ecology Section of Ecological Society of America, a founder of Statistics and Environment Section of American Statistical Association, and a founder of the International Society for Risk Analysis, International Society for EcoHealth, Society for Syndromic Surveillance, and Digital Government Society of North America. He is founding editor-in-chief of the international journal *Environmental and Ecological Statistics* and founding director of the Penn State Center for Statistical Ecology and Environmental Statistics.

Dr Patil has published 30 volumes and 300 research papers. He has received several distinguished awards which include Distinguished Statistical Ecologist Award of the International Association for Ecology, Distinguished Achievement Medal for Statistics and the Environment of the American Statistical Association, Best Paper Award of the American Fisheries Society, and the Best Paper Award of the American Water Resources Association.

He was a member of the UNEP Science Advisory Panel with Nobel Laureate Mario Molina for the UNEP Division of Environmental Assessment and Early

Warning. He recently served on the NSF Panel for Homeland Security and Geographic Information Systems. He has been on the Science Advisory Board of the Spatial Accuracy Symposia. In the recent past, he has served on the EPA Science Advisory Board Regional Vulnerability Assessment Panel and chaired a UNEP Expert Panel for Human Environment Index.

Dr Patil has been recently principal investigator of a large NSF project on digital governance and surveillance hot spot geoinformatics for monitoring, etiology, early warning, and sustainable development. This has involved upper level set scan-based geospatial and spatiotemporal hot spot detection and partial order theory-based multicriteria ranking and prioritization with several national and international live case studies.

Chapter 1
Why Prioritization, Why Ranking

1.1 Motivating Issues and Situations

Let us begin with examples.

1.1.1 Chemicals

Chemicals can be as harmful to humans and the environment as they are useful. Therefore, it appears rather clear that only those chemicals should be used in the market that do not have an adverse impact on humans and the environment. The list of chemicals in the market of the European Union between 1971 and 1981 (EINECS list, http://chemicalwatch.com/927) contains 1,00,000 chemicals and almost 1,000 chemicals newly enter the market yearly, see, e.g., Bruggemann and Drescher-Kaden (2003), van Leeuwen et al. (1996), and Ahlers (1999). How do we find out whether they are hazardous? There are many time-consuming and expensive investigations necessary to perform a risk assessment. Hence the question is: With which chemicals to begin at first? Thus ranking is needed to give the more involved investigations a reasonable operating sequence (Newman, 1995). Once accepted that a ranking is needed, we discover that there is no intrinsic property of a chemical which tells us that it is hazardous. Still worse, one needs to know the hazard of chemicals in different scenarios. Hence, several aspects of a chemical need to be simultaneously considered. And thus the final and central question arises: How to rank chemicals characterized by several attributes?

Examples related to chemicals are given in Chapter 11.

1.1.2 Child Well-Being

In a report of UNICEF, a ranking of 21 rich nations was performed with respect to child well-being. For this purpose, 40 attributes were identified characterizing each country. From these 40 attributes, 6 were constructed by which the countries were ranked. It is clear that each of these six rankings need not be the same. Therefore, a

R. Brüggemann, G.P. Patil, *Ranking and Prioritization for Multi-indicator Systems*, Environmental and Ecological Statistics 5, DOI 10.1007/978-1-4419-8477-7_1,

composite indicator was defined, giving each of the six indicators the same weight. How far is this justified? What influence does this kind of aggregation have on the final result? Italy, for example, could get a better position if the indicator "family" would get more weight on the index. How can we analyze the role of weights? We discuss this in more detail in Chapter 12.

1.1.3 Regional Pollution

Geographical sites can be ranked with respect to their pollution. The natural question is then: What constitutes pollution, and how to measure it? For example, the Environmental Protection Agency (EPA) in Baden-Wuerttemberg, Germany, performed over years a careful monitoring study and included many possible targets, like herb layer and tree leaves. One may think of highly polluted regions as "high spots or hot spots." How to find them becomes an issue if there is a joint pollution by several chemical elements (see Chapter 11).

1.1.4 Integrity of Watersheds

Scientists of the Atlantic Slope Consortium (ASC) developed three levels of indicators to describe the health of watersheds. The indicators of the three levels increase in quality and accuracy of the data as well as the amount of cost and efforts needed to obtain the data. An important question is about how well level one or level two indicators perform compared with level three indicators. Partial order may help with this question (Chapter 14).

1.1.5 Surface Water Management Strategies

High concentration of nutrients such as phosphorus or nitrogen in surface waters is of much concern for environmental protection agencies. What could be done to improve the situation? Clearly one has to study the release paths by which nutrients enter the surface waters. Then one has to develop strategies to control these and limit the emissions into surface waters. How well do such strategies work? In Chapter 11, we analyze 15 management strategies developed to reduce the concentration of nitrogen in the surface waters of the river Elbe basin. Each strategy is characterized by eight indicators according to the path through which nitrogen enters the surface water. Is there a best strategy? Can we compare, for example, rural and technical strategies? Unfortunately they turn out to be incomparable when partial order is applied. However, we use tools to facilitate the comparison without having to develop weights for all the eight indicators.

1.2 Composite Indicators

Composite indicators are applied and constructed everywhere. Saltelli et al. (2008) characterize the issue of composite indicators as follows: "Composite indicators tend to sit between advocacy (when they are used to draw attention to an issue) and analysis (when they are used to capture complex multidimensional phenomena)." The construction of composite indicators (OECD, 2008) can be described in the following six steps:

(1) Aim: What is to be indicated?
(2) Do we have a measure for that aim? If not already measurable, one mostly needs a set of several scalar indicators as proxies to describe the aim. Depending on the inherent complexity of the aim and the information available, the set of indicators may be pretty large or small.
(3) How to select these indicators which can serve as a basis for construction of the composite indicator?
(4) If the initial set of indicators is large, then it is convenient as an interim step to aggregate them as per commonalities. These interim aggregations are called pillars, from which the composite indicator is built. How do we construct the pillars? How far do we accept contextual overlapping, i.e., that one indicator describes partially the same aspects as another? Beyond this, orientation aspects are assessed.
(5) How to obtain the composite indicator from the pillars? If conceptual simplicity prevails at this stage, one may combine the values of the pillars by a weighted sum.
(6) Since weights often come under scrutiny and controversy, it is a good practice to test the composite indicator for its robustness and sensitivity to results in response to varying weights.

For any of these six steps, concepts and methods are available to assess and use them. Besides expert judgments, univariate methods and multivariate methods are available. It is imperative that composite indicators deliver not only rankings but also satisfactory metrics.

1.3 What Does Partial Order Offer with the Composite Indicator Given?

In order to understand why and where partial order can be of help with the above steps, we provide a preliminary explanation of partial order: Partial order theory is a discipline associated with discrete mathematics and its subdiscipline, graph theory. In the case of a suitable binary relation between two objects, partial order theory is the theory by which objects, characterized by multiple indicators, can be compared and ordered, (see Chapter 2). The order relations can be displayed as in graph theory. Therefore, partial order and graph theories have many common topics.

Using composite indicators, objects of interest can be compared and an important application is to deduce through the scalar values of the composite indicators a ranking of the objects. Partial order as the theory of order is applied to the set of objects and it delivers insights into the six steps which result in ranking of objects. Besides helpful scientific insights into the above six steps, partial order renders results which help clarify the roles and consequences of indicators and their weights.

Let us now describe what partial order offers for the six steps:

(a) We can derive a measure by which the set of indicators can be checked for its appropriateness and completeness as a proxy for a non-measurable nevertheless important aim. We call this measure an "ambiguity graph" and introduce it in Chapter 4.
(b) The composite indicator depends on the functional form and especially if a linear combination is selected, it depends on the weights. Independent of whether there is uncertainty about the functional form or about the weights, partial order can derive subsets of objects whose relative rankings are invariant with respect to the functional form selected or the weights. In this connection, a key concept in partial order theory is that of a chain. We introduce the concept in Chapters 2 and 3. It appears almost everywhere in the monograph.
(c) Because of the averaging process in the weighted sum, the individual role of a single indicator cannot be easily traced back. Partial order theory offers some tools to overcome this difficulty. These tools are developed within the context of stepwise aggregation: Start with an indicator, add the next, see what happens until the composite indicator is finally attained. In Chapter 7, devoted to stepwise aggregation, several tools are explained, such as "comparability acquisition profile" (Patil, 2001).
(d) The averaging process, mentioned in (c), may affect objects in different ways if weights are uncertain. Uncertainty concerning the weight values results in a rank interval indicative of ambiguity in the ranks of objects. Partial order theory provides an upper limit for the ranges of ranks of objects ("rank ambiguity") due to a set of possible weight vectors (Bruggemann et al., 2001; Patil and Taillie, 2004). We discuss this point in Chapter 3 and we revisit this ambiguity concept in Chapter 7. There, we conduct a Monte Carlo simulation in changing the weights and in observing the corresponding rank frequency distributions for the objects in response to the varied weights.
(e) The crucial role and consequence of weights are well known. Therefore, we offer a method to deduce weights from the data matrix alone, where the rows are defined by the objects and the columns by the indicators (Patil, 2001). We discuss this method in a case study about watersheds in Chapter 14.
(f) Partial order theory also offers several methods to obtain linear orders of objects (with or without ties). Therefore, one of these partial order methods could be selected if a ranking is wanted that does not need to weight the indicators. One may even compare the ranking due to a composite indicator with that obtained from partial order theory if there are no uncertainties. We discuss how to obtain a ranking from partial order in Chapter 9 and how to compare different partial orders in a rather general setting in Chapter 10.

Table 1.1 Data matrix with indicators of different scaling levels

	q_1 (continuous in concept)	q_2 (linguistic description)	q_3 (ordinal indicator)
x_1	0.3	Good	2
x_2	0.35	Medium	3
x_3	0.2	Bad	1

(g) Partial order can work even if the data matrix consists of indicators of different scaling levels as shown below. This kind of a situation occurs often in scientific fields where quantitative measures are difficult to obtain (Table 1.1).

Chapters 3, 4, 7, 9, and 10 and to some extent Chapter 14 help enlighten with steps (1)–(6) to construct composite indicators.

1.4 What Does Partial Order Offer More Generally?

Partial order, in its own right, delivers results, some of which may not be restrictive to steps (1–6) but nevertheless help understand the impacts of indicators on the objects in a multi-indicator system.

Such results are important, especially when crunching the indicators into a composite indicator is not an option, as it was the case in a study of pollution in a state of Germany. There the measurements of single indicators were so expensive that an averaging into a composite indicator was seen to be too disadvantageous (see Chapter 11).

The Hasse diagram, which is a graph theoretical visualization of a partially ordered object set, is an ideal tool if the number of objects is not too large. Striking feature in Hasse diagrams is the concept of incomparability, which appears if the order of objects due to one indicator contradicts the order of another indicator. Chains can be easily identified from a Hasse diagram. If the Hasse diagram is too messy to get chains by inspection, software tools help find chains. Many concepts can be motivated just by discussing them within a simple Hasse diagram but are still valid even when the Hasse diagram loses its visual appeal, because it is too complex and messy. These important concepts follow.

1.5 Important Questions and Concepts Involving Partial Order

(a) *Where is an object, and why is it where it is?* This question aims at the position of an object in a Hasse diagram, identifies its minimum rank, its maximum rank, and the objects which are incomparable to the object under consideration. Subsets of objects can be characterized by their pattern of indicator values as shown in Fig. 1.1. There a Hasse diagram is constructed of regions in a state in

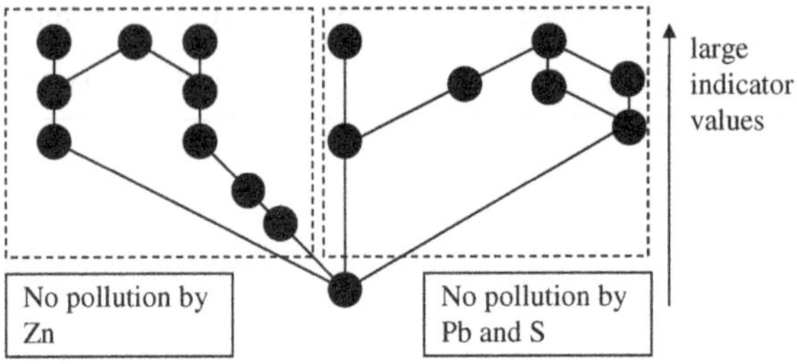

Fig. 1.1 Example of a Hasse diagram, where parts of it can be characterized by certain indicator values

Germany, polluted by lead (Pb), cadmium (Cd), zinc (Zn), and sulfur (S). The vertices are representing the regions and the lines comparabilities.

In many cases, formal concept analysis (Chapter 8), which is part of partial order theory, provides a powerful visualization where the information about the indicator values and the positions of objects is simultaneously available. Formal concept analysis allows a "symmetric analysis" of the data matrices (Annoni and Bruggemann, 2008).

(b) *Which indicators influence the positions of objects?* Although this question is not in the foreground of the construction of composite indicators, the sensitivity of indicators to a Hasse diagram and hence to the objects in it throws also a light on the selection and interpretation of the indicators. For example, in a study about fish communities in wetlands, it turns out that the indicator describing the population of a certain fish species has a high impact on the Hasse diagram displaying the impacts of the indicator on the positions of the objects. This is directly related to the strategies of that fish species to survive under competition and bad water quality.

(c) *How to model ordinally – a fuzzy approach in partial order?* Partial orders appear in many facets, depending on how the order relation is defined. As we use partial order to rank objects described by a tuple of indicator values, we must use an appropriate order relation, the product order (Chapter 2). Often data matrices contain indicators continuous in concept so that even small numerical differences can influence the partial order. In Chapter 6 we discuss several techniques to perform "ordinal modeling," i.e., how far we can ignore numerical differences which seem to be too small for being interpreted as an order relation. An important concept therefore is that of fuzzy partial order. A fuzzy membership function is introduced which describes as to how to rate an object above or below another even when their data profiles crisscross. We apply fuzzy partial order to a data matrix concerning the effects of biomanipulation and we see how biological competitions among phytoplankton species suppress the basic information about biomanipulation.

So, our answer to "why partial order?" can be summarized as follows.

Partial order delivers analytical tools to better interpret and understand how from a multi-indicator system a composite indicator is built and what can be said about relative rankings of objects without the need of specifying weights or even the functional form of aggregation.

This monograph describes the partial order concepts, methods, and tools within the first ten chapters and applies them to the case studies in subsequent five chapters. We now consider some choice examples of interesting issues and questions.

1.6 Pertinent Issues and Questions

1.6.1 Weights and Indicator Values

Could Italy improve its ranking just by scrutinizing the weights? We render in Chapter 12 how the indicators of interest can be found and that in the case of Italy a higher weight for the indicator "family" would improve the position of Italy in the final ranking. Can Germany do the same and try to be better in the final ranking than Netherlands? Our analysis shows: No chance! Germany must improve its values of the indicators. Change in weights will not help. Does Germany have a chance to get a better ranking position in comparison to some other nations? Yes, since Germany is incomparable to some other nations, changing weights would influence the final ranking position of Germany relative to these nations. Must we rely on different trials of weights to see what can happen? No, since we can show that the possible ranking interval of each object depends on a simple characteristic of the partial order as discussed in Chapter 3.

1.6.2 Problems with Averaging

Within a study of bridge stability crossing channels, bridge 17 got a worse evaluation in comparison with bridge 57. As proxies for "bridge stability," indicators are defined which have influence on the bridge stability, such as channel alignment, local channel characteristics, and bank stability.

Analysis by partial order tools shows that because bridge 17 is incomparable to bridge 57, bridge 17 must have at least one indicator where bridge 17 is better than bridge 57, which is classified as an "excellent" bridge/stream system. We can now identify which property makes bridge site 17 better than bridge site 57: It is the channel alignment. Although the ordinal way of consideration of objects implies loss of some information, we see that some important information is not lost. The remaining information is crucial. It is, however, unavailable if only the composite indicator is considered.

1.6.3 Associations and Implications of Indicators

During the investigation of the environmental performance indicator (EPI), the interest lies in how differently nations of different regions of the world are ranked. As

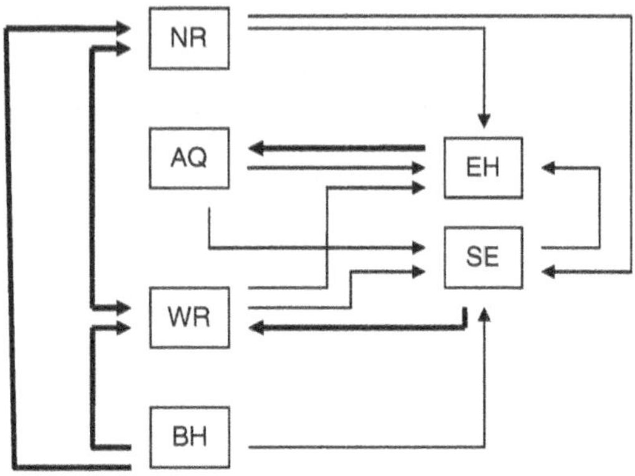

Fig. 1.2 Association and implication network among the indicators of the EPI study. The *simple arrows* represent associations or implications found for nations of the EU and the *bold arrows* represent those of the nations of ASEAN

examples, we selected ASEAN and EU nations. Partial order applied to the nations as objects does not yield useful results. There is too high a degree of incomparabilities. This throws light on why weights are needed, but at the same time on problems with them. On the one hand, without weights a ranking would mean to fight losing battles because of too many incomparabilities. However, on the other hand, any incomparability implies a compensation: Good values in one indicator may average out bad values of other indicators and vice versa in getting a composite indicator.

So instead, we studied the association and implication structure of the indicators of the ASEAN group and EU and we found rather different associations (see Fig. 1.2, where we present the results as a joint network).

Note that in ASEAN the resource aspect is more pronounced (natural resources are associated with water resources and vice versa), whereas in the EU, this striking fact is not observed. Details, see Chapter 15.

1.6.4 Prioritization and Ranking for a Subset of Objects ("Hot Spots")

We may not always be interested in a comparative analysis of all objects of an object set. Instead we may want to put our fingers on those objects which have, for example, high values in some indicators. Such objects may serve as candidates for a more detailed scrutiny. It could be, for example, because we want to study them further by using more information about them. A very simple transformation applied to any single indicator may do that job. However, we have a multi-indicator system and a partial order in our hand and we must ask: Is the transformation compatible with the partial order and how does the simultaneous application of the transformation affect the objects? In Chapter 6, we show that the transformation is compatible with the partial order and derive an equation which estimates the fraction of relevant and irrelevant objects.

1.6.5 *How Do We See the Role of Indicators in Terms of Single Objects?*

How does the minimum rank of an object vary with the cumulation of indicators in a canonical sequence? In Chapter 4, we see that some characteristic partial order quantities of an object, such as its number of incomparable elements or the number of elements below it, vary with the canonical sequence and apply these ideas to child well-being (Chapter 12), bridge stability (Chapter 13), and watersheds (Chapter 14). As can be expected, some objects will vary strongly, whereas some others may not.

1.6.6 *Proximity Analysis*

For a robustness study of a composite indicator relative to weights, a distance measure is needed. We introduce proximity analysis (Chapter 10) and apply it to watersheds, where three levels of sophistication are considered. It is of interest to know as to how far indicators of a level of low degree of sophistication can serve as proxies for indicators of a level of high sophistication. We show that the low-cost indicators (level one) are better proxies for high-cost indicators (level three) than are level two indicators.

1.6.7 *What to do with supervised classification?*

Often the object set is partitioned into disjoint subsets using external information. We need to compare the resulting classes with each other. In order to do this, we employ concepts of dominance and separability (Restrepo et al., 2008). Whereas dominance is conceptually a generalization of an order relation, separability measures the degree of incomparabilities among two disjoint object subsets (Chapter 5).

Dominance: A typical question is: What are the dominances among European nations, classified due to their geographical positions, when, for example, the Human Environment Index (HEI) is considered. The dominance analysis shows that nations of south Europe are dominating almost all the others. This kind of a question with its potential to simplify complex Hasse diagrams serves as an attractive application of dominance analysis.

Separability: If the separability gets by definition its maximum value of 1, a natural question arises as to which indicators are responsible for the fact that no object of one object set is comparable with an object of another object set. If, for example, it turns out that regions of high agricultural density are separated from those of high industrial activity when pollution is of concern, then the question is: Which pollution indicators are responsible for the separatedness? We introduce an important concept, namely that of antagonistic

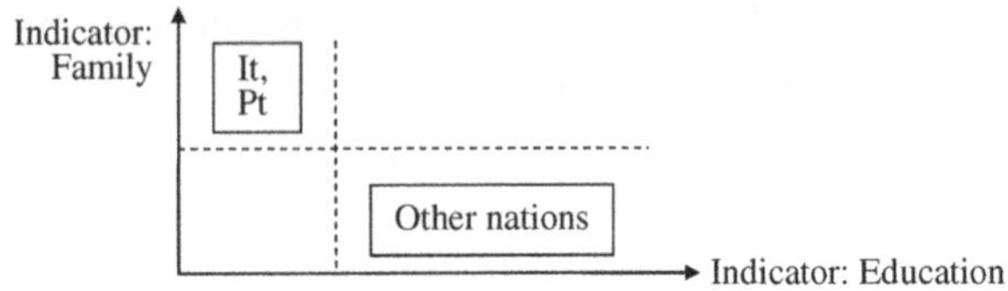

Fig. 1.3 Indicators "family" and "education" are antagonistic with respect to the set {Italy (It), Portugal (Pt)} and the set of other nations

indicators: A minimum set of indicators needed to explain the separation of two object subsets. In Chapter 12, child well-being, the indicators "family" and "education" are antagonistic in their role of explaining the separation of two subsets of nations. Italy and Portugal are good in "family" whereas less good in "education." For the multitude of other nations, the reverse is true (Fig. 1.3).

1.6.8 Visualization in Multi-indicator Systems

Statistics provides powerful methods to visualize even large data matrices. Does partial order with its focus on comparison provide visualization tools? An important graphical representation is the Hasse diagram. However, Hasse diagrams lose in general their appealing charm if the number of objects is too large. Myers and Patil (2010) developed visualization alternatives. Another well-known visualization tool is POSAC (partial order scalogram analysis with coordinates) described in Chapter 3. POSAC is applied on Internet sources about drinking water quality in Germany (Chapter 11), where partial order dimension analysis is also of help. In Chapter 14, watershed evaluation, weights are derived from the data matrix using POSAC.

1.7 Organization of Our Book

This monograph focuses on partial order and its applications in different scientific fields:

- We first explain what a partial order is and then provide a graphical display, called a Hasse diagram, where the objects to be ranked are positioned in a network-like graph.
- We discuss how far we can help with the selection of attributes helpful for ranking.
- We show the intricate role of attributes and the positions of objects in the Hasse diagram.
- We find data-driven rankings without the intervention of stakeholders.

Finally, we will focus on different examples.

The monograph consists of four parts:

(I) a basic theoretical part;
(II) illustrative case studies;
(III) live case studies;
(IV) appendix with data matrices and additional material.

References

Ahlers, J. (1999). The EU existing chemicals regulation. ESPR-Environ. Sci. Pollut. Res., 6(3), 127–129.

Annoni, P. and Bruggemann, R. (2008). The dualistic approach of FCA: A further insight into Ontario Lake sediments. Chemosphere, 70, 2025–2031.

Bruggemann, R. and Drescher-Kaden, U. (2003). Einfuehrung in die modellgestuetzte Bewertung von Umweltchemikalien – Datenabschaetzung, ausbreitung, verhalten, wirkung und Bewertung. Berlin: Springer.

Bruggemann, R., Halfon, E., Welzl, G., Voigt, K. and Steinberg, C. (2001). Applying the concept of partially ordered sets on the ranking of near-shore sediments by a battery of tests. J. Chem. Inf. Comput. Sci., 41(4), 918–925.

EINECS. http://chemicalwatch.com/927

Myers, W.L. and Patil, G.P. (2010). Partial order and rank range runs for compositional complexes in landscape ecology and image analysis, with applications to restoration, remediation, and enhancement. Environ. Ecol. Stat., 17, 411–436.

Newman, A. (1995). Ranking pesticides by environmental impact. Environ. Sci. Technol., 29(7), 324A–326A.

OECD (Nardo, M., et al.). (2008). Handbook on Constructing composite indicators -methodology and user guide (pp. 1–158). Ispra: OECD.

Patil, G.P. (2001). Penn State environmetrics and ecometrics, cross-disciplinary classroom notes. Center for Statistical Ecology and Environmental Statistics, Penn State University.

Patil, G.P. and Taillie, C. (2004). Multiple indicators, partially ordered sets, and linear extensions: Multi-criterion ranking and prioritization. Environ. Ecol. Stat., 11, 199–228.

Restrepo, G., Bruggemann, R., Weckert, M., Gerstmann, S. and Frank, H. (2008). Ranking patterns, an application to refrigerants. MATCH Commun. Math. Comput. Chem., 59, 555–584.

Saltelli, A., Ratto, M., Andres, T., Campolongo, F., Cariboni, J., Gatelli, D., et al. (2008). Global sensitivity analysis – the primer. Chichester: Wiley.

van Leeuwen, C.J., Bro-Rasmussen, F., Feijtel, T.C.J., Arndt, R., Bussian, B.M., Calamari, D., et al. (1996). Risk assessment and management of new and existing chemicals. Environ. Toxicol. Pharmacol., 2, 243–299.

Chapter 2
Partial Order and Hasse Diagrams

2.1 Data Matrix

Suppose there are five objects. Think of them as sediment samples a, b, c, d, e which we would like to rank. The first and main question is: What is the aim of ranking? We can rank the five sediment samples according to their age, or according to their content of a mineral, etc. If we know the aim of ranking, we need to identify properties that are relevant. In the case of ranking according to their age, it may be simple. Just order the samples according to their age!

In other cases, it may not be as simple. If, for example, the hazard for humans is of concern, then how to define the hazard caused by sediments to humans? One way of doing this is to determine properties like acute toxicity, or hygienic aspects, or potential carcinogenicity. Even hygienic aspects have several facets which need to be considered. Thus we come up with some properties, say q_1, q_2, q_3, which define the columns of a data matrix, whereas its rows represent the objects.

The next question we are concerned with is the orientation. Do all the properties q_1, q_2, and q_3 contribute to the aim of the ranking in the same way? This means: Is an increasing value for each property associated with an increasing hazard? For example, toxicity q_1 is measured as that concentration, where for a fraction of test species a well-defined adverse effect can be observed. A large value of the (acute) toxicity is less hazardous than a low value. On the other hand, the hygienic aspect q_2 is measured by the number of fecal coliforms. Here a large value of fecal coliforms is more of hygienic concern than is a low value. The two properties of a sediment sample are not similarly oriented. Therefore we must transform the properties so that they have a common monotonicity with the aim. Without knowing the aim and without checking the correct orientation of the attributes, a partial order analysis is meaningless.

The question of orientation is closely connected with another problem which is more a matter of convention: Should large values of (transformed) properties always mean "bad" or should they mean "good"? Here we do not follow a general rule; the important point is that the same orientation is considered for all properties for ranking. The consequence is that for every study, the kind of orientation and its meaning in terms of "good" and "bad" must be explicitly given.

R. Brüggemann, G.P. Patil, *Ranking and Prioritization for Multi-indicator Systems*, Environmental and Ecological Statistics 5, DOI 10.1007/978-1-4419-8477-7_2,

Having clarified the two basic questions, we can begin to compare each object with another. The comparison has to be based on the data matrix. So, let us assume that sediment sample a has values (2.0, 7.3, 1.0) and sediment sample b has values (3.1, 8.4, 1.5). Let us furthermore think of "high values" indicating a bad state. Then examining the three properties of sediment samples a and b, we conclude that sediment sample b is worse than sediment sample a, because all values of sample b are simultaneously larger than those of sample a. Let us now consider sediment sample c: (4.2, 8.1, 2.3). We see that c is worse than a but c cannot be compared with b because two properties favor b (q_1 and q_3) but the property q_2 favors c.

Adding two more sediment samples d (1.7, 2.6, 0.1) and e (5.8, 12.3, 3.7), we see that d is better than a, a is better than b, and hence d is better than b. There are still some comparisons to be performed and the reader should realize that even for small data matrices and only for some few properties, the statement which object is better (or worse) than another is not difficult, but troublesome. What we have established among the objects is a partial order, because we cannot give each pair of objects an order.

In the next section, we will explain the partial order more thoroughly and introduce some useful notation.

2.2 Characteristics of Partial Order

2.2.1 Axioms

Let us suppose that an "object set" X (in technical terms also called a "ground set") consists of our objects of interest. Suppose that X is a finite set (we do not mention it further). In our example above, X consists of objects a, b, c, d, e. We also write $X = \{a, b, c, d, e\}$. Furthermore, recall that we wish to compare objects of the object set. Therefore we use the symbol $\leq$ as a binary relation among the objects. The role of this relation is now fixed up by axioms:

$$\text{Axiom 1:} \quad \text{Reflexivity:} \quad x \in X : x \leq x \tag{2.1a}$$

$$\text{Axiom 2:} \quad \text{Anti-symmetry:} \quad x \leq y, y \leq x \text{ implies } y = x \tag{2.1b}$$

$$\text{Axiom 3:} \quad \text{Transitivity:} \quad x \leq y \text{ and } y \leq z \text{ implies } x \leq z \tag{2.1c}$$

Reflexivity: An object can be compared with itself.

Anti-symmetry: If both comparisons are valid, i.e., y is better than x and at the same time, x is better than y, then this axiom requires that x is identical with y. Later we will see that this requirement is very restrictive.

Transitivity: Transitivity is present if the objects are characterized by properties which are at least ordinal scaled. Any measurable quantity like height, length, and price implicitly bears the transitivity. There are also properties, like "color," where the meaning for ordering is unclear. If color is just a category like "red," "blue" by which objects can be labeled, then color is not a property relevant for ranking. If, however, color is given an order like red $\leq$ green $\leq$ blue, then objects can be ordered. It is a question of design of the matrix, availability of this kind of information, and use for the ranking aim.

2.2.2 *Quotient and Object Sets*

In applications, it is convenient to relax slightly the requirements concerning partial order. Several objects may have the same numerical values but are certainly different individuals (ties). So we consider the objects as equivalent, expressing that they have identical rows in the data matrix, but must nevertheless be considered as different items. These objects form an equivalence class and one may take one object out of the equivalence class and let it represent all the others. In such cases we proceed as follows (Patil and Taillie, 2004): We consider only one of the objects of any equivalence class as a representative and perform all operations which can be done in partial order theory. We keep in our memory, or in the computer memory, all the other objects being represented. We insert them whenever needed.

To make a clear distinction:

The set of equivalence classes under an equivalence relation $\mathfrak{R}$ is called quotient set, denoted, e.g., by $X/_{\mathfrak{R}}$.

From any equivalence class, one element is selected as representative. (2.2a)

When, however, all objects, even the equivalent ones, are to be taken into consideration, then we speak of the object set. (2.2b)

2.3 Product Order

2.3.1 *Notation*

How do we arrive at a partial order if a data matrix is at hand?

Let x, y be two different objects of the object set X. Let Q be the space of measurements (of different scaling levels). If, for instance, data are continuous in concept, then $Q \subset R^m$ (the m-dimensional space of real numbers). Let $q(x)$ be the data row for x and $q(y)$ for y, i.e., $q(x) \in Q$. We say

$$\begin{aligned} x \leq y, &\text{ if and only if } q(x) \leq q(y), \\ q(x) \leq q(y), &\text{ if and only if } q_i(x) \leq q_i(y), \text{ for all } i \end{aligned} \tag{2.3}$$

The space of measurements, Q, having the order relation property allows us to define order relations of the object set.

If x, y are different objects but $q(x) = q(y)$, i.e., $q_i(x) = q_i(y)$, for all i, then the objects x and y are called equivalent and the equivalence relation in (2.2a) is the equality. Equivalence is denoted as

$$x \cong y \tag{2.4}$$

If we want to exclude equivalence, then we also write

$$x < y \tag{2.5}$$

Consequently

$$\begin{aligned} &x < y, \text{ if and only if } q(x) \leq q(y), \\ &q(x) \leq q(y), \text{ with at least one } q_i^*, \\ &\text{for which } q_i^*(x) < q_i^*(y) \text{ is valid.} \end{aligned} \tag{2.6}$$

Sometimes it is necessary to specify the $\leq$ or $<$ relation for a set. In that case, $\leq$ or $<$ gets an appropriate subscript, e.g., $\leq_{\{q1,\, q2\}}$ or $\leq_{\{q1,\, q3\}}$ indicates that different partial orders are considered, one with the attributes q_1 and q_2, and the other one with q_1 and q_3.

The order among the objects based on Eqs. (2.3) and (2.6) is called "product order" or "component-wise order." Product order is our method to obtain a partial order from a data matrix and the focus of the monograph is on the partial order analysis (PoA) of data matrices. With $x <_{\{qi,\, qj\}}$ or $x \parallel_{\{qi,\, qj\}} y$ (for $\parallel$, see below) we indicate that the relation between x and y is based on a certain subset of attributes.

In our example above, the condition (2.6) cannot be established for the sediment samples b and c. It is convenient to express this fact by $b \parallel c$. The symbol $\parallel$ expresses that "b is incomparable to c" or that there is a conflict among the attribute values of b and c. When for the objects x, y it is valid that $q(x) \leq q(y)$ or $q(x) \geq q(y)$, then x and y are comparable. If the comparability between two objects is to be indicated without defining the orientation, then we write $x \perp y$.

When the object set X is equipped with a partial order, meaning that the objects of X are related to each other by a relation, which obeys the above-mentioned axioms, then we write $(X, \leq)$. If no confusion is possible, we also use bold symbol for the object set X to denote the corresponding partial order and add indices if necessary. For example, $\mathbf{X}_i = (X_i, \leq)$. An object set equipped with a partial order is often called a poset (partially ordered set). Our analysis is based on a data matrix, and we see from Eq. (2.3) that $x \perp y$ or $x \parallel y$ depends on the attributes used. It is convenient to speak of an attribute set. Bruggemann et al. (1995) introduced the concept information base (IB) which is the set of attributes used in the data matrix. Therefore, we will write either $(X, \{q_1, q_2, \ldots\})$ if it is important to refer to the attributes or (X, IB). As (X, IB) is the basis for an ordinal analysis of the data matrix, we introduce the following definition.

(X, IB) is the partial order based on Eq. (2.3), where

$$q_i \in \mathrm{IB} \text{ and } x \in X \tag{2.6a}$$

$(X/\cong, \mathrm{IB})$ is the partial order based on Eq. (2.6), where $q_i \in \mathrm{IB}$ and we take from each equivalence class exactly one element x, the representative (see Eq. (2.2)).

$$\text{Thus } (X/\cong, \mathrm{IB}) \text{ is the partial order of representatives} \tag{2.6b}$$

Furthermore, we denote the number of elements of a set A as usual as $|A|$. The set A may be either X or IB or subsets of them. In the following, we use the terms "attributes" when we are speaking of the columns of the data matrix without specifically referring to partial order, whereas we use the term "indicator" when their use for an ordinal analysis is to be stressed. As the focus of the monograph is the ordinal analysis, we will be using "attributes" and "indicators" interchangeably. The data rows are identified by the objects. Sometimes, if we stress that the objects belong to some set, we also speak of them as "elements of a set X."

2.3.2 Example

In Section 2.1, we have an example, so we will fix the concepts and notation just with that (Table 2.1).

The object set is $X = \{a, b, c, d, e\}$. Let us introduce $\mathrm{IB} = \{q_1, q_2, q_3\}$. If we would like to know whether $a \leq b$, we have to check q_1, q_2, and q_3 for a and b. Generally, taken the whole set of objects, there are $|X|^*(|X| - 1)^*|\mathrm{IB}|/2$ single attribute comparisons.

In our example, we find that

$$a < b, a < e, a < c, b < e, c < e, d < a, d < b, d < e, d < c$$

With this list, everything is said! However, it is convenient to explicitly state that $b \parallel c$.

2.4 Some Basic Concepts

1. Data matrices having the same rank matrix have the same partial order.

Table 2.1 Illustrative example

	q_1	q_2	q_3
a	2	7.3	1
b	3.1	8.4	1.5
c	4.2	8.1	2.3
d	1.7	2.6	0.1
e	5.8	12.3	3.7

2. If there is no incomparability, then we speak of a complete, total, or linear order. In the case of a complete order, the objects $x \in X$ can be arranged in a sequence $x_1 < x_2 < \ldots < x_n$, i.e., a ranking is found.
3. *Chain*: If a subset $X' \subset X$ can be found such that for all $(x, y) \in X' \times X'$ a complete order can be found, then this subset, together with the partial order relation, is a chain.
4. When for a chain C, no element $\in X$ can be found to extend C, then C is called maximal. There may exist a maximum chain.
5. *Weak order*: Representative elements of equivalence classes are in a chain, but there are nontrivial equivalence classes.
6. *Antichain*: If a subset $X' \subset X$ can be found such that for no $(x, y) \in X' \times X', x \perp y$ holds, then this subset, equipped with the partial order relation, is called an antichain.
7. When for an antichain (AC), no element ∈ X can be found, by which AC can be extended, then AC is maximal. There may exist a maximum antichain.
8. In finite data matrices, chains and antichains contain a finite number of objects. Therefore, we can speak of chains or antichains having a certain length, according to the number of elements they contain. Within a partial order in general, there can be several maximal chains and several maximal antichains.
9. *Height*: Number of elements of the longest chain is called the height of the poset.
10. *Width*: The number of elements of the maximum of antichains is called the width of the poset.
11. Maximal, minimal, greatest, least, isolated elements of a poset:

    A maximal element $x \in X$ is an element for which no relation $x \leq y$ can be found.

    The set of maximal elements of (X, IB) is denoted as MAX(X, IB) or if no confusion is possible, we write simply MAX.

    A minimal element $x \in X$ is an element for which no relation $y \leq x$ can be found.

    The set of minimal elements of (X, IB) is denoted as MIN(X, IB) or if no confusion is possible, we write simply MIN.
12. *Greatest /least element*: There is only one maximal/minimal element (quotient set).
13. *Isolated element*: An element $x \in X$ which is at the same time a maximal and a minimal element is called an isolated element.

    Let us call an isolated element i, then for all x ∈ X-{i}: i || x.

    The set of isolated elements of (X, IB) is denoted as ISO(X, IB) or if no confusion is possible, we write simply ISO.
14. *Proper maximal/minimal element*: A maximal/minimal element $x \in X$ which is not isolated.
15. *Cover relation*: x is covered by y if there is no element $z \in X$ for which $x < z$ and $z < y$. We write this as $x \leq: y$.

We may examine points 1–15 on the basis of the partial order list. However, it is far simpler to apply the graphical display of a partial order! Therefore this is introduced next.

2.5 Hasse Diagram

With the cover relation at hand, we can get a diagrammatic representation of the partially ordered set (poset).

Let us consider x and y, and assume that $x \leq: y$. Then we draw x in a vertical plane below y and connect both with a straight line. This is repeated for every ordered pair, i.e., for all pairs of two objects for which $\leq:$ relation holds. The resulting diagram is denoted as Hasse diagram (sometimes partial order set diagram, order diagram, line diagram, or simply the diagram) after the German mathematician Hasse, who made this kind of visualization popular.

In our example, $X = \{a, b, c, d, e\}$ (Fig. 2.1).

There are many remarks to be made:

1. Differently drawn Hasse diagrams may nevertheless graphically represent the same partial order. In that case we speak of isomorphic Hasse diagrams.
2. As the Hasse diagram allows the overview about the order relation in a very convenient way, it is very important to draw the Hasse diagram carefully. Aeschlimann and Schmid (1992) have given many recommendations. Nevertheless, there are many degrees of freedom to draw a Hasse diagram.
3. The objects are located vertically in the drawing plane in order to get them organized in "levels." For example, object d forms the first level, object a the second, objects b and c the third, and finally object e the fourth level. If an object could be located in several vertical positions, the highest possible one is selected (see Fig. 2.2 for a demonstration).

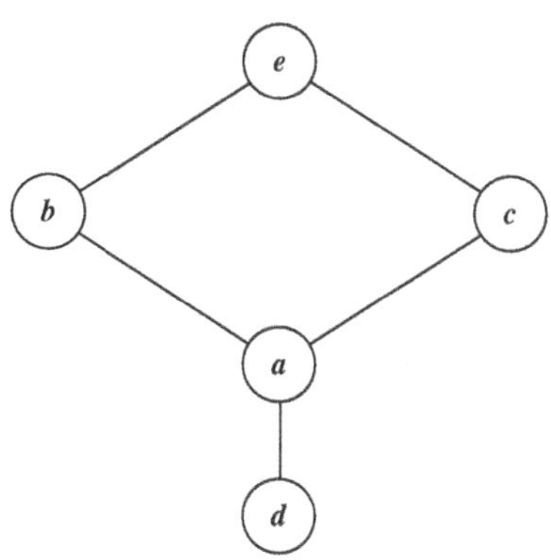

Fig. 2.1 Hasse diagram based on data of Table 2.1

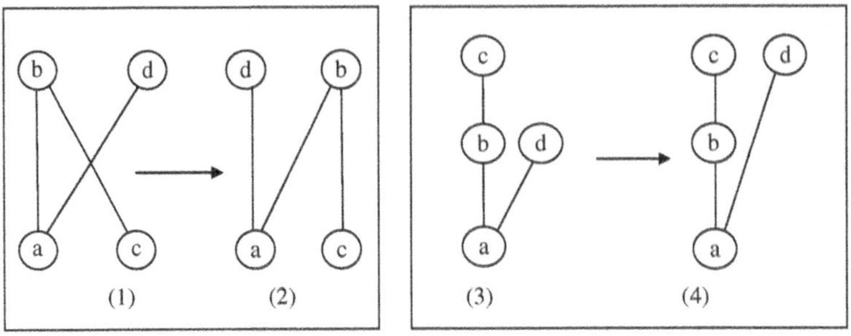

Fig. 2.2 Drawing rules of Hasse diagrams

4. If avoidable, the lines should not cross each other in locations which are not those of objects (see Fig. 2.2 for a demonstration).
5. There should be as few different slopes as possible for the single lines which represent the cover relations.
6. Most software realizations locate the objects symmetrically. The next five items refer to Fig. 2.1.
7. The fact that $d \leq b$ can be easily deduced from the Hasse diagram because of transitivity; no line appears for $d \leq b$.
8. There is one maximal element, namely the object *e*. There is one minimal element, namely the object *d*. Object *d* is the only one minimal element, therefore object *d* is the least element and similarly object *e* is the greatest element.
9. A chain is, for example, $d < a < b$. This is not the maximal chain, because we could add *e*.
10. The set $\{b, \ c\}$ is an example for an antichain. The width of the partial order is 2.
11. The height of the poset is 4 (counting the objects *d*, *a*, *b*, *e*).

Figure 2.2 shows examples of "crossings" and how convention 2 is working.

In Fig. 2.2, the four Hasse diagrams (1) and (2) on the one side and (3) and (4) on the other side are order theoretically correctly drawn (they are isomorphic). However, in (1) there is an avoidable crossing and (4) follows the remark 3, whereas diagram (3) does not.

Sometimes it is convenient to refer to the "fence relation" and to a "dual" poset or "dual" Hasse diagram. An example may be sufficient for an explanation (Fig. 2.3).

On top of Fig. 2.3, objects *x* and *y* are in a "fence relation." Fences or "zigzag posets" are often denoted by $F(n)$, according to the number of objects. Objects in a fence relation are connected (in the ordinary graph theoretical sense, but not necessarily comparable). At the bottom, an example of duality between posets, i.e., between Hasse diagrams, is shown.

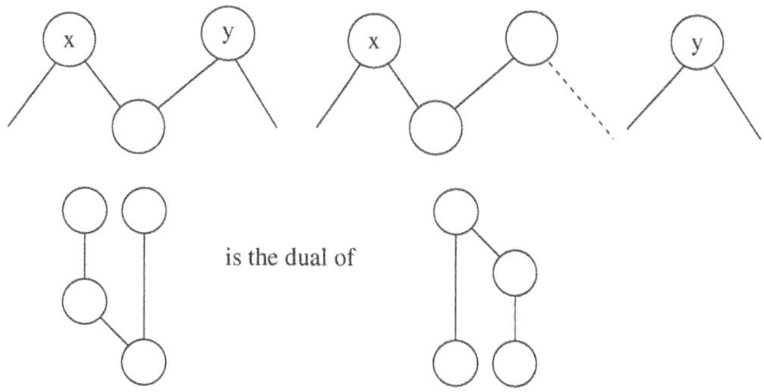

Fig. 2.3 Fences and dual Hasse diagrams

2.6 Components

Let us assume the object set $X = \{a, b, c, d\}$ and the Hasse diagram of its partial order in Fig. 2.4.

A partially ordered set can be considered a directed graph (digraph) without cycles. We speak of a weak connection if its underlying graph is connected. In Fig. 2.2, object c and d are weakly connected, because the underlying graph contains a sequence of edges (an edge in this case) between c and d. The maximal weakly connected components, where there is no outside object which can be included, such as $(\{a, b\},\ \text{IB})$ and $(\{c, d\},\ \text{IB})$ in Fig. 2.4, we simply call components of the partially ordered set. Isolated elements can also be considered as components ("trivial components").[1] The appearance of components is exciting, because their presence indicates interesting data structures and a high sensitivity to any weights of a composite indicator (see Chapter 5). Components of partially ordered sets are maximal, because no element $\in$ X can be found to extend components. In Chapter 5, we call subsets of components with the inherited order relation "separated subsets."

Fig. 2.4 Hasse diagram of (X, IB). $\text{IB} = \{q_1, q_2\}$, see table

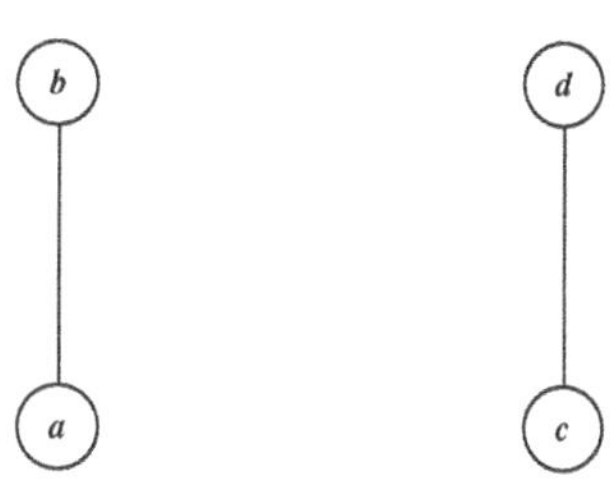

	q_1	q_2
a	3	2
b	4	4
c	1	5
d	2	5

[1] In former publications often called "hierarchy."

2.7 ζ Matrix and Other Representations of Partial Order

A convenient way to code a partial order is the ζ matrix: The rows and columns of this matrix are labeled with the object names. If $a < b$, then the corresponding cell gets a 1, in all other cases a 0.

Let

$$x, y \in X, \text{ then } \zeta(x, y) = 1 :\Leftrightarrow x < y \tag{2.7}$$

For example, the partial order represented in Fig. 2.1 obtains the following ζ matrix:

$$\zeta = \begin{matrix} \\ a \\ b \\ c \\ d \\ e \end{matrix} \begin{matrix} a\,b\,c\,d\,e \\ \begin{pmatrix} 0&1&1&0&1 \\ 0&0&0&0&1 \\ 0&0&0&0&1 \\ 1&1&1&0&1 \\ 0&0&0&0&0 \end{pmatrix} \end{matrix}$$

Note that transitive relations are coded by giving the corresponding cell a 1. So the entry, belonging to row d and column b, gets a 1. A variant of the matrix ζ is the cover matrix, which we will not use in this book. The main diagonal of the matrix ζ contains 1 if in Eq. (2.7) the $\leq$ relation is used.

Another possibility to represent a partial order is to describe it as a set of ordered pairs, X^2: Let $(x, y) \in X^2$ be an ordered pair, then

$$(x, y) \in (X, \text{ IB}) : \Leftrightarrow x < y \tag{2.8}$$

as defined in (2.6).

The set of ordered pairs consists of all pairs of comparable elements except the diagonal of X^2. Hence

$$|(X, \text{ IB})| = \sum \sum \zeta_{ij} \tag{2.9}$$

The Hasse diagram (Fig. 2.1) would therefore get the following representation (suppressing the reflexivity relation):

$$(X, \text{ IB}) = \{(d, a), (d, b), (d, c), (d, e), (a, b), (a, c), (a, e), (b, e), (c, e)\}$$

This kind of representation will be useful in Chapter 10 and is useful for programming purposes. Now we know a lot about posetic characteristics of the data matrix. But how does this help in our ranking problem? This we discuss in Chapter 3.

2.8 Summary and Commentary

The evaluation of a data matrix by partial order needs the following: (i) a ranking aim, (ii) orientation, and (iii) comparison of objects according to (i). The graphical display by a Hasse diagram allows one an easy way to identify the concepts mentioned in Section 2.4. How far are they helpful for interpretation? Let us go back to the ideas discussed in Section 2.1: The analysis of a set X with respect to prioritization and ranking means (1) establishing a partial order, (2) clarifying how far equivalence classes (ties) appear and how to handle them (by analyzing the quotient set), (3) finding out the chains and antichains, and (4) finding the maximal, minimal, and isolated elements.

Maximal or *minimal* elements are priority elements, which most often are of special concern. *Isolated* elements can be considered as elements which are maximal and minimal elements simultaneously. So far they are also priority elements. However – as we will see later – isolated elements indicate peculiarities of the data matrix. *Chains*: Elements are in a chain if their attributes vary simultaneously either (weakly) increasing or (weakly) decreasing. Often, there is a positive rank correlation among the elements of a chain. We will later see that under a weighting scheme, i.e., a set of weights to construct a composite indicator, elements of a chain will keep their mutual order, whereas elements of an antichain can get very different positions in the final ranking.

References

Aeschlimann, A. and Schmid, J. (1992). Drawing orders using less ink. Order, 9, 5–13.

Bruggemann, R., Schwaiger, J. and Negele, R.D. (1995). Applying Hasse diagram technique for the evaluation of toxicological fish tests. Chemosphere, 30(9), 1767–1780.

Patil, G.P. and Taillie, C. (2004). Multiple indicators, partially ordered sets, and linear extensions: Multi-criterion ranking and prioritization. Environ. Ecol. Stat., 11, 199–228.

Chapter 3
Simple Combinatorial Structures

3.1 Order Preserving Maps

It is of interest to compare two partially ordered sets (more about this topic, see Chapter 10). We may, for example, ask whether all $\leq$ relations in one poset are reproduced in the other. In technical terms, we are asking whether or not

$$\text{a "mapping" } g \text{ from } X_1 \text{ to } X_2 \text{ is order preserving,} \tag{3.1a}$$

i.e., whether $(x \leq y)$ in X_1 implies $(g(x) \leq g(y))$ in X_2.

Consider, for example, six sampling sites {Id-no: 6, 8, 9, 22, 23, 30} in the German State Baden-Wuerttemberg, where the concentration of the metals lead (Pb), cadmium (Cd), zinc (Zn), and sulfur (S) (mg/kg dry weight) was measured, once in tree leaves (LHS of Fig. 3.1) and once in the herb layer (RHS of Fig. 3.1). Following the notation of Chapter 2, the object set X is $X = \{6, 8, 9, 22, 23, 30\}$ and there are two information bases $\text{IB}_1 = \{\text{Pb, Cd, Zn, S: in tree leaves}\}$ and $\text{IB}_2 = \{\text{Pb, Cd, Zn, S: in herb layer}\}$. Hence, we obtain two posets (X, IB_1) and (X, IB_2).

In Fig. 3.1 (RHS), we observe that some circles contain more than one object label. The corresponding objects are equivalent (see Section 3.2). There arises a natural question: Can we avoid the measurements in the herb layer if we know the results based on tree leaves? Translated into a posetic question: Does a relation $x \leq y$ for the tree leaves imply a corresponding relation $x \leq y$ for the herb layer? If yes, this can save enormous time and money. Unfortunately, in this case, the mapping g between the two empirical partial orders is not order preserving: See the following:

$$6 \leq 8 \rightarrow g(6) \leq g(8), 6 \leq 23 \rightarrow g(6) \leq g(23), 30 \leq 8 \rightarrow g(30) \leq g(8), 30 \leq 23 \\ \rightarrow g(30) \leq g(23), 9 \leq 23 \rightarrow g(9) \parallel g(23)$$

$9 \leq 23$ for tree leaves corresponds to $9 \parallel 23$ in the herb layer. Therefore the mapping is not order preserving. We now have the following three comments concerning order preserving maps:

R. Brüggemann, G.P. Patil, *Ranking and Prioritization for Multi-indicator Systems*, Environmental and Ecological Statistics 5, DOI 10.1007/978-1-4419-8477-7_3,

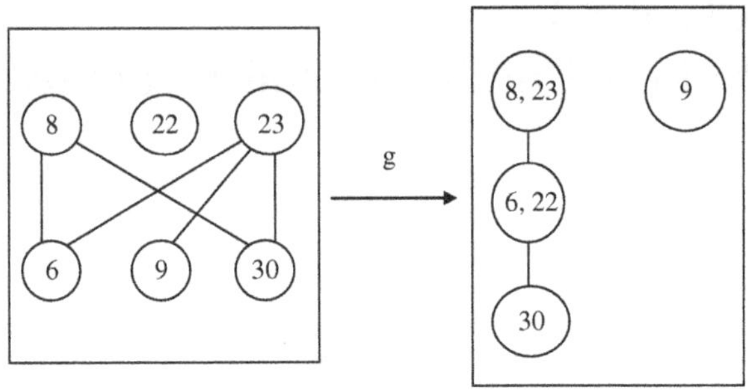

Fig. 3.1 Comparison of two Hasse diagrams as visualizations of (X, IB_1) (*LHS*) and (X, IB_2) (*RHS*)

1. Order preserving map is a sharp and restrictive tool. If it can be established for a mapping from one object set to itself, then the order preserving map is an enrichment of orders. This is always a very favored result. Many decision support tools (see Chapter 1) try to enrich the original order relations. Enrichment of orders is the leading concept in Chapters 6, 7, and 9.
2. If exceptions are ignored, an order preserving map may be said to hold to a certain degree. Here, for example, above, it holds for four out of five order relations.
3. A most important application of order preserving maps lies in their application to obtain linear orders.

The third comment relates to the heart of prioritization and ranking: If we can obtain a linear order for all objects just from the data matrix (i.e., without additional weighting, see below and Chapter 7), this will provide the stakeholder with an alternative ranking, and he may check the role and consequence of subjective preferences. Section 3.2 is a step toward this end.

3.2 Linear Extensions

Important order preserving maps are those which relate a partial order to a linear order, especially those where the object set is the same. In that case, the order preserving map enriches the number of comparability relations, and the linear order is called a linear extension.

A linear extension is a linear order,

$$\text{which preserves the order relations of a poset.} \tag{3.1b}$$

For example, the partial order shown in Fig. 3.1 has the linear extension (Fig. 3.2).

The linear extension shown in Fig. 3.2 (RHS) is not the only one. In order to present them, it is not always convenient to draw them as Hasse diagrams, but as linear sequences, beginning with the bottom element, ending with the top element.

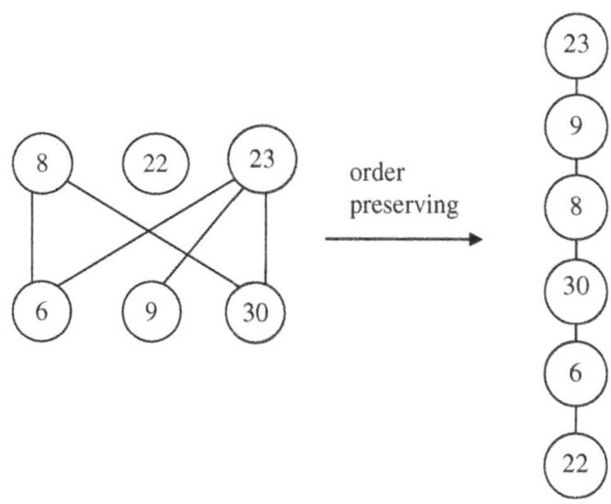

Fig. 3.2 Finding a linear extension from an empirical poset

Table 3.1 Some other linear extensions found for the Hasse diagram in Fig. 3.1 (LHS)

Linear extension 1	(9	30	6	22	23	8)
Linear extension 2	(9	6	30	23	22	8)
Linear extension 3	(30	9	6	8	22	23)
Linear extension 4	(30	6	9	8	22	23)

So the linear extension shown in Fig. 3.2 will also equivalently be presented as (22 < 6 < 30 < 8 < 9 < 23) or even simpler (22, 6, 30, 8, 9, 23).

Some more linear extensions, taken from the Hasse diagram of Fig. 3.1 (LHS), are shown in Table 3.1.

We introduce two new concepts.

The number of all linear extensions of (X, IB): LT(X, IB): If no confusion is possible, then we simply write LT. The number of all linear extensions of a poset (*X*, IB), LT(*X*, IB) is very important as it appears in almost every application of linear extensions.

The height of an object x in a linear extension:
$h_{\text{le}(i)}(x)$ is the count of elements $\leq x$. (3.2)

Each object *x* has a well-defined "height," $h(x)$, in each of the linear extensions. For example, object 30 has height 3 and object 6 has height 2 in the linear extension shown in Fig. 3.2, RHS. The height $h(x)$ for object *x* varies over the linear extensions, therefore the index le(i) refers to the *i*th linear extension.

The set of all linear extensions of a partially ordered set *X*, LE(*X*), allows the following applications:

(1) Let *x* be an element of the partially ordered set $(X, \leq)$. Compare the number of linear extensions where *x* has a certain height *h* with the total number of linear extensions, LT. This may be interpreted as the probability for *x* to have height *h*,

i.e., prob($h_{\mathrm{le}(i)}(x) = h$), le($i$) $\in$ LE. If there is no confusion possible, we write simply $h(x)$.

$$\text{Height (or rank) probability: prob}(h(x) = h) = \#\text{LE}(h(x) = \text{h})/\text{LT} \tag{3.3}$$

Varying h, we obtain the height probability function of object x (for examples, see Section 3.3).

(2) Let $x \parallel y$ in $(X, \leq)$. The number of linear extensions in which $x > y$ is #LE($x > y$). The proportion #LE($x > y$)/LT is called the mutual probability of x to have a higher height than

$$y\,(\text{probm}(x > y)). \tag{3.4}$$

(3) By taking the average (or the median) of all heights of an object x over all linear extensions, we obtain the "averaged height (rank)", hav(x), by which for all objects a linear or a weak order can be found. Also the symbol Rkav(x) for averaged rank is used in the literature. For the concept of averaged heights, see Winkler (1982):

$$\text{hav}\ (x) = \sum h_{\mathrm{le}(i)}(x)/\text{LT} \tag{3.5}$$

We now illustrate the above with Figs. 3.3 and 3.4.

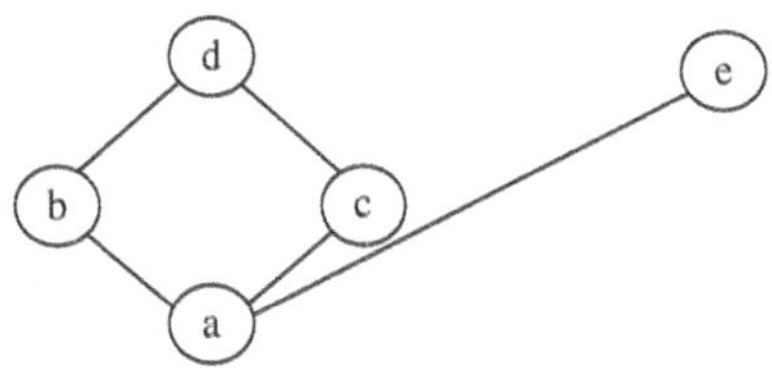

	q1	q2
a	1	1
b	2	1
c	1	2
d	3	3
e	0	4

Fig. 3.3 Hasse diagram and the data matrix as example to derive the linear extensions

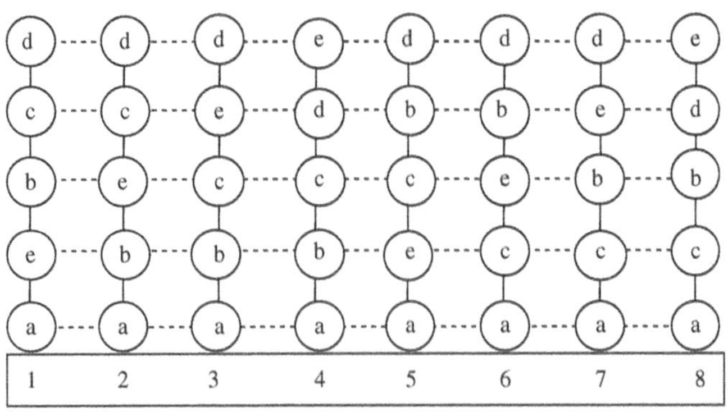

Fig. 3.4 The eight linear extensions drawn in a Hasse diagram manner

Trotter (1992), Atkinson and Chang (1986), and Edelman et al. (1989) describe methods to construct linear extensions. Patil and Taillie (2004) show a "linear extension decision tree." Here we can easily derive the eight linear extensions, observing that b can only be above or below c. In either case, we get a chain of four elements $a < b < c < d$ or $a < c < b < d$. Object e can get all positions above a. The linear extensions are seen in Fig. 3.4.

The linear extensions in Fig. 3.4 (their enumeration is shown in the box below and the heights 1–5 are indicated by horizontal broken lines) are the result of order preserving maps applied to the partial order in Fig. 3.3 and observing the condition of linearity. We see that some of the objects take different positions in the linear extensions. For example, object e has in the first linear extension the height 2, whereas in the fourth one the height 5. Other objects like object a are invariant and have height 1 throughout.

Now we are going to illustrate the three applications:

1. We select a height $h = 3$, and the object e, and count the number of linear extensions, in which the height of object e is $h = 3$. The number of linear extensions with $h(e) = h = 3$ is 2. Comparing with the total number of linear extensions, we obtain

$$\text{prob}(h(e) = h = 3) = 2/8 = 0.25$$

2. Object d is incomparable with e. How often is object $d >$ object e? This question is meaningful if we reformulate it in the following manner: How many linear extensions can we find in which object d has a higher position than e. We count six linear extensions, where $d > e$. These are all linear extensions except nos. 4 and 8. Hence

$$\text{probm}(d > e) = 6/8 = 0.75$$

3. Let us now look for object b. Object b has the heights 3, 2, 2, 2, 3, 3, 4, 4. Hence the averaged height $\text{hav}(b) = (3 + 2 + 2 + 2 + 3 + 3 + 4 + 4)/8 = 2.875$.

The map g^*: $(X, \text{IB}) \rightarrow (X, \{\text{hav}\})$ is order preserving and is of special interest: It provides us with a linear or a weak order of the objects of X. Because $(X, \{\text{hav}\})$ is an alternative to the common use of composite indices, we call this ranking a canonical order (see Chapter 9). $(X, \{h_{\text{le}(i)}\})$ induces a linear order:

$$(X, \{\text{hav}\}) \text{ induces a canonical order.} \tag{3.6}$$

3.3 Real-Life Example

This example comes from the monitoring study in the south-western state Baden-Wuerttemberg in Germany (Kreimes, 1996). We consider a subset of sampling sites and the information basis IB = {Pb, Cd}, with Pb and Cd being the concentrations of Pb (lead) and Cd (cadmium), respectively, measured in the herb layer (mg/kg dry weight). Figure 3.5 shows the Hasse diagram. It consists of two non-connected parts, two components (see Chapter 2).

As an illustrative example for Eq. (3.3), in Section 3.3, see Fig. 3.6.

It is not helpful to write down all 882 linear extensions to trace the position of any object. Instead the graphics in Fig. 3.6 shows how the frequency of height from 1 to 9 is varying. Note that we draw a continuous line for a better readability.

The diagram shows, for example, that heights above 7 are more probable for object 57 over objects 34 and 12, whereas heights below 5 are more probable for object 12 over objects 57 and 34. The graphs prob($h(x) = h$) vs h can also be non-monotonous, with unimodality somewhere in the middle (see Fig. 3.7).

As an example for Eq. (3.5), we will now calculate all averaged heights (Table 3.2).

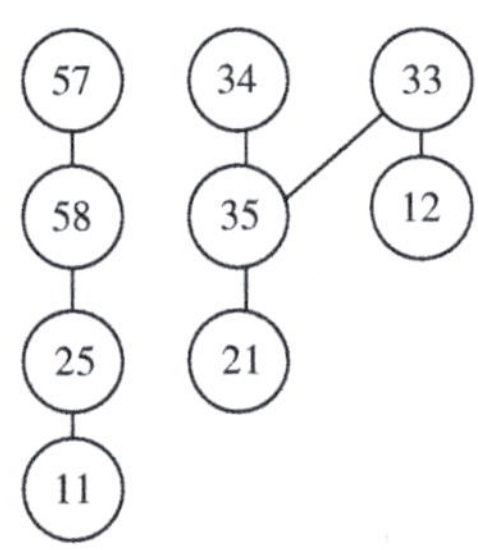

Fig. 3.5 Evaluation of sampling sites by the concentration of lead (Pb) and cadmium (Cd) (mg/ kg dry mass) in the herb layer. The objects are labeled as 11, 25, 58, etc

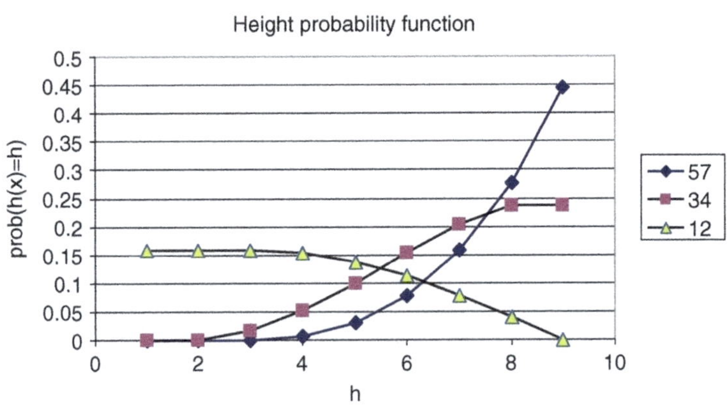

Fig. 3.6 Height (rank) probability function for some objects of the poset in Fig. 3.5

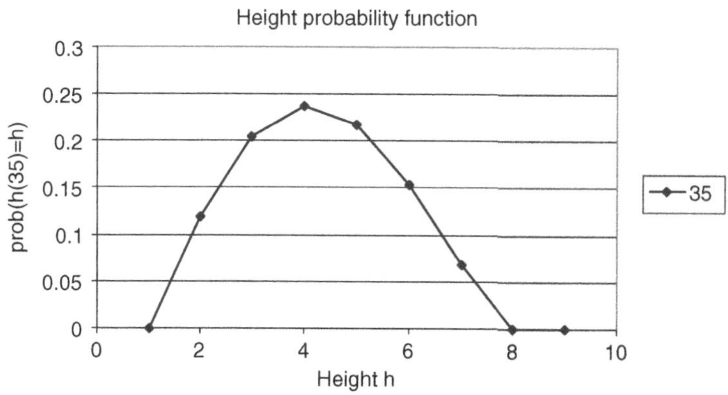

Fig. 3.7 The same as in Fig. 3.6. However, only sampling site 35 is drawn

Table 3.2 Averaged heights hav(x)

Object x	hav(x)	Object x	hav(x)
57	8	35	4.3
58	6	21	2.14
25	4	34	7.14
11	2	12	3.14
33	7.62		

Based on hav(x) in Table 3.2, the objects can be ordered as

$$11 < 21 < 12 < 25 < 35 < 58 < 34 < 33 < 57$$

providing an alternate ranking to any empirical index-based ranking.

We do not claim that this ranking is "the truth." It is based solely on the ordinal properties of the data matrix. Nevertheless, providing such an alternative is of great help in identifying deviations from the empirical index-based ranking, and hence in examining the role of subjective weightings (see also the discussion in Section 10.7). Finally, as an example for Eq. (3.4) in Section 3.2 (Fig. 3.8), we calculate probm $(57 < x)$ for all $x \in X$, with $x \parallel 57$.

Linear extensions offer important tools to examine the data matrix in matters that have to do with individual ranking and mutual positioning of the objects. However, we are faced with a computational problem: The number of linear extensions goes with $n!$, the number of objects being n. Therefore, even for medium sized data matrices, theoretical results and approximations are necessary. We will discuss them later in this monograph.

Some readers may ask for methods to calculate the number of linear extensions. For empirical data matrices and the resulting Hasse diagrams, most often there is no method at hand except for the computer to do the combinatorial exercise (see Chapter 9).

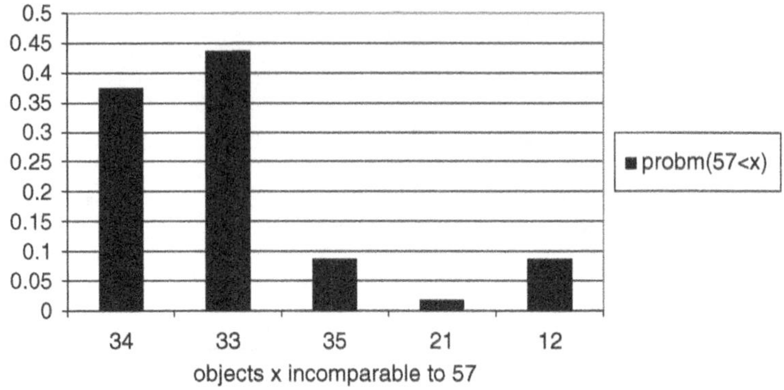

Fig. 3.8 probm($57 < x$), based on the Hasse diagram in Fig. 3.5

3.4 Dimension

3.4.1 Motivation

Given a poset (X, IB) and its visualization by a Hasse diagram, a question arises: Can we find a smaller set of attributes from which we can get the same Hasse diagram? This question directs toward a possible representation of the ordinal properties of the data matrix in a lower dimensional space. Let us imagine that a data matrix has five attributes. If we can find two attributes, which generate the same Hasse diagram, i.e., which lets the original order relations invariant, then we can represent the objects in a two-dimensional scatter plot. This will considerably simplify the ordinal analysis.

We illustrate this consideration by a real-life example.

In the wetlands southeast of Berlin in Germany, there are creeks, which are of interest because of their fish community (Bruggemann and Fredrich, 1997). For the development of a wetland management plan, it was of interest to recognize creeks as hot spots based on their striking fish communities. The experts selected nine fish species and the number of individuals of every fish species was determined for all creeks. For the sake of brevity, let us look at four of these creeks, F, M, K, and T. The data matrix contains four rows and nine columns. Their Hasse diagram is shown in Fig. 3.9 and is rather simple.

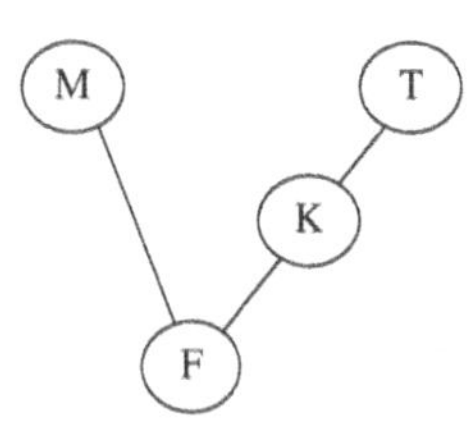

Fig. 3.9 Hasse diagram of four creeks in the wetlands southeast of Berlin

Table 3.3 New attributes for the Hasse diagram in Fig. 3.9

Creek	q_1	q_2
T	3	0
K	2	0
M	1	2
F	0	0

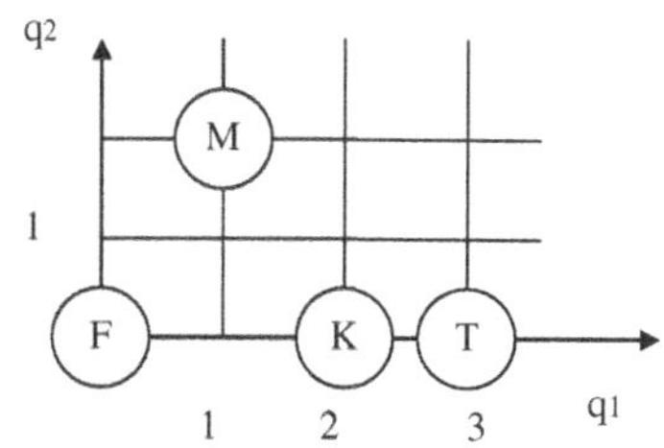

Fig. 3.10 Model of an embedding of the poset of Fig. 3.9 into a two-dimensional coordinate system

This poset, however, can also be represented by only two attributes. For example, attributes with values as given in Table 3.3 will do the job.

That means for an ordinal presentation it is sufficient to use only two attributes. In other words, the poset of Fig. 3.9 can be embedded into a two-dimensional space (see Fig. 3.10 for one of many possibilities). This resembles the concept of latent variables in multivariate statistics: Even if the data matrix is made of m attributes, it may be sufficient to represent the partial order by some fewer latent variables.

See Chapter 11 for more details about the wetlands and their fish communities.

3.4.2 Theoretical Conceptualization

We come back to our originally stated question: Can we replace the original data matrix of m columns by a data matrix which has $m' < m$ (especially $m' = 2$) columns without changing the ordinal information in it. If the dimension of the poset dim(X, IB) is m', then the answer is "yes." Finding dim(X, IB), however, is difficult. Theoretical results can be found in Stanley (1986) and Trotter (1992). Of practical value is the theorem of de Fraysseix and De Mendez (1996):

$$\begin{aligned}&(1)\ \text{If } (X,\ \text{IB}) \text{ has a greatest and a least element, and}\\&(2)\ \text{If } (X,\ \text{IB}) \text{ can be drawn in a plane without crossings,}\\&\quad\ \text{then } \dim(X,\ \text{IB}) = 2.\end{aligned} \tag{3.7}$$

If (X, IB) has no greatest or least element, include these as fictitious objects and apply Eq. (3.7) on this extended poset.

If dim (X, IB) $= 2 < m$, the number of attributes of the data matrix being m, then we know an embedding into a plane, a scatter plot, is possible. However, how do we find the needed two attributes, which we call in analogy to multivariate statistics latent order variables (LOVs)? The partial order scalogram analysis (POSAC) discussed in Section 3.5 finds LOVs by approximation. When one intends to use POSAC, it may be a good idea to check dim(X, IB) (Annoni and Bruggemann, 2009, 2011; Bruggemann et al., 2001).

3.5 POSAC

3.5.1 Overview

For convenience, we introduce POSAC following Patil (2005). For more details, see Borg and Shye (1995), Voigt et al. (2004a, b), and Bruggemann et al. (2003). For software POSAC, see http://ca.huji.ac.il/bf/Hudap-Info.pdf. POSAC is a method to reduce the attributes into a smaller number of dimensions, with the goal of correctly preserving as many of the comparabilities that exist in the original model as possible. The goal of the POSAC method is to graphically represent a data matrix with m columns in a two-dimensional space. The two-dimensional coordinate representation of objects with observed profiles, the data row of object x, $(q_1(x), q_2(x), \dots, q_m(x))$, should best preserve profile order relations. POSAC constructs new axes, which together correctly present as many of the order relations as possible. POSAC is similar to principal component analysis (PCA) in that both are dimension reduction methods, but while PCA tries to preserve distances, POSAC tries to preserve comparabilities.

3.5.2 A Perceptive Introduction

There are three possible order relations in a two-dimensional Cartesian coordinate space. The possibilities are indicated in Fig. 3.11. A given object a divides the attribute space into four quadrants. The objects $y \in X$ that fall in the first quadrant are intrinsically better than a (i.e., $y > a$), and those that fall in the third quadrant are intrinsically worse than a ($y < a$). We call the quadrant (i) the upward shadow and (iii) the downward shadow of object a. Shadows are subsets of Q and should not be confused with down sets or up sets (see Section 3.6.2). The second and fourth quadrants are regions of ambiguity; objects falling here are incomparable with object a, i.e., $y \parallel a$.

In a data matrix of m columns, we want to form a partially ordered set by comparing their profiles, provided by the rows of the data matrix. In the partially ordered set, some pairs of profiles may be ordered or comparable, while some pairs of profiles are incomparable. Consider an example of three profiles with four attributes: 3142, 3242, and 1118. Here 3142 implies that the first attribute has value 3, the second attribute has value 1, etc.

Profiles 3142 and 3242 are ordered with 3242 greater than 3142, but 3242 and 1118 are incomparable, since the first attribute is better for the first profile (as $3 > 1$),

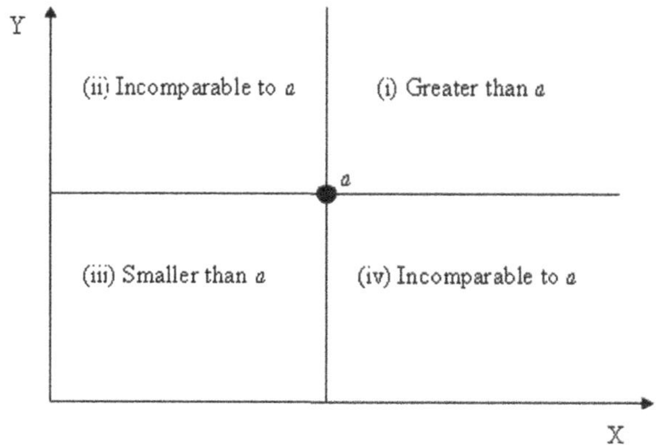

Fig. 3.11 Two-dimensional ordering

and the fourth attribute is better for the third profile (as 2 < 8). If two profiles are comparable, say 3142 and 3242, then it can be represented (or preserved) if we assign just a single score to every profile in the pair. For example, let us assign 1 to 3142 and 2 to 3242. Then 2 > 1 reflects the fact that 3242 > 3142. Let now two profiles be incomparable, say 3242 and 1118. Assigning just one numerical value to each profile cannot represent the fact that they are incomparable, because the set of all numerical values is totally ordered. However, the set of all pairs of numerical values is a partially ordered set. So, let us assign two values to each profile of the incomparable pair to represent their incomparability. Let us first locate the comparable profiles in the plot. For example, assign to 3142 the shorter profile (1, 1) to represent that 3242 is greater than 3142; it needs to be assigned somewhere in the upper right square to (1, 1), say (2, 2). Now, we add profile 1118 to the plot. Since this profile is incomparable to both profiles 3142 and 3242, it must be assigned within the intersection of regions that are incomparable to both (1, 1) and (2, 2). That is the shaded area in Fig. 3.12. For example, we can pick the point (3, 0) to represent profile 1118. The incomparability of (3, 0) with (1, 1) and (2, 2) represents that of 1118 with 3142 and 3242.

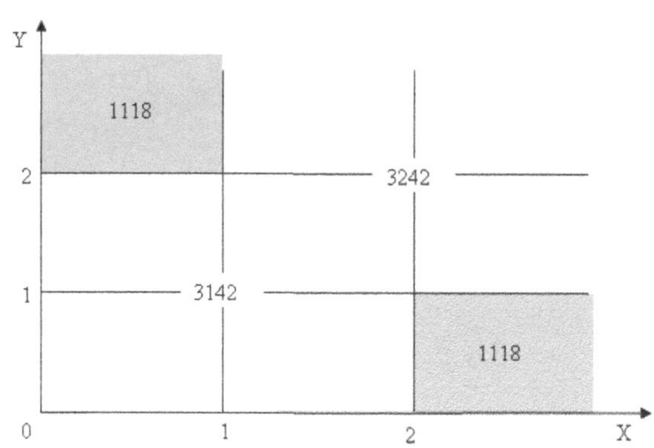

Fig. 3.12 Ordering of three objects

The POSAC algorithm can result in some profiles being unable to be accurately located in the two-dimensional coordinate space. With a large number of profiles, misrepresentation becomes a potential liability of POSAC. In order to measure how well POSAC retains comparabilities from the original data set, we compute the proportion of comparabilities correctly represented; if a pair of objects were comparable in the original data set, then they would have to be comparable with the correct orientation in the POSAC diagram in order to be considered correctly represented. Similarly, if a pair of objects is incomparable in the original data set, then they would have to be incomparable in the POSAC diagram as well. We would like the proportion of comparabilities correctly represented to be as high as possible, and a proportion above 0.75 is considered rather good for large data sets. Therefore, knowledge of the dim (X, IB) helps to evaluate the approximations of POSAC (see Chapter 11).

Here we use the program package SYSTAT 11 (http://www.systat.com) in the feature of Analysis in the toolbar, under Scale. The POSAC program produces a two-dimensional diagram with the objects represented and also provides the proportion of comparabilities that are correctly represented (see Section 11.3 for a pitfall of SYSTAT 11).

3.6 Down Sets and Up Sets

3.6.1 Complex Hasse Diagrams

Often we have to analyze data matrices, which have many rows (i.e., many objects) and many columns (i.e., many attributes). Hence the corresponding Hasse diagrams have many objects and many connecting lines.

An example of a complex Hasse diagram is shown in Fig. 3.13 (pollution in regions of Baden-Wuerttemberg, Germany).

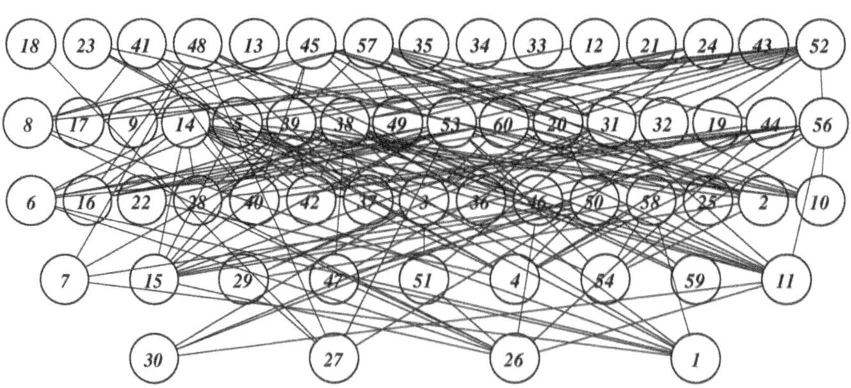

Fig. 3.13 Hasse diagram of 59 objects

Table 3.4 Methods to analyze complex ("messy") Hasse diagrams

No.	Methods	Remark	See section ...
1	Down sets, Up sets, and intervals	The data matrix remains unchanged	This section, see below
2	Selection of a subset of attributes	As we will discuss more thoroughly, deleting attributes from the data matrix will enrich the order relations. The Hasse diagram will get more chains and therefore simpler to analyze	Chapter 4
3	Discretization	Attributes continuous in concept may be classified	Chapter 6
4	p-Algorithm	Concentrate on the most important objects	Chapter 6
5	Aggregate attributes	...step by step, see METEOR	Chapter 7
6	Calculate the linear order	Either by analyzing the set of linear extensions or by application of approximate methods	Chapter 9
7	Contextual subsets	Taking a subset out of the whole set of objects with a common feature. For example, instead of 59 regions of Baden-Wuerttemberg, select only the regions with a common property, for example, granitic rock material	Chapter 11

How does a messy Hasse diagram in Fig. 3.13 help us? Generally a Hasse diagram provides an insightful, picturesque analysis and visualization to the problem. Even such a messy Hasse diagram reveals the extent of ambiguity due to incomparabilities and complexity due to the data matrix itself involved in the ordinal analysis of the data matrix. Some tools to analyze such Hasse diagrams are listed in Table 3.4.

Method 1: As we will see, the method of analyzing down sets, up sets, or intervals needs a selection of objects of interest. The data matrix is not changed. It is just an order theoretical selection of some rows of the data matrix. Down sets, up sets, and intervals allow us to "navigate" through the Hasse diagram.

Method 2: The data matrix is not transformed. However, there is a selection of columns.

Method 3: An order preserving transformation is applied. Such a transformation can certainly be justified, but it is a step away from the given data material.

Method 4: A transformation of the data matrix is performed, which helps to focus on priority objects.

Method 5: Columns of the data matrix are combined. For example, by a weighted sum of some attributes.

Method 6: A complete chain is obtained and the aim of ranking is fulfilled. However, considered from the point of view of Hasse diagrams, a chain does not tell us much about the objects themselves.

Method 7: Here a supervised selection of some rows of the data matrix is done. For example one may select all regions of Baden-Wuerttemberg, which are located at river Rhine. The information to select a subset of objects is an external one.

3.6.2 Principal Down Sets and Up Sets, and Successors and Predecessors

Let us select an object x. We investigate objects that have all attributes with smaller values. Following Chapter 2, we are seeking those elements y of the partially ordered set for which $y \leq x$ holds. In technical terms

$$O(x) := \{y \in X : y \leq x\} \tag{3.8}$$

As $O(x)$ depends on the element x, $O(x)$ is called the principal down set, generated by x:

$$y \in O(x) - \{x\} \text{ is a successor.} \tag{3.9a}$$

$$S(x) := O(x) - \{x\} \text{ is the set of successors.} \tag{3.9b}$$

Similarly, it is of interest to select an element x and find elements y with $x \leq y$.

$$\text{In technical terms, } F(x) := \{y \in X : y \geq x\}. \tag{3.10}$$

As $F(x)$ depends on the element x, $F(x)$ is called the principal up set, generated by x:

$$y \in F(x) - \{x\} \text{ is a predecessor.} \tag{3.11a}$$

$$P(x) = F(x) - \{x) \text{ is the set of predecessors.} \tag{3.11b}$$

Finally, it is of interest to select two elements x and y, $x \leq y$, and to determine element z with $x \leq z \leq y$. The set

$$I(x, y) := \{z : z \in X, x \leq z \leq y\} \tag{3.12}$$

is called the interval of x and y.

Down sets, up sets, and intervals are interesting, because they

- provide order theoretical tools to get simpler Hasse diagrams (as mentioned above, we speak of "navigation through a Hasse diagram") and
- are needed for several counting tools.

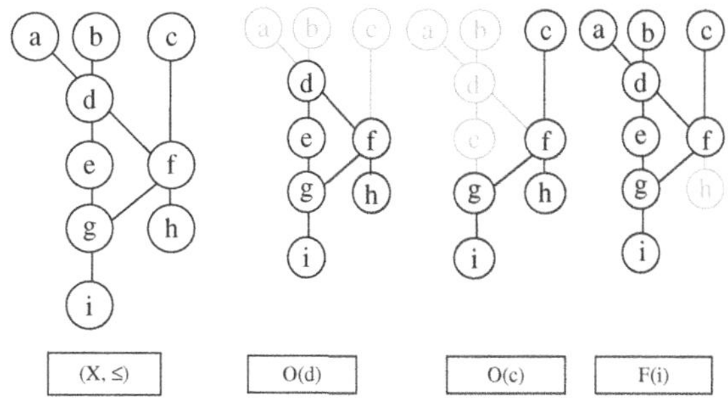

Fig. 3.14 Two principal down sets and one principal up set, taken from the poset $(X, \leq)$

$|O(x)|$, $|F(x)|$, $|I(x, y|$ can be easily determined by evaluating their definitions. In Fig. 3.14, the concepts of down sets and up sets are exemplified.

3.7 Ranking Interval

3.7.1 Index

To get linear or weak orders we can

1. rank objects using the information from the Hasse diagram and its parameters like $|F(x)|$, and $|O(x)|$, without introducing weights. We call this a canonical order and discuss this in Chapter 9;
2. introduce an index and try to get information about the possible range of positions of an object in the ranking due to that index.

We call an index Γ, a function based on the attributes of the information base.

Most often an index is just a weighted sum of column-wise normalized attributes. In that case, the weights are numbers between 0 and 1, their sum is 1, and the aggregation function is called an index.

The following observation holds.

Let $x, y \in X$ and $q(x)$ and $q(y)$ be the rows of normalized and correctly oriented attributes for objects x and y:

$$x \leq y \Rightarrow q(x) \leq q(y) \Rightarrow \Gamma(x) \leq \Gamma(y) \tag{3.13}$$

Therefore the mutual position of two comparable objects in a Hasse diagram will be reproduced in the index-based ranking, see Fig. 3.15.

3.7.2 A Relation Between (X, IB) and $(X, \{\Gamma\})$

When we refer to different orders (one due to (X, IB) and one due to $(X, \{\Gamma\})$, we will write O_{poset} and O_Γ. Due to O_Γ, the object x must at least get the height $|O(x)|$.

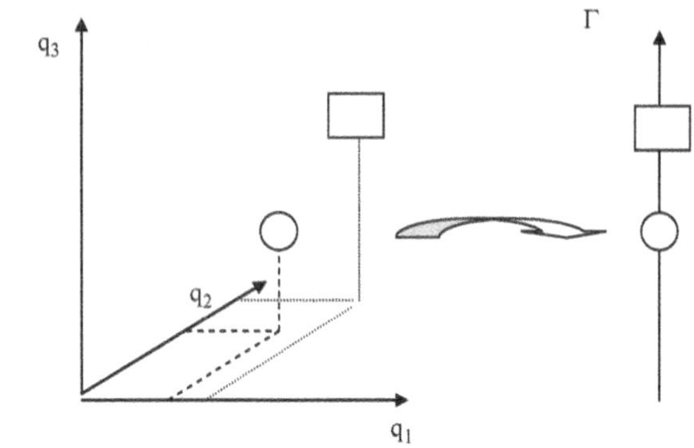

Fig. 3.15 Two comparable objects, "*circle*" < "*rectangle*," are characterized by values of three attributes: q_1, q_2, q_3. The index Γ maps them order preservingly into a one-dimensional coordinate

Let us now introduce the set $U(x)$:

$$U(x) := \{y \in X, y \parallel x \text{ in } (X, \text{IB})\} \tag{3.14}$$

Let $x \in X/_{\cong}$. Index Γ generally maps $y \in U(x)$ to positions below or above x, because for them, Eq. (13.3) does not hold. The maximal possible height for object x is

$$\text{Max}(h_\Gamma(x)) = |O(x)| + |U(x)| \tag{3.15}$$

All $y \in U(x)$ are imagined in positions below x, hence x gets the maximal possible height. The minimal possible height for object x is

$$\text{Min}(h_\Gamma(x)) = |O(x)| \tag{3.16}$$

Therefore maximal height – interval, $\text{Max}(h_\Gamma(x)) - \text{Min}(h_\Gamma(x))$, for any object x in O_Γ is

$$|O(x)| \leq h_\Gamma(x) \leq |O(x)| + |U(x)| \tag{3.17}$$

Hence the maximal height–interval $\Delta h_\Gamma^{\max}(x)$, the "ambiguity in ranking" is

$$\Delta h_\Gamma^{\max}(x) = n + 1 - (|O(x)| + |F(x)|), \; n \text{ being} |X/_{\cong}| \tag{3.18}$$

The right-hand side of Eq. (3.18) is $|U(x)|$. Hence Eq. (3.18) can also be written as

$$\Delta h_\Gamma^{\max}(x) = |U(x)| \tag{3.19}$$

We call $\Delta h_\Gamma^{\max}(x)$ the ranking interval of x in O_Γ and Eq. (3.19) tells us that the interval $\Delta h_\Gamma^{\max}(x)$ does not depend on Γ but on $|U(x)|$, which is a property of (X, IB).

For more details and examples, see Chapter 7. Also see Bruggemann et al. (2001) and Patil and Taillie (2004).

3.8 Summary and Commentary

Chapter 3 provides us with some concepts, like

- order preserving maps
- linear extensions
- average heights, ranking probability, and mutual rank probability
- dimension
- POSAC
- down sets and up sets

Order preserving maps are needed to define linear extensions. These in turn allow us to calculate average heights of objects and are a means to obtain a canonical order.

When the data matrix has more than three columns, a presentation as a series of scatter plots becomes troublesome; nevertheless, the Hasse diagram allows a graphical display of the objects in their ordinal relation to each other. Down sets, up sets, and intervals allow "navigation" through a Hasse diagram by focusing on the order relations of the generating elements.

POSAC goes a step further: POSAC helps the stakeholder by representing the objects in a two-dimensional plane, however by a more or less severe approximation, because some order relations will be ignored. The poset dimension can help to predict whether by POSAC an exact presentation in a two-dimensional plane is possible.

References

Annoni, P. and Bruggemann, R. (2009). Exploring partial order of European countries. Soc. Indicators Res., 92, 471–487.

Annoni, P., Bruggemann, R. and Saltelli, A. (2011). Partial order investigation of multiple indicator systems using variance – based sensitivity analysis. Environ. Model. Softw., 26, 950–958.

Atkinson, M.D. and Chang, H.W. (1986). Extensions of partial orders of bounded width. Congressus Numerantium, 52, 21–35.

Borg, I. and Shye, S. (1995). Facet theory – form and content. Thousand Oaks, CA: Sage.

Bruggemann, R. and Fredrich, F. (1997). Eine mathematische Analyse der Fischgesellschaften im gosener Feuchtwiesengebiet. In IGB (Ed.), Berichte des IGB 4 (pp. 93–94). Berlin: IGB.

Bruggemann, R., Halfon, E., Welzl, G., Voigt, K. and Steinberg, C. (2001). Applying the concept of partially ordered sets on the ranking of near-shore sediments by a battery of tests. J. Chem. Inf. Comput. Sci., 41(4), 918–925.

Bruggemann, R., Welzl, G. and Voigt, K. (2003). Order theoretical tools for the evaluation of complex regional pollution patterns. J. Chem. Inf. Comput. Sci., 43, 1771–1779.

De Fraysseix, H. and De Mendez, P.O. (1996). Planarity and edge poset dimension. Eur. J. Combinatorics, 17, 731–740.

Edelman, P., Hibi, T. and Stanley, R.P. (1989). A recurrence for linear extensions. Order, 6, 15–18.

Kreimes, K. (1996). Oekologisches Wirkungskataster Baden-Wuerttemberg – Bewertung und zusammenfassende Darstellung von Untersuchungsergebnissen. In: U. Arndt, A. Fomin, and S. Lorenz (Eds.), Bio-indikation; neuere Entwicklungen – Nomenklatur – Synoekologische Aspekte; Beitraege und Diskussion 1. Hohenheimer Workshop zur Bioindikation am Kraftwerk Altbach-Deizisau, 1995 (pp. 160–169). Ostfildern: Guenter Heimbach.

Patil, G.P. (2005). Cross-disciplinary class room notes. Center for Statistical Ecology and Environmental Statistics, Penn State University.

Patil, G.P. and Taillie, C. (2004). Multiple indicators, partially ordered sets, and linear extensions: Multi-criterion ranking and prioritization. Environ. Ecol. Stat., 11, 199–228.

POSAC. See http://ca.huji.ac.il/bf/hudap

Stanley, R.P. (1986). Enumerative combinatorics volume I. Monterey: WadsworthandBrooks/Cole.

SYSTAT. http://www.systat.com/.

Trotter, W.T. (1992). Combinatorics and partially ordered sets dimension theory. Baltimore, MD: The Johns Hopkins University Press.

Voigt, K., Bruggemann, R. and Pudenz, S. (2004b). Chemical databases evaluated by order theoretical tools. Anal. Bioanal. Chem., 380, 467–474.

Voigt, K., Welzl, G. and Bruggemann, R. (2004a). Data analysis of environmental air pollutant monitoring systems in Europe. Environmetrics, 15, 577–596.

Winkler, P. (1982). Average height in a partially ordered set. Discr. Math., 39, 337–341.

Chapter 4
Sensitivity and Ambiguity

4.1 Tasks

The fundamental basis of our ordinal analysis is the data matrix: The attributes define its columns and the objects its rows. We pose two questions:

1. What role does any single attribute play? Can we, for example, save time and money, because some attribute has little comparative power?
2. What can be said about the attribute set from the partial order point of view? Should we delete any attribute? Should we add more attributes to the data matrix?

We attempt to answer these two questions in this chapter. In Section 4.2, we consider impacts to the partial order when reducing the information base (attribute-related sensitivity) and in Section 4.3, we introduce a measure for the ambiguity of partial order in response to the set of attributes.

4.2 Attribute-Related Sensitivity

4.2.1 Concept

The intention behind an attribute-related sensitivity measure is not to contextually evaluate the attributes. Here it is of interest to examine as to how an attribute influences the position of objects in a Hasse diagram. We want to know the impact of the removal of a column from the data matrix.[1] Hence we have to compare the partial order, induced by the original data matrix, with that of the modified data matrix in order to find out the impact of the modification (i.e., the sensitivity to a Hasse diagram). We will measure the sensitivity by defining a suitable distance measure:

[1] We could also define as sensitivity of the (Spearman) correlation among indicators. This, however, is of no interest here.

R. Brüggemann, G.P. Patil, *Ranking and Prioritization for Multi-indicator Systems*, Environmental and Ecological Statistics 5, DOI 10.1007/978-1-4419-8477-7_4,

Large impact of the removal of a column of the data matrix will need large distance between initial poset and modified poset. The distance will be conceptualized by counting the ordinal change (mismatch) between the pairs $(x, y) \in (X, \text{IB})$ and $(x, y) \in (X, \text{IB}(i))$, with $\text{IB}(i) = \text{IB} - \{q_i\}$. (See Chapter 2 and especially Eqs. (2.8) and (2.9).) There are several methods counting the pairwise mismatch: (a) using down sets or up sets (see Chapter 3) or (b) using the ζ matrix (see Section 2.7).

4.2.2 Counting the Mismatches Using Down Sets

We restrict our analysis to down sets; using up sets would follow the same logic.

There are two information bases, the original one (IB) and the modified one which is called IB(i). $\text{IB}(i) \subset \text{IB}$, hence any comparability of (X, IB) must be reproduced in $(X, \text{IB}(i))$. Therefore

$$(X, \text{IB}(i)) \supseteq (X, \text{IB}) \text{ and } O(x, \text{IB}(i)) \supseteq O(x, \text{IB})$$

(As different information bases are of concern we extend the notation of down sets appropriately.) (4.1)

To count the ordinal mismatch between the two down sets, we use the symmetric difference of sets $\Delta(A \; \Delta \; B := (A \cup B) - (A \cap B), A, B$ being two arbitrary sets), count its content, and call the result $W(x, \text{IB}, \text{IB}(i))$[2]:

$$W(x, \text{IB}, \text{IB}(i)) = |O(x, \text{IB}(i)) \; \Delta \; O(x, \text{IB})| \tag{4.2}$$

As the complete object set X is of interest, we sum up

$$W(X, \text{IB}, \text{IB}(i)) = \sum W(x, \text{IB}, \text{IB}(i)), \quad x \in X \tag{4.3}$$

One can show that $W(X, \text{IB}, \text{IB}(i))$ is indeed a "distance" between both posets.

$$W(X, \text{IB}, \text{IB}) = W(X, \text{IB}(i), \text{IB}(i)) = 0, W(X, \text{IB}, \text{IB}(i)) = W(X, \text{IB}(i), \text{IB})$$

and the triangle inequality is fulfilled. Equation (4.2) can be simplified applying simple set-algebraic relations:

$$W(x, \text{IB}, \text{IB}(i)) = |O(x, \text{IB}(i))| - |O(x, \text{IB})| \geq 0 \tag{4.4}$$

Furthermore $W(X, \text{IB}, \text{IB}(i))$ can be normalized by the denominator $n^*(n-1)/2$, n being the number of objects:

---

[2] Note that the notation $W(X, \text{IB}, \text{IB}(i))$ has nothing to do with weights or weighting schemes.

$$\sigma(X, \text{IB}, \text{IB}(i)) = W(X, \text{IB}, \text{IB}(i))/(n^*(n-1)/2) \tag{4.5}$$

Generally $W(q_i)$ is used and we call this quantity the sensitivity measure of the partial order to the attribute q_i deleted from the data matrix.

4.2.3 Counting the Mismatches Using ζ Matrices

The method of down sets has some intuitive charm; the method by using ζ matrices, however, is computationally simpler. Let $\zeta(X, \text{IB})$ be the matrix ζ related to the original poset, (shorthand notation: ζ_1) and $\zeta(X, \text{IB}(i))$ (shorthand notation: ζ_2) related to the modified one. Then the (squared Euclidian) distance of ζ_1 from ζ_2 can be defined as follows:

$$D^2_{\zeta_1, \zeta_2} = \sum_i \sum_j (\zeta_{2,\,i,\,j} - \zeta_{1,\,i,\,j})^2 = \sum_i \sum_j |(\zeta_{2,\,i,\,j} - \zeta_{1,\,i,\,j})| \tag{4.6}$$

As before, we write simply $D^2(q_i)$ if there is no confusion possible.

4.2.4 Relation Between $W(q_i)$ and $D^2(q_i)$

The content of a down set $|O(x, \text{IB})|$ or $|O(x, \text{IB}(i))|$ can be calculated from the ζ matrix:

$$|O(x, \text{IB})| = \sum \zeta_{\text{IB}}(j, x)$$

(where we indicate the information base IB by a subscript and perform the sum over $j = 1, \ldots, n$). Hence Eq. (4.3) can also be written in terms of the ζ matrix: $W(x, \text{IB}, \text{IB}(i)) = \Sigma\zeta_{\text{IB}(i)}(j, x) - \Sigma\zeta_{\text{IB}}(j, x) = \Sigma(\zeta_{\text{IB}(i)}(j, x) - \zeta_{\text{IB}}(j, x))$, with $(\zeta_{\text{IB}(i)}(j, x) - \zeta_{\text{IB}}(j, x)) \geq 0$.

Changing to the complete object set X, we arrive as

$$W(X, \text{IB}, \text{IB}(i)) = \sum \sum (\zeta_{\text{IB}(i)}(j, x) - \zeta_{\text{IB}}(j, x))$$

which is the same as Eq. (4.6), in a slightly different notation.

4.2.5 Remarks

(1) If two posets have the same object set X but are of different contextual origin, then the methods presented in Sections 4.2.3 and 4.2.4 can be easily extended. See Bruggemann et al. (2001) or Bruggemann and Carlsen (2006).

(2) A further generalization is possible in selecting a subset $X' \subset X$ instead of X. For example, the down set-based sensitivity measure would read as follows (with (X, IB_1) and (X, IB_2) as two posets having the object set X in common):

$$W(X', \mathrm{IB}_1, \mathrm{IB}_2) = \sum_{x \in X'} (|O(x, \mathrm{IB}_1)| - |O(x, \mathrm{IB}_2)|) \tag{4.7}$$

(3) Originally the sensitivity measure based on down sets was of special interest, because the objects located at the top of a Hasse diagram were priority elements and their reaction on deleting attributes from the data matrix was to be modeled.

4.2.6 Illustrative Example

In Table 4.1, a data matrix with five objects and three attributes is displayed. We want to know the importance of q_i to the Hasse diagram.

Besides (*X*, IB), we need to analyze three other posets, namely $(X, \mathrm{IB}(1))$, $(X, \mathrm{IB}(2))$, and $(X, \mathrm{IB}(3))$ (Fig. 4.1).

4.2.6.1 Method Using Down Sets

The comparison of (*X*, IB) with $(X, \mathrm{IB}(1))$, $(X, \mathrm{IB}(2))$, and $(X, \mathrm{IB}(3))$ gives the following values for $W(q_i)$:

$$W(X, \mathrm{IB}, \mathrm{IB}(1)) = 0, W(X, \mathrm{IB}, \mathrm{IB}(2)) = 3, \text{and } W(X, \mathrm{IB}, \mathrm{IB}(3)) = 1$$

So we conclude that deletion of attribute q_2 has the most impact on the Hasse diagram.

In Table 4.2 we render in detail the calculation of $\mathrm{W}(X, \mathrm{IB}, \mathrm{IB}(2))$: columns *A*:=..., *B*:=... demonstrate the calculation of the contents of the down sets, generated by the elements of the first column; the remaining three columns show the steps to obtain for every generating element the symmetric difference. As finally a sum over all generating elements is to be performed, and the cell of the sixth column and last row represents the final result. The tie $a \cong b$ is considered as $a > b$ and at the same time $b > a$.

Table 4.1 Illustrative data matrix

	q_1	q_2	q_3
a	1	1	1
b	1	4	1
c	2	3	2
d	3	3	5
e	4	5	3

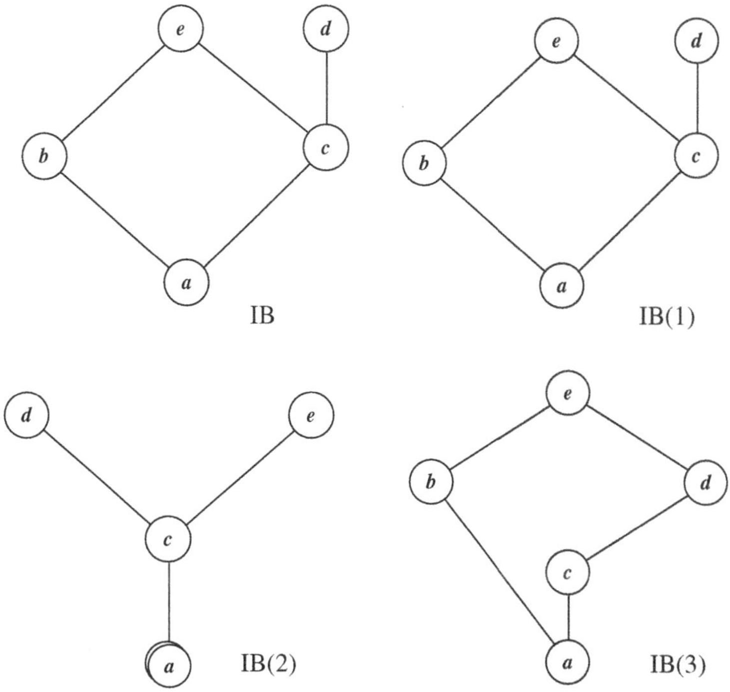

Fig. 4.1 Hasse diagrams of (X, IB) and three $(X, \mathrm{IB}(i))$. Note in $(X, \mathrm{IB}(2))$, there is an equivalence (tie): $a \cong b$

Table 4.2 Evaluation of $W(X, \mathrm{IB}, \mathrm{IB}(2))$

x	$A := O(x, \mathrm{IB})$	$B := O(x, \mathrm{IB}(2))$	$A \cup B$	$A \cap B$	$A \Delta B$
a	a	a, b	a, b	a	b
b	a, b	a, b	a, b	a, b	$\emptyset$
c	a, c	a, b, c	a, b, c	a, c	b
d	a, c, d	a, b, c, d	a, b, c, d	a, c, d	b
e	a, b, c, e	a, b, c, e	a, b, c, e	a, b, c, e	$\emptyset$
Σ					3

4.2.6.2 Method Using ζ Matrices

The calculation of $D^2(X, \mathrm{IB}, \mathrm{IB}(i))$ with $i = 1, 2, 3$ would need to determine the differences $\Delta\zeta := \zeta_{\mathrm{IB}(i)} - \zeta_{\mathrm{IB}}$, and then summing over all elements of $\Delta\zeta$. As $(X, \mathrm{IB}(2))$ not only is the most impacted poset but contains a tie ($a \cong b$), we select once again $D^2(X, \mathrm{IB}, \mathrm{IB}(2))$ as example. As in the down set-based method, we replace the tie $a \cong b$ by $a > b$ and $b > a$. Rows and columns are labeled as a, b, c, d, e and an entry 1 indicates that the row-determining element is greater than the column-determining element:

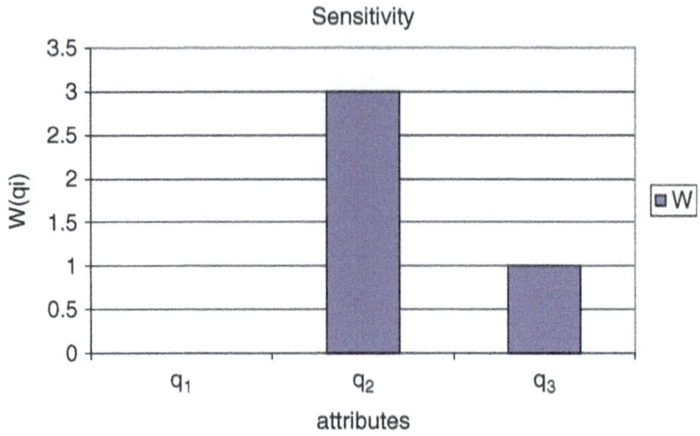

Fig. 4.2 Attribute-related sensitivity of the Hasse diagram (data matrix, see Table 4.1)

$$\varsigma_{\mathrm{IB}(2)} = \begin{pmatrix} 0&1&0&0&0 \\ 1&0&0&0&0 \\ 1&1&0&0&0 \\ 1&1&1&0&0 \\ 1&1&1&0&0 \end{pmatrix}, \varsigma_{\mathrm{IB}} = \begin{pmatrix} 0&0&0&0&0 \\ 1&0&0&0&0 \\ 1&0&0&0&0 \\ 1&0&1&0&0 \\ 1&1&1&0&0 \end{pmatrix}, \Delta\varsigma = \begin{pmatrix} 0&1&0&0&0 \\ 0&0&0&0&0 \\ 0&1&0&0&0 \\ 0&1&0&0&0 \\ 0&0&0&0&0 \end{pmatrix}$$

Equation (4.5) requires that summation be performed over all entries of the matrix $\Delta\xi$: Hence we arrive at $D^2(X, \mathrm{IB}, \mathrm{IB}(2)) = 3$.

Figure 4.2 shows the typical attribute-related sensitivity.

4.3 Ambiguity Due to Augmentation of Indicator Sets

4.3.1 Concept

Ranking ambiguity is caused by incomparabilities that appear in a poset. Hence we define

$$\begin{aligned} &U(X, \mathrm{IB}') = \{(x, y), x, y \in X \text{ with } x\|_{\mathrm{IB}'}y\}, \mathrm{IB}' \subseteq \mathrm{IB} \text{ and} \\ &U(X/\cong, \mathrm{IB}') := \{(x, y), x, y \in X/\cong \text{with } x\|_{\mathrm{IB}'}y\}, \mathrm{IB}' \subseteq \mathrm{IB} \end{aligned} \tag{4.8}$$

as measures of ambiguity in ranking (see Section 3.7, Eqs. (3.18) and (3.19)). In order to obtain a measure in the scale [0, 1], we normalize $|U(X, \mathrm{IB}')|$ by $n^*(n-1)/2n$ being the number of objects and $|U(X/\cong, \mathrm{IB}')$ by $n_K{}^*(n_K - 1)/2$, n_K

being the number of elements in the quotient set,[3] and call these quantities the ambiguity $\mathrm{Am}(X, \mathrm{IB}')$ of the poset (X, IB').

When $\mathrm{IB}' = \mathrm{IB}$, all indicators of the multi-indicator system are considered and Am(IB) becomes a characteristic quantity of the poset (X, IB) (formerly called P(IB)). We note that when the set of indicators $\{q_1, q_2, \ldots\}$ is augmented by a further indicator q', then $\mathrm{Am}(X, \{q_1, q_2, \ldots\}) \leq \mathrm{Am}(X, \{q_1, q_2, \ldots\} \cup \{q'\})$ (Halfon and Reggiani 1986).

4.3.2 Illustrative Example

In Fig. 4.3, a Hasse diagram together with its data matrix is depicted.

Although software is doing the job of counting $|U(X, \mathrm{IB})|$, it may be helpful to perform the counting "by hand." Following Fig. 4.3 and Table 4.3, the denominator $n^*(n-1)/2 = 28$, $|U(X, \mathrm{IB})| = 15$, hence $\mathrm{Am(IB)} = 0.536$. Let us add an attribute q_5, with values $q_5(a) = 8, q_5(b) = 7, q_5(c) = 6, q_5(d) = 5, q_5(e) = 4$, $q_5(f) = 3, q_5(g) = 2$, and $q_5(h) = 1$, then the partial order becomes a complete antichain (not shown), demonstrating the maximum possible ambiguity of $(X, \{q_1, \ldots, q_5\})$.

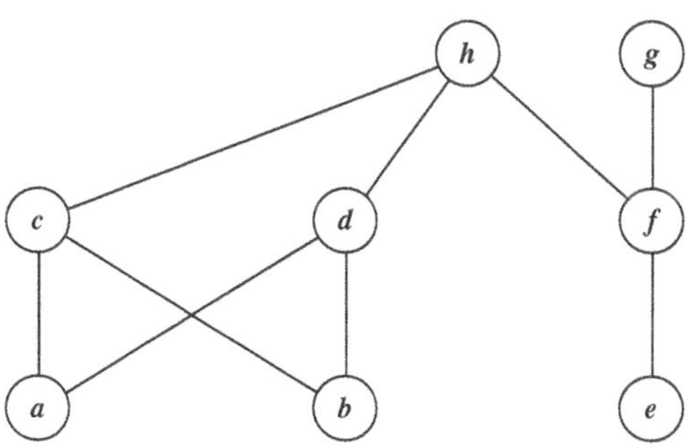

	q_1	q_2	q_3	q_4
a	1	4	2	1
b	2	5	1	2
c	3	6	4	3
d	4	7	3	4
e	5	1	5	5
f	6	2	6	6
g	7	3	7	8
h	8	9	8	7

Fig. 4.3 Illustrative example $X = \{a, b, c, d, e, f, g, h\}$, $\mathrm{IB} = \{q_1, q_2, q_3, q_4\}$

Table 4.3 Counting incomparabilities (Fig. 4.3). After checking a, c, e, f, g, no new incomparable pairs can be found

Object	Incomparable pairs	$\lvert U(x)\rvert$ (see Chapter 3)
g	$(g, h), (g, c), (g, d), (g, a), (g, b)$	5
f	$(f, d), (f, c), (f, a), (f, b)$	4
e	$(e, c), (e, d), (e, a), (e, b)$	4
c	(c, d)	1
a	(a, b)	1
Σ		15

[3] Although the difference between object set X and the quotient set $X/\cong$, and the set of representants, respectively, is very important, we write in the following simply X.

4.4 Graphs of Characteristic Properties of a Poset

4.4.1 Concept

Canonical sequence: We wish to define a cumulative set of indicators $\{q_1\} \subset \{q_1, q_2\} \subset \ldots \{q_1, q_2, \ldots, q_m\} = \text{IB}$ and call this series of attribute sets a canonical sequence. Because (IB, $\subset$) is a partial order, we can select several chains starting with a single indicator and ending up in the complete set of indicators, IB. We use the sensitivity $W(q_i)$ to order the subsets of IB. The order of accumulating the indicators in the canonical sequence follows the decreasing order of the $W(q_i)$ values. When the sensitivities are tied, we order arbitrarily and document this appropriately. We call the serial count of the cumulative subsets natt.

Cumulative ambiguity graph: The ambiguity $\text{Am}(X, \text{IB}')$ can be considered as a function of natt, Am(natt). As such, Am(natt) indicates the following: (i) $\text{Am(natt)} = 0$: the indicators do not yield conflicting rankings, weights are not needed; (ii) $\text{Am(natt)} = 1$: no comparability remains and without weights no ranking can be obtained; (iii) $0 < \text{Am(natt)} < 1$: comparabilities can be found in the poset and a relative ranking of some objects is possible. If nevertheless a ranking of all objects is wanted, then canonical orders can be determined. (iv) When $\text{Am}(X, \text{IB}')$ approaches $\text{Am}(X, \text{IB})$ with cumulation of indicators, the poset (X, IB′) may be considered as an approximation for (X, IB) and the chains and other quantities of interest can be identified. The corresponding reduced set IB′ plays the role of IB in subsequent ranking studies. (v) Whereas a high value of Am(X, IB) indicates that additional indicators will not have much of influence on the poset (X, IB), it is not possible to make further statements about additional indicators.

Decomposition of IB: Consider a certain value of natt, say natt* with $1 < \text{natt}^* < m$. Then a set $\text{IB}^{(1)}$ of the first natt* indicators and a set $\text{IB}^{(2)}$ of the residual indicators can be obtained. When we follow the device of ordering the indicators due to decreasing sensitivity, the set $\text{IB}^{(1)}$ has the indicators which mainly contribute to conflicts, whereas $\text{IB}^{(2)}$ has the indicators of less conflicting potential. Therefore, $\text{IB}^{(2)}$ may be considered as the set of "fine-tuning" indicators.

CAM: Am(natt) has its maximal value if $\text{natt} = m$, and as discussed above, is a characteristic quantity of the poset (X, IB) related to the multi-indicator system. Therefore, we call Am(m) the "cumulative ambiguity maximum" (CAM). If CAM is "near" 1, the partial order has only few comparabilities in comparison to $n^*(n-1)/2$. So an additional indicator will not have a large impact on the Hasse diagram. Removing an indicator from the multi-indicator system, however, may induce many changes.

Local ambiguity graph: $|U(x, \{q_1, q_2, \ldots\})|$: $|U(x)|$ as function of natt allows a "local" view, because the graph is related to a single object. The shape of the curve deviates sometimes characteristically from that of Am(natt), because the focus is on a single object instead of the whole object set. In view of Section 3.7, the curve shows how the maximum ranking interval, $\Delta h_\Gamma^{\max}$, of object x varies with natt. The resulting graph is called local ambiguity graph.

Minimum rank graph: Because $|O(x)|$ indicates the minimum rank of x in any composite indicator Γ, the function $|O(x)| = f(\text{natt})$ is of interest. Its graphical display is called the minimum rank graph and makes the variation of the minimum rank position of x evident, while starting with the most important attribute and accumulating one attribute after another according to the canonical sequence until the complete set of attributes is obtained.

$|F(x)| = f(\text{natt})$: $|F(x)|$ as a function of natt shows how the number of predecessors varies with natt. This curve is rarely used. Therefore, it has no name.

Relation among $|O(x)|, |U(x)|$, and $|F(x)|$: Changes in $|O(x)|$ or $|F(x)|$ imply changes in $|U(x)|$ because

$$|U(x)| + |O(x)| + |F(x)| = n + 1 \tag{4.9}$$

holds, n being $|X/\cong|$. (See also Chapter 6.) Hence

$$\begin{aligned} &|A(x)|\,(\text{natt} = k) \leq |A(x)|\,(\text{natt} = k+1), A \text{ being } O, S, F, \text{ or } P \\ &\Rightarrow |U(x)|\,(\text{natt} = k+1) \geq |U(x)|\,(\text{natt} = k) \end{aligned} \tag{4.10}$$

4.4.2 Remarks

(1) Basically all characteristics of partial order can be considered as a function of natt. For example, the width of a poset could equally well be used. However, up to now the characteristics mentioned above seem to be the most useful ones.

(2) Sometimes it is useful to explain the graphs of the characteristics of a partial order with model partial orders. For example, Am(natt) may increase, whereas $|O(x)|$ remains constant. A partial order model would then be as shown in Fig. 4.4.

4.4.3 Illustrative Example

The Hasse diagram together with its data matrix is shown in Fig. 4.5.

Figure 4.6 represents the results of the attribute-related sensitivity.

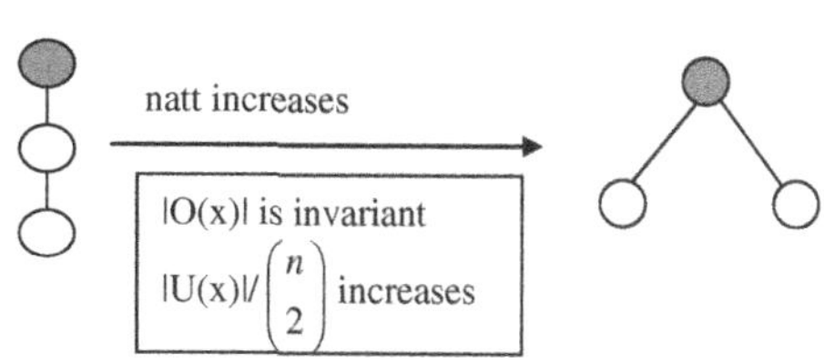

Fig. 4.4 Model poset explaining the graphs of characteristics of the poset. Object x, grey circle

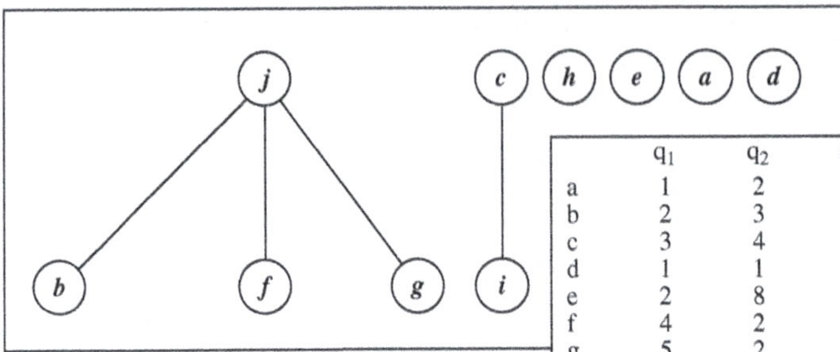

	q_1	q_2	q_3	q_4	q_5
a	1	2	3	4	5
b	2	3	1	6	5
c	3	4	4	2	5
d	1	1	5	4	7
e	2	8	6	5	2
f	4	2	2	5	6
g	5	2	1	5	6
h	6	3	8	2	7
i	2	4	3	1	3
j	8	5	2	9	9

Fig. 4.5 Example $X = \{a, b, c, d, e, f, g, h, i, j\}$, $\text{IB} = \{q_1, q_2, \ldots, q_5\}$

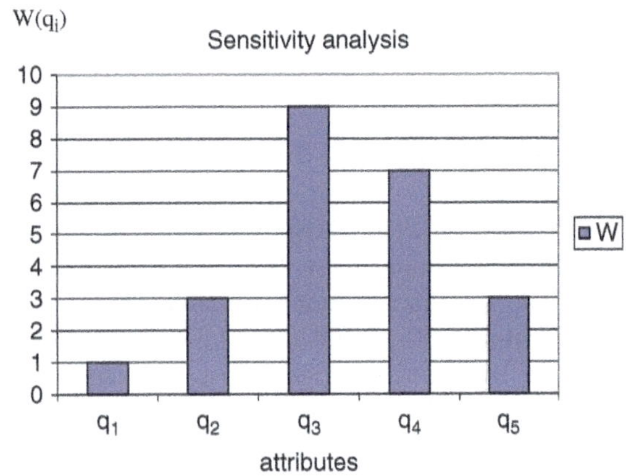

Fig. 4.6 Results of attribute-related sensitivity

We order the indicators as follows: $q_3 > q_4 > q_2 > q_5 > q_1$, with $q_2 > q_5$ as arbitrary choice. Hence we get five attribute sets and find the canonical sequence:

$$\{q_3\} \subset \{q_3, q_4\} \subset \{q_3, q_4, q_2\} \subset \{q_3, q_4, q_2, q_5\} \subset \{q_3, q_4, q_2, q_5, q_1\} = \text{IB}$$

Am(natt) is shown in Fig. 4.7.

One may consider the first two indicators (following the canonical sequence) as $\text{IB}^{(1)}$ and the residual ones as $\text{IB}^{(2)}$. Here the decomposition does not lead to striking differences in the two partial orders, because the cumulative ambiguity graph reaches CAM with a pretty smooth slope.

The graphs $|O(x)|$, $|U(x)|$ vs natt with objects c and f are shown in Fig. 4.8.

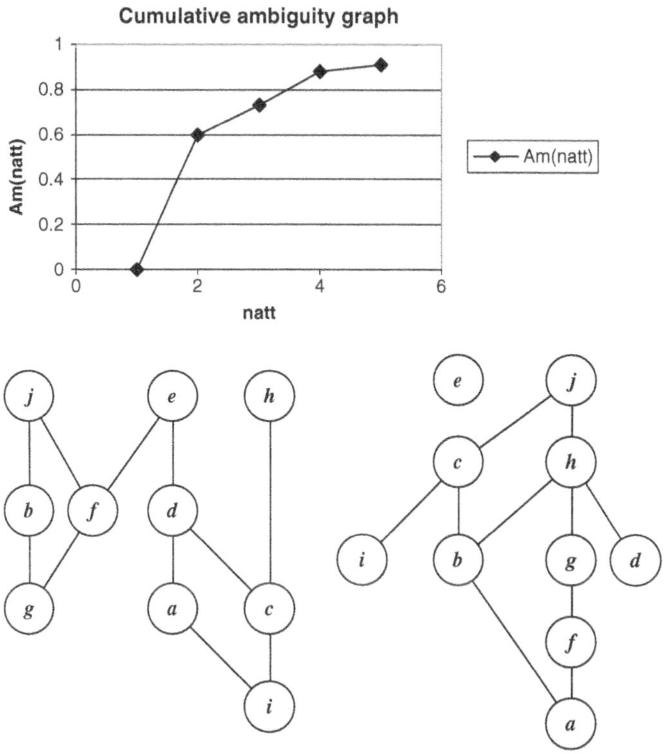

Fig. 4.7 *Top*: Cumulative ambiguity graph, based on the data of Fig. 4.5. *Bottom*: (*LHS*) The partial order due to $\text{IB}^{(1)} = \{q_3, q_4\}$, with $|U(X, \text{IB}^{(1)})| = 27$, and (*RHS*) $\text{IB}^{(2)} = \{q_1, q_2, q_5\}$, with $|U(X, \text{IB}^{(2)})| = 25$

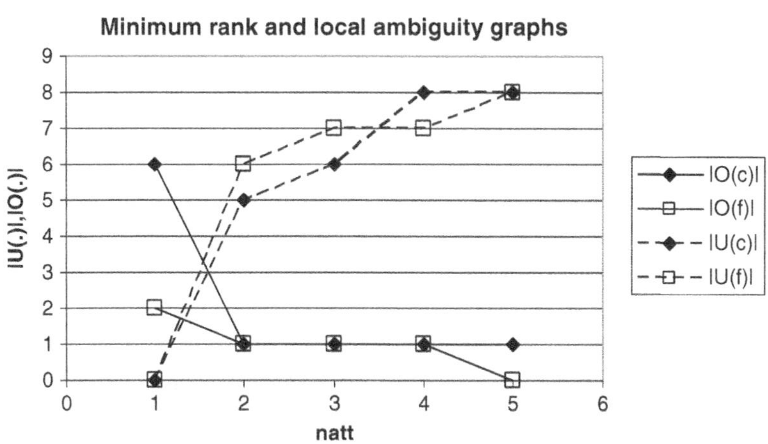

Fig. 4.8 $|O(x)|$ and $|U(x)|$ of objects c and f as functions of natt

Minimum rank graph:

(a) *Object f*: The rather low number of successors of object *f* is slightly reduced; finally, object *f* becomes a minimal element.
(b) *Object c*: This object has many successors if the order O_{q3} is considered. The next attribute q_4 reduces the number of successors; the remaining three attributes do no more influence the number of successors and therefore the minimum rank.

Local ambiguity graph:

(a) *Object f*: The addition of q_4 remarkably increases its incomparabilities; the remaining attributes have less influence on $|U(f)|$.
(b) *Object c*: The function $|U(x)|$(natt) is approximately linear. Any new attribute has the same importance to the position of object *c* in the overall order O_Γ.

4.5 Summary and Commentary

In Chapter 4, we developed the concepts (i) sensitivity measure, (ii) ambiguity, (iii) cumulative ambiguity graph, and (iv) minimum rank graph, and other graphs depending on the canonical sequence of attributes.

Sensitivity helps to find out influential attributes for the whole object set. Due to the design of the sensitivity measure, the sensitivity for a single object can be investigated. Future work should stress the multivariate character of the sensitivity analysis as several characteristics of a partial order must be examined simultaneously. Methods suggested and developed by Saltelli (http://en.wikipedia.org/wiki/Sensitivity; Saltelli and Annoni, 2010) may be a good basis. This may suggest possibilities of where improvements by stakeholders are possible in the data matrix.

CAM sounds more academic. However, it is important to know as to whether the attribute set or a part of it is sufficient to characterize the problem, or whether it exceeds the needs of an evaluation. Sensitivity and ambiguity (called earlier stability) were introduced pretty early in the literature. See Bruggemann et al. (2001), Bruggemann and Voigt (1996), and Voigt et al. (2004a, b).

A large positive slope of the cumulative ambiguity graph can be indicative of the initial attributes being sufficient to perform the ranking. This will enable future investigations with smaller set of attributes, thus saving time and money. Furthermore Am(natt) provides an overview of the whole object set. If an individual object is of more interest, the minimum rank graph or other similar line graphs like the local ambiguity graph support the analysis. A steep decrease in the minimum ranking graph, for instance, indicates that the additional indicators have a major influence on the position of the object. In case of ties, then canonical sequence is not uniquely defined and different graphs may be obtained. Therefore, the actually selected sequence should be documented. In the future, we will add a tie-breaking rule.

References

Bruggemann, R. and Carlsen, L. (2006). Partial order in environmental sciences and chemistry (p. 406). Berlin: Springer.

Bruggemann, R., Halfon, E., Welzl, G., Voigt, K. and Steinberg, C. (2001). Applying the concept of partially ordered sets on the ranking of near-shore sediments by a battery of tests. J. Chem. Inf. Comput. Sci., 41(4), 918–925.

Bruggemann, R. and Voigt, K. (1996). Stability of comparative evaluation, – example: Environmental databases. Chemosphere, 33, 1997–2006.

Halfon, E. and Reggiani, M.G. (1986). On ranking chemicals for environmental hazard. Environ. Sci. Technol., 20, 1173–1179.

Saltelli, A. http://en.wikipedia.org/wiki/Sensitivity.

Saltelli, A. and Annoni, P. (2010). How to avoid a perfunctory sensitivity analysis. Environ. Model. Softw., 25, 1508–1517.

Voigt, K., Bruggemann, R. and Pudenz, S. (2004a). Chemical databases evaluated by order theoretical tools. Anal. Bioanal. Chem., 380, 467–474.

Voigt, K., Welzl, G. and Bruggemann, R. (2004b). Data analysis of environmental air pollutant monitoring systems in Europe. Environmetrics, 15, 577–596.

Chapter 5
Structures of Partial Orders

5.1 Motivation

While visualizing a poset (*X*, IB) with a Hasse diagram, it is initially interesting to observe the following:

1. Whether or not there is a messy system of lines.
2. Whether the Hasse diagram resembles a
   a. triangular shape or
   b. rectangular shape.
3. Whether there are different components or approximate components.

As (*X*, IB) is based on a data matrix, we want to relate these three aspects in the Hasse diagram with the properties of the data matrix. That is, we want to discover properties of the data matrix through the structure of Hasse diagrams. Therefore, Chapter 5 is organized as follows: (1) we revisit the concept of levels, (2) we show how down sets and up sets are related to attribute properties, (3) the concept of separation of object subsets is introduced, (4) we explain why and how far structures of a poset and properties of a data matrix are related. Finally, (5) the concept of dominance of object subsets is discussed.

5.2 Levels and Shapes of a Hasse Diagram

5.2.1 Width and Height

In Chapter 2, height and width of a poset have been introduced. Both numbers describe the shape of a Hasse diagram by inscribing it into a rectangle with height and width. The determination of width may be difficult (at least in complex Hasse diagrams) as the following example (Fig. 5.1) shows.

In Fig. 5.1, the height is 3, and following the drawing protocol of Hasse diagrams (by different software packages like WHASSE and PyHasse, see Chapter 17) we

R. Brüggemann, G.P. Patil, *Ranking and Prioritization for Multi-indicator Systems*, Environmental and Ecological Statistics 5, DOI 10.1007/978-1-4419-8477-7_5,

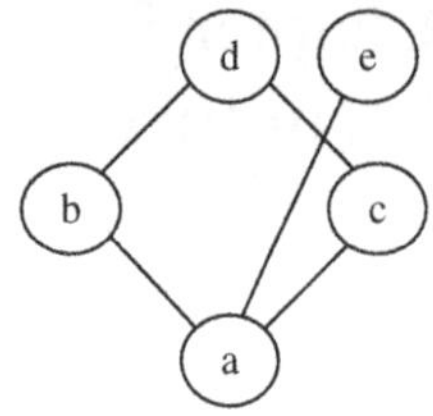

Fig. 5.1 Width and antichains

identify the antichains $\{b, c\}$, $\{d, e\}$ both having two elements. However, the width of the poset in Fig. 5.1 is 3, because the maximum antichain is $\{b, c, e\}$. In messy Hasse diagrams, it is difficult to identify the maximum antichain by visual inspection. Therefore, we use the concept of levels as a visual proxy for the discussion of shapes of the Hasse diagrams.

5.2.2 Level

The concept of levels is very useful:

- Due to the level concept, a weak order can be found among the objects.
- Levels are descriptive tools as they allow a partitioning of the objects even in messy Hasse diagrams.
- Levels are the starting point for a visualization technique, developed by Myers and Patil (2008), suitable for a huge number of objects.

5.2.2.1 Construction

$$\text{Let MAX} \subseteq \text{X be the set of maximal elements of a poset (see Chapter 2).} \tag{5.1}$$

$$\text{lg} = \text{number of cover relations in the maximum of all maximal chains.} \tag{5.2}$$

$$\text{An element } x \in \text{MAX gets the level number lev}(x) = \text{lg} + 1 = \text{height.} \tag{5.3}$$

Now perform a partitioning of X as follows.

Eliminate MAX from X and determine the new MAX. This new set gets a level number reduced by 1.

Continue the elimination process until X is exhausted.

The level sets are the equivalence classes under the equivalence relation:

$$\text{lev} = \text{lev}(x) = \text{lev}(y), \text{ with lev} \in \{1, 2, \ldots, \text{height}\} \tag{5.4}$$

$$\text{Notation: level}_{\text{lev}} \text{ is the level set with the level number lev.} \tag{5.5}$$

In Fig. 5.2, an example follows.

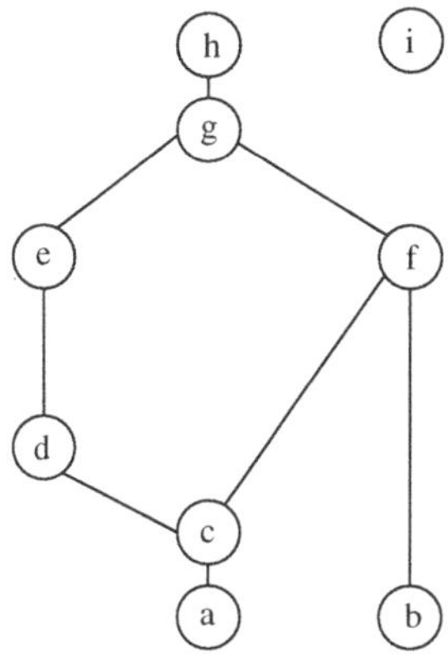

Start
lg = 5
because the maximum of the maximal chains is a ≤ : c, c ≤ :d, d ≤ :e, e ≤ : g, g ≤ : h.

MAX = {h, i} and gets as level set:
Level_6 = {h,i}

Elimination process:
After elimination of Level_6 from X the new MAX is: {g}, and gets level number 5.
Hence level_5 = {g}
The next elimination renders {e,f} as the set with level number 4.

Levels (as sets):
level_6 = {h,i}
level_5 = {g}
level_4 = {e,f}

Level numbers:
lev(c) = 2
lev(e) = lev(f) = 4
lev(a) = 1
lev(b) = 3

Fig. 5.2 Illustrative example of the concept "level"

By the number lev, the levels are enumerated from the bottom to the top of a Hasse diagram. By introducing the equivalence relation among objects "having equal lev" (RL), the quotient set $X/_{\text{RL}}$ consists of the levels and the levels are strictly ordered due to increasing lev. In terms of the object set *X*, we obtain a weak order.

5.2.3 Shapes of Hasse Diagrams

5.2.3.1 Motivation

Roughly, we can identify the following types of shapes of Hasse diagrams:

1. With increasing level number, $|\text{level}_{\text{lev}}|$ is constant: rectangular shape. The number of incomparabilities is approximately constant.
2. With increasing level number, $|\text{level}_{\text{lev}}|$ is increasing: The vertex of the triangle is at the bottom of the Hasse diagram. The incomparabilities are increasing with lev.
3. With increasing level number, $|\text{level}_{\text{lev}}|$ is decreasing: The vertex of the triangle is at the top of the Hasse diagram. The incomparabilities are decreasing with lev.

For most practical purposes, these three basic shapes are sufficient.

In order to motivate the role of shapes, let us think of a class of students, being evaluated with respect to different disciplines:

- *Rectangular shape*: Independent of the level of skill, the disparity in the performance in single disciplines remains the same.
- *Triangle with the vertex at the bottom*: With increasing skill, the students show more and more disparity in the performance in single disciplines.
- *Triangle with the vertex at the top*: The better, in general, the student, the lesser the disparity in the performance in different disciplines.

5.2.3.2 Sharpening the Concept

Incomparabilities are not only among the elements of the levels but also between those of different levels such as the objects *b* and *e* in Fig. 5.2:

$$U(\text{level}_i) := \sum_{x \in \text{level}_i} |U(x)| \tag{5.6}$$

From Eq. (5.6), we can calculate the average number of incomparabilities of the *i*th level:

$$\overline{U}(\text{level}_i) = \frac{U(\text{level}_i)}{|\text{level}_i|} \tag{5.7}$$

Applying mainHD16.py of the PyHasse (see Chapter 17) delivers three histograms (Fig. 5.3).

The outcomes shown in Fig. 5.3 confirm that its Hasse diagram can be considered as having a triangular shape.

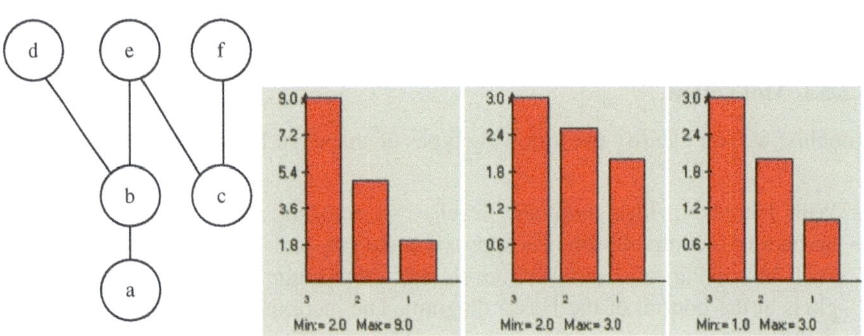

Fig. 5.3 *Top*: Hasse diagram; *bottom*: (*LHS*) $U(\text{level}_i)$, (*middle*) $\overline{U}(\text{level}_i)$, and (*RHS*) $|\text{level}_i|$ as function of the lev

5.2.4 Shapes and Weak or Linear Orders

The shape of a Hasse diagram allows to establish a relation

- through $\overline{U}(\text{level}_i)$ between lev and $\Delta h_\Gamma^{\max}(x)$, $x \in \text{level}_{\text{lev}}$, i.e., between lev and the ranking intervals and
- between lev(x) and $\min(h_\Gamma(x))$ (Chapter 3) because in general $|O(x)|$ increases with lev(x)

as follows:

Rectangular shape: Increasing lev(x) has no strong influence on $\Delta h_\Gamma^{\max}(x)$, $x \in \text{level}_{\text{lev}}$, because $\overline{U}(\text{level}_i)$ does not change much with lev.
Triangular shape (vertex at the bottom): Increasing lev(x) implies increasing $\Delta h_\Gamma^{\max}(x)$, $x \in \text{level}_{\text{lev}}$ and $\min(h_\Gamma(x))$, because $\overline{U}(\text{level}_i) < \overline{U}(\text{level}_{i+1})$ and in general $|O(x)|$ becomes larger with lev.
Triangular shape (vertex at the top): Increasing lev(x) implies decreasing $\Delta h_\Gamma^{\max}(x)$, $x \in \text{level}_{\text{lev}}$ but increasing $\min(h_\Gamma(x))$, because $\overline{U}(\text{level}_i) > \overline{U}(\text{level}_{i+1})$ and $|O(x)|$ increases with lev.

5.3 Down Sets and Up Sets Related to Properties of the Data Matrix

5.3.1 Idea

So far down sets and up sets are introduced to (i) simplify the Hasse diagram and (ii) relate $\Delta h_\Gamma^{\max}(x)$ with $|U(x)|$.

In this section, we render a relation between principal down sets and principal up sets and properties of the data matrix.

5.3.2 Realization

Through Eqs. (2.3) and (2.6)

$$y \in O(x) \Rightarrow q_i(y) \leq q_i(x) \text{ and } y \in F(x) \Rightarrow q_i(y) \geq q_i(x) \tag{5.8}$$

and

$$y \in \cap\, O(x_i) \Rightarrow q_j(y) \leq \min(q_j(x_i)) \text{ and } y \in \cap\, F(x_i) \Rightarrow q_j(y) \geq \max(q_j(x_i)) \tag{5.9}$$

Equations (5.8) and (5.9) couple properties of a poset (down sets and upsets) with some properties of the data matrix. Hence, navigation through a Hasse diagram, keeping Eqs. (5.8) and (5.9) in mind, renders some insights into the data matrix:

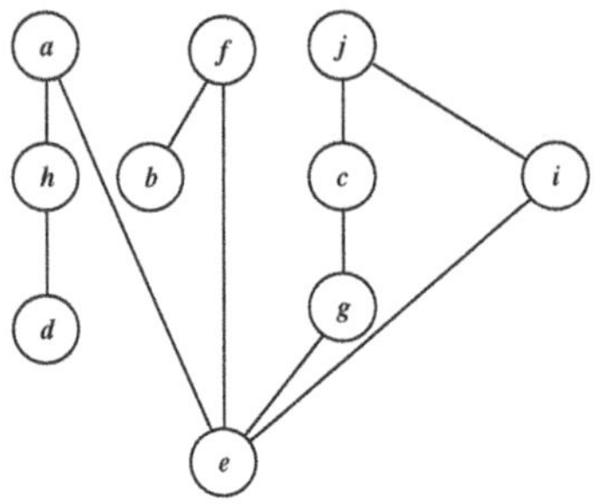

	q_1	q_2	q_3	q_4
a	8	4	2	2
b	1	3	7	2
c	2	8	1	3
d	8	0	1	1
e	2	4	0	1
f	2	4	8	3
g	2	7	1	2
h	8	3	2	1
i	7	5	0	2
j	7	8	2	5

Fig. 5.4 Hasse diagram of (X, IB), $X = \{a, b, c, d, e, f, g, h, i, j\}$, $\text{IB} = \{q_i : i = 1, \ldots, 4\}$

Application of Eqs. (5.8) and (5.9) is best done for minimal or maximal objects (Chapter 2) in order to obtain useful, nonempty down sets and up sets.

5.3.3 Illustrative Example

In Fig. 5.4, a Hasse diagram together with its data matrix is shown.

- *Object j*: $q_3(j) = 2$. The range of $q_3(x)$ is $0, \ldots, 8$. Equation (5.8) tells us that every object in $O(j)$ must have values in q_3 which are less than or equal to 2.
- *Object f*: $q_1(f) = 2$. The range of $q_1(x)$ is $1, \ldots, 8$. Equation (5.8) tells us that for objects *b* and *e* (being elements of $O(f)$), $q_1 \leq 2$.
- *Object a*: $q_4(a) = 2$. The range of $q_4(x)$ is $1, \ldots, 5$. Equation (5.8) tells us that for objects *h*, *e*, and *d* (being elements of $O(a)$), $q_4 \leq 2$.
- *Object e*: $e \in (O(f) \cap O(j) \cap O(a))$. Equation (5.9) tells us that e must have low values simultaneously in q_1, q_3, and q_4. Especially $e \in O(i)$, hence $q_3(e) = 0$ as $q_3(i) = 0$.
- *Object e*: $q_2(e) = 4$. Equation (5.8) tells us that $q_2(x) \geq 4$ for all elements $x \in F(e) = \{e, a, f, g, c, j, i\}$.

5.4 Separation of Object Subsets

5.4.1 Motivation

By a Hasse diagram, an ordinal representation of an $n \times m$ matrix in a plane is possible, even if *m* (the number of attributes (columns of the matrix)) is larger than 2. As such, it is a convenient visualization taking care of the order relations among the objects due to Eq. (2.3) or (2.6). However, the data profiles (Section 3.5) cannot directly be seen. Even if POSAC allows an approximate two-dimensional scatter plot based on latent order variables, the relation to the original attributes is difficult to establish. So, why not try a projection of object subsets to a two-dimensional plane based on the original attributes preserving order theoretical information as much as possible? Hence the questions are the following:

(1) Which projection? and (2) Which object subsets?

We begin with the second question, give then an answer to the first one. Finally we discuss an intimate relation between the Hasse diagram and the data matrix.

5.4.2 Separated Subsets, an Illustrative Example

Figure 5.5 shows the Hasse diagram of 11 objects and three attributes.

Naturally the following questions arise:

(1) Why are all the objects of the subset $X_1 = \{m_{34}, m_{33}, m_{32}, m_{31}, m_3\}$ not comparable with all those of the subset $X_2 = \{m_1, m_2, m_{12,1}, m_{12,2}, m_{12,3}\}$? What are the common properties of X_1 and X_2 responsible for their separation in the Hasse diagram?

Beyond this, the second question in Section 5.4.1 is still open: How do we find such separated subsets in a messy Hasse diagram?

5.4.3 Articulation Points and Separated Object Subsets

Here we are going to answer the second question of Section 5.4.2.

Let n_{H1} be the number of components in poset (X, IB) and x_a be an element of $X/\cong$ such that $(X/\cong - \{x_\mathrm{a}\}, \mathrm{IB})$ has n_{H2} components with $n_{\mathrm{H2}} > n_{\mathrm{H1}}$, then x_a is called an articulation point. (5.10)

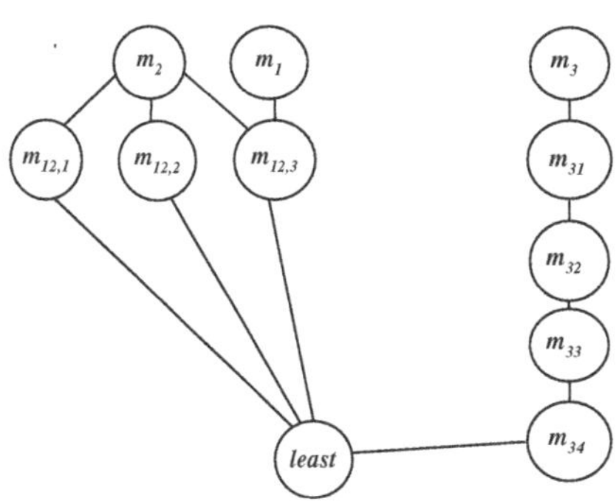

	q_1	q_2	q_3
m_1	8	9	1
m_2	9	8	2
m_3	2	6	8
$m_{12,1}$	6	7	2
$m_{12,2}$	7	6	2
$m_{12,3}$	7	7	1
least	1	1	1
m_{31}	2	6	7
m_{32}	1	5	7
m_{33}	1	4	6
m_{34}	1	3	6

Fig. 5.5 (*LHS*) Hasse diagram of the data matrix (*RHS*)

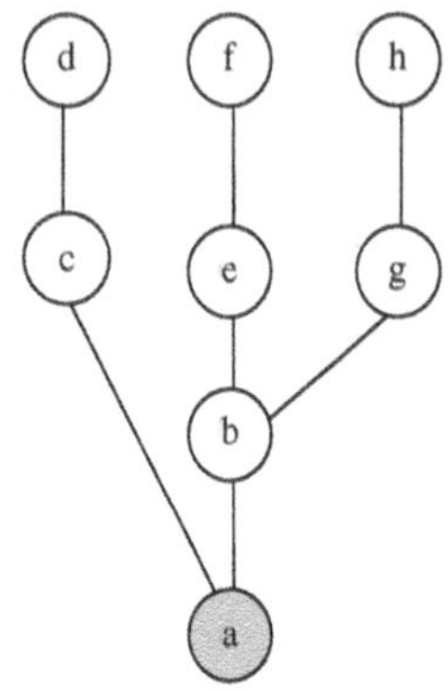

Fig. 5.6 Hasse diagram exemplifying the concept "articulation point"

In Fig. 5.5 the object "least," in Fig. 5.6 object a is an articulation point. By deletion of the row of object a (Fig. 5.6) in the data matrix, we obtain two disjoint subsets $X_1 = \{d, c\}$ and $X_2 = \{b, e, f, g, h\}$ which are components in the partial order. However, object b is not an articulation point, because $\{g, h\}$ and $\{e, f\}$ are still connected with object a through the transitivity of order relations (Chapter 2).

Let us identify two disjoint subsets X_1 and X_2 such that for all $x \in X_1$ and all $y \in X_2$, $x \mid\mid y$. We call such disjoint object subsets separated object sets and the identification of articulation points is a tool to find separated object subsets, because their presence is the reason for what we called "approximate components."

In Fig. 5.6, the subsets $\{c, d\}$ and $\{b, e, f, g, h\}$ are approximate components. Deletion of the articulation point (object a) generates two components.

5.4.4 Separability

5.4.4.1 Motivation

The concept of separability goes the other way round: Instead of trying to find separated subsets, it is supposed that two candidate subsets are found, and we want to assess their degree of separation.

5.4.4.2 Concept

Let us identify two disjoint subsets of $X/\cong$: X_1 and X_2. The possible number of relations (i.e., of $<$ or $\mid\mid$ relations) $N(X_1, X_2)$ between X_1 and X_2 is

$$N(X_1, X_2) = |X_1|^* |X_2| \tag{5.11}$$

Let $x \in X_1$ and $y \in X_2$, then $x \mid\mid y$ or $x < y$ or $y < x$. We count the $\mid\mid$ relations as follows:

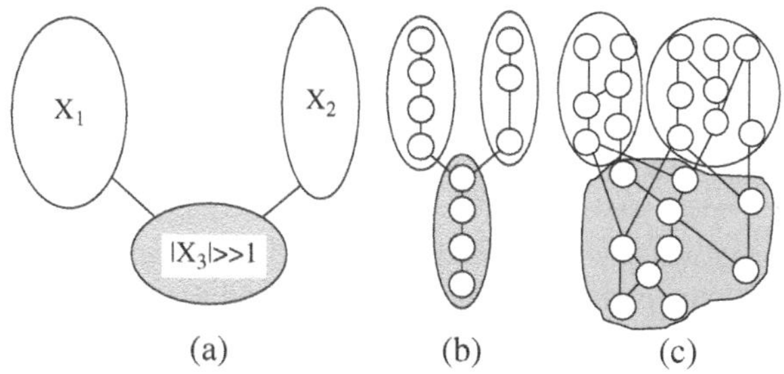

Fig. 5.7 (**a**) Separated subsets in a schematic presentation of Hasse diagrams. (**b**) and (**c**) Examples for which the scheme (**a**) may stand

$$U(X_1, X_2, \mathrm{IB}') = \{(x, y) : x \ ||_{\mathrm{IB}'} y, \ x \in X_1, \ y \in X_2, \ X_1 \cap X_2 = \emptyset\}, \ \mathrm{IB}' \subseteq \mathrm{IB} \quad (5.12)$$

We define the separability, $\mathrm{Sep}(X_1, X_2, IB')$, as follows:

$$\mathrm{Sep}(X_1, X_2, \mathrm{IB}') := |U(X_1, X_2, \mathrm{IB}')| / N(X_1, X_2) \quad (5.13)$$

We note that $\mathrm{Sep}(X_1, X_2, \mathrm{IB}') = \mathrm{Sep}(X_2, X_1, \mathrm{IB}')$.

The separability allows us to characterize any disjoint pair of subsets $X_i, X_j \subset X$ and to find separated subsets without checking the Hasse diagram for articulation points (Fig. 5.7).

5.4.4.3 Illustrative Example

Figure 5.8 shows a Hasse diagram together with three subsets X_1, X_2, and X_3, $X_i \subset X$. We demonstrate the calculation of Sep $(X_\mathrm{i}, X_\mathrm{j})$[1]:

$$|X_1| * |X_2| = 4, |U(X_1, X_2)| = 4, \mathrm{Sep}(X_1, X_2) = 1$$
$$|X_1| * |X_3| = 6, |U(X_1, X_3)| = 6, \mathrm{Sep}(X_1, X_3) = 1$$
$$|X_2| * |X_3| = 6, |U(X_2, X_3)| = 4, \mathrm{Sep}(X_2, X_3) = 4/6 = 0.666$$

In the first two cases, the subsets X_1 and X_2 are separated, whereas subsets X_2 and X_3 are not separated.

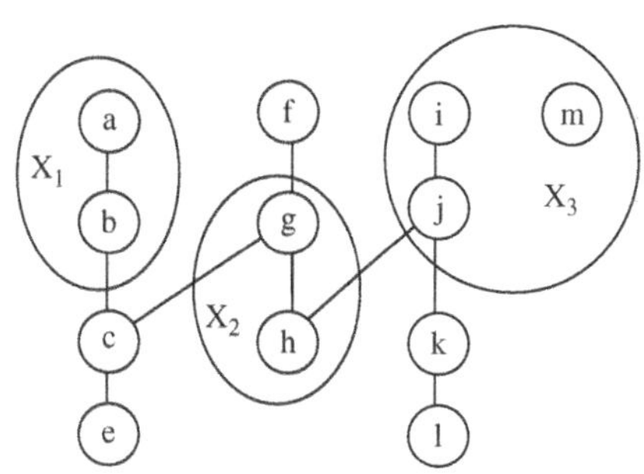

Fig. 5.8 Hasse diagram to demonstrate the calculation of separability

[1] We sometimes simplify the notation by omitting the reference to IB'.

5.5 Data Matrix and Separation of Object Subsets in Partial Order

5.5.1 Motivation

So far we have discussed how to find separated subsets. These subsets are found by applying partially ordered object set and are not necessarily an expression of external classification. For example, by inspection of a Hasse diagram, two separated subsets may be identified which consist of both countries of Asia and Europe. Thus the interest is in properties of the data matrix that are responsible for this separation.

In this section, our focus is to find a best projection (question 1 in Section 5.4.1) and how we can find approximate solutions.

5.5.2 Antagonism

5.5.2.1 Concept

It should be possible to relate structural properties of the Hasse diagram, like the appearance of separated object subsets to properties related to the data matrix.

Let us consider $x, y \in X$ and $x \,||\, y$. The singletons $\{x\}$ and $\{y\}$ are the simplest example of separated object subsets. In case of $x \,||\, y$, there are two attributes q_i and q_j, $i \neq j$ such that $q_i(x) < q_i(y)$ and $q_j(x) > q_j(y)$. We say, the separation of x and y is due to q_i and q_j. Let us now consider two separated object subsets X_1 and X_2 with $|X_1|$ or $|X_2| > 1$, then it may be possible that not just one pair of attributes breaks all comparabilities simultaneously among the (unordered) pairs of $X_1 \times X_2$. Hence, we have to search for the smallest subset of attributes which simultaneously breaks all comparabilities of $(x, y) \in X_1 \times X_2$.

If IB' exists such that $x \,||_{IB'} y$ for all $x \in X_1$ and all $y \in X_2$ with $X_1, X_2 \subset X$ and $\text{Sep}(X_1, X_2) = 1$ and IB' $\neq \emptyset$, IB' $\subseteq$ IB, then we call IB' the set of antagonistic attributes/indicators and abbreviate it by AIB(X_1, X_2) (antagonistic information base) and we often write AIB if there is no confusion possible (Simon, 2003; Simon et al., 2004a, b). AIB contains those attributes which are causing the separation of subsets X_1 and X_2: While some attributes of AIB may have large values for objects of X_1 and small values for those of X_2, some other attributes have low values for objects of X_1 and large ones for X_2. The attributes of AIB separate X_1 and X_2 because they are "antagonistic."

The smallest possible AIB is a pair $\{q_i, q_j\}$ such that for all $x \in X_1$ and all $y \in X_2$, we obtain $x \,||\, y$. (5.14)

1. This is the most desirable result of antagonism study because then a reasonable graphical display by a two-dimensional scatter plot may be possible. We also write that the attributes of AIB "explain" the separation of X_1 and X_2. The search for AIB is a computational task and is a tool in the software WHASSE (Bruggemann et al., 1999), as well as in PyHasse (Bruggemann and Voigt, 2009).

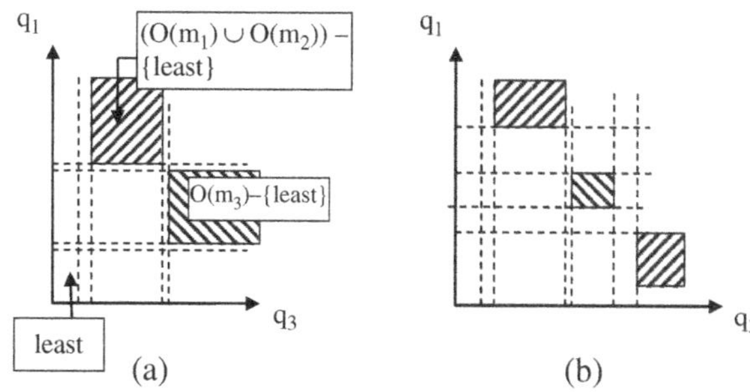

Fig. 5.9 |AIB| = 2. (**a**) A scatter plot of X_1 and X_2 (Fig. 5.5); (**b**) a more complex pattern of two separated subsets

Example 1: Two attributes are sufficient to explain the separation of two subsets.

We return to the Hasse diagram of Fig. 5.5 and select the subsets $X_1 = \{m_{34}, m_{33}, m_{32}, m_{31}, m_3\}$ and $X_2 = \{m_1, m_2, m_{12,1}, m_{12,2}, m_{12,3}\}$. We note that $\text{Sep}(X_1, X_2) = 1$. Indeed AIB contains only two attributes q_1 and q_3, so we are able to construct a scatter plot (Fig. 5.9).

Figure 5.9 demonstrates the usefulness of the concept of antagonistic attributes: We see that q_1 has large values for X_2 and low values for X_1, whereas q_3 has low values for X_2 but large values for X_1, thus explaining the separation of the two subsets.

It may however be possible that we need more than two attributes to explain the separation of object subsets (Example 2), and it is possible that even with $|\text{AIB}| = 2$, the pattern of the separated subsets X_1 and X_2 is more complex (Fig. 5.9b).

Example 2 (real-life example):

Scientists of the Canadian Center of Inland Waters (CCIW) have developed a test battery (see Dutka et al., 1986). The responses of this test battery (our indicators) indicate the status of water samples or sediment samples with respect to their adverse impact on humans and on the environment.

The test battery includes as attributes (i) one fecal test (fecal coliforms, FC), (ii) two hygienic tests (test for coprostanol and coliforms *Escherichia coli*), CP and CH, (iii) one test for acute toxicity, MT (Microtox® test), and (iv) a genotoxicity test. Fifty sediment sites, labeled by numbers, were analyzed by applying this test battery. Figure 5.10 shows the Hasse diagram.

By inspection, we select two subsets X_1 and X_2 with $\text{Sep}(X_1, X_2) = 1$:

$$X_1 := \{5,\ 25,\ 27,\ 31,\ 95\} \text{ and } X_2 := \{7,\ 9,\ 18,\ 23,\ 32\}$$

How many and which attributes out of the five responses of the test battery explain that separation? Figure 5.11 shows how $\text{Sep}(X_1, X_2, \text{IB}_i)$ increases, depending on the number of attributes.

Figure 5.11 demonstrates that four out of five attributes are necessary to explain the separation of X_1 and X_2. Therefore in Section 5.5.3, we pose the question: "if $|\text{AIB}| > 2$, then what?"

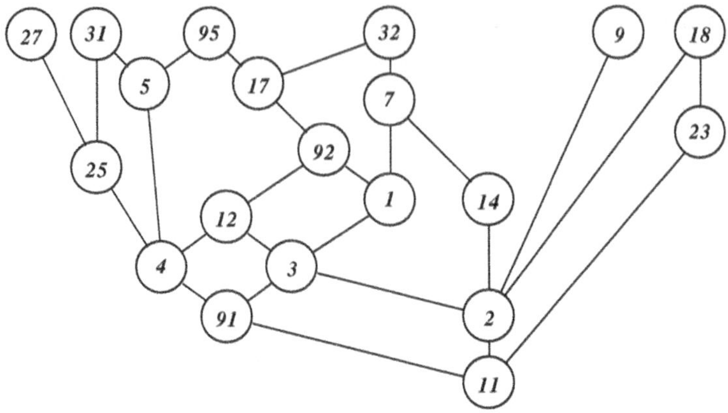

Fig. 5.10 Hasse diagram of sediment samples of Lake Ontario, based on a test battery

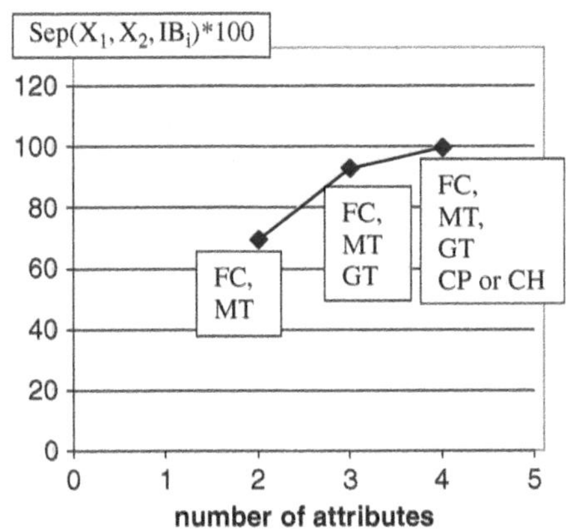

Fig. 5.11 Antagonism of attributes, Lake Ontario. *Ordinate* explained separation in % when IB_i is increasing, according to natt

5.5.3 *If |AIB| > 2, Then What?*

5.5.3.1 Motivation

In the case of $|\text{AIB}| = 2$, there is often a nice pictorial representation possible, like that shown in Fig. 5.9a. We recover diagrams of this kind several times in the application part of this monograph. However, if $|\text{AIB}| > 2$, then a 2D scatter plot allows only an insufficient view on the properties of the data matrix. Nevertheless, some general insights are possible even if $|\text{AIB}| > 2$: Let us assume that $|\text{AIB}| = 3$ and $1 > \text{Sep}(X_1, X_2, \{q_1, q_2\}) > 0.5$.

We see that $\{q_1, q_2\}$ does not completely explain the separation of X_1 and X_2. However, the separability degree is large enough to assume that a scatter plot based on q_1 and q_2 is a good starting point. Obviously, some few object pairs (one object taken from X_1 and the other one from X_2) are only incomparable if a third attribute is introduced. So, one may find graphical techniques to indicate the role of the third attribute to break the remaining comparabilities. We will present several examples in the application part (for example, we will construct a 3D scatter plot in the watershed case study, Chapter 14).

In the following, we will not display possible visualization techniques but demonstrate by an example that the appearance of separated subsets in the partial order implies some constraints on the attributes of the data matrix.

5.5.3.2 Structures in the Hasse Diagram Imply Constraints on the Data Matrix

Let us think of a scatter plot where the separation is not complete, like in Fig. 5.12.

There are the subset $X_2 = X_{20} \cup X_{21} \cup X_{22}$ and the subset X_1. The subsets X_1 and X_{20} are large in comparison to X_{21} and X_{22}. X_1 and X_{20} alone would be completely separated by the attributes q_1 and q_2. However, X_{21} and X_{22} contain objects which are comparable with some of X_1, thus causing an incomplete separation of X_1 and X_2. The third attribute q_3 has to break these comparabilities. A scatter plot (Fig. 5.12) will serve as an example.

The following observations are based on the assumption that a geometrical configuration as in Fig. 5.12 holds. In our experience, this kind of scatter plot is quite common. We define

$$X_i < X_j :\Leftrightarrow, \text{ for all } x \in X_i, \text{ for all } y \in X_j : x < y$$
$$X_i \parallel X_j :\Leftrightarrow, \text{ for all } x \in X_i, \text{ for all } y \in X_j : x \parallel y$$

To accomplish a complete separation by one and only one attribute q_3, the attribute must necessarily lead to the following order relations:

$$X_{21} >_{q3} X_1 \text{ and } X_{22} <_{q3} X_1 \tag{5.15}$$

Before we show how the structure of the Hasse diagram (existence of separated subsets) implies constraints on the data matrix, we need a compact notation:

$$q_3(X) := \{q_3(x), x \in X\} \text{ and } q_3(X_1) > q_3(X_2) :\Leftrightarrow, \text{ for all } x \in X_1 \text{ and all } y \in X_2 : q_3(x) > q_3(y)$$

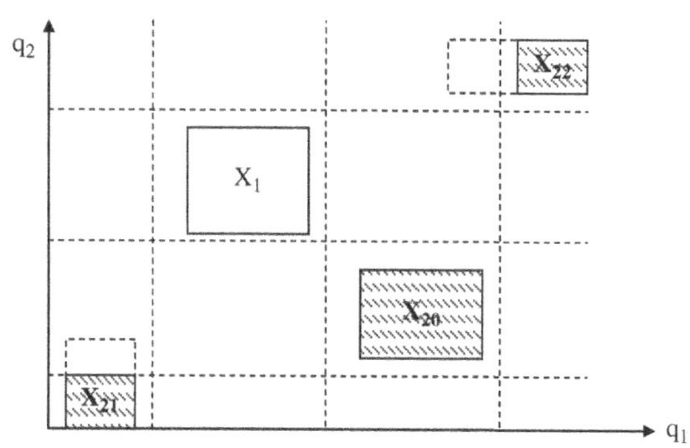

Fig. 5.12
$X_2 = X_{20} \cup X_{21} \cup X_{22}$. X_1 is separated from X_{20} completely. There may be some overlap of X_{20} with X_{21} and X_{22} (indicated by *broken lines*)

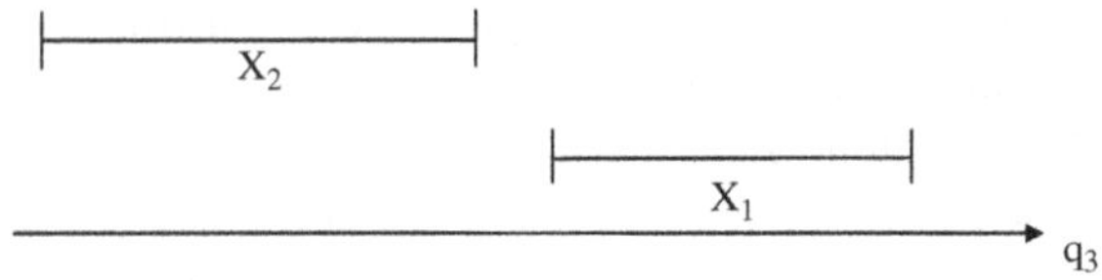

Fig. 5.13 Presentation of the order relation with respect to q_3 on the line of real numbers: $q_3(X_2) < q_3(X_1)$

We can represent $q_3(X_1) > q_3(X_2)$ as closed intervals on the line of real numbers (Fig. 5.13).

We show that the assumption (a) $q_3(X_1) > q_3(X_{20})$ or (exclusively (b) $q_3(X_1) < q_3(X_{20})$) together with Eq. (5.15) leads to a contradiction of the assumption $|\mathrm{AIB}| = 3$.

In the case of (a), we find $X_{21} >_{q_3} X_1, X_{21} <_{q_1} X_1, X_{22} <_{q_3} X_1, X_{22} >_{q_1} X_1, X_{20} <_{q_3} X_1$ and $X_{20} >_{q_1} X_1$. Hence $X_1 \,||_{\{q1,q3\}}\, (X_{21} \cup X_{22} \cup X_{20})$.

Similarly in the case of (b), we find $X_1 \,||_{\{q2,q3\}}\, (X_{21} \cup X_{22} \cup X_{20})$.

Assumptions (a) and (b) imply that only two attributes would explain the separation to 100% which contradicts $|\mathrm{AIB}| = 3$.

Therefore

$$|\mathrm{AIB}| = 3 \Rightarrow q_3(X_1) \cap q_3(X_{20}) \neq \emptyset \text{ or } q_3(X_{20}) \cap q_3(X_1) \neq \emptyset \tag{5.16}$$

Together with Eq. (5.15), we arrive at Fig. 5.14, which summarizes the result.

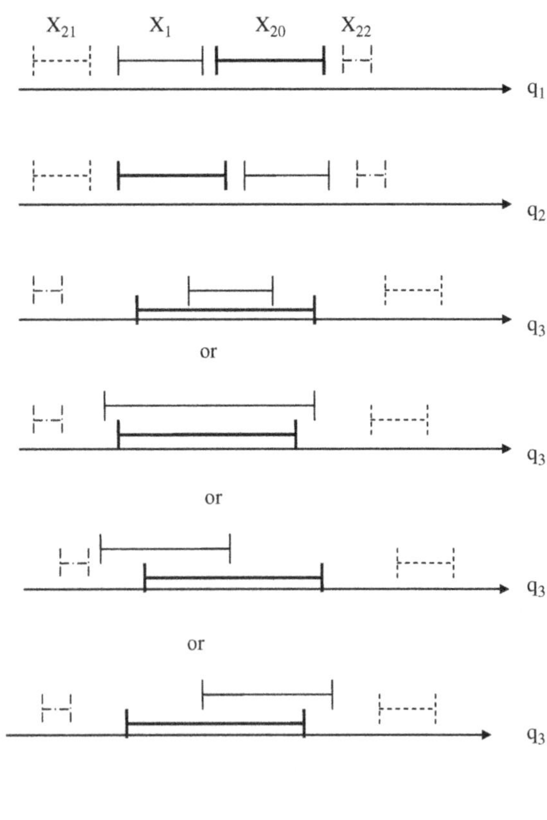

Fig. 5.14 Schematic representation of the intervals of the object sets if $|\mathrm{AIB}| = 3$

Assuming the geometrical configuration such as in Fig. 5.12, we see that separated subsets with |AIB| = 3 imply that $q_3(X_{20})$ or $q_3(X_1)$ must be within an interval, with an upper limit by the minimum value of $q_3(X_{21})$ and a lower limit by a maximum value of $q_3(X_{22})$, and that the intervals $q_3(X_1)$ and $q_3(X_{20})$ must have a common intersection.

A 3D model within a real case study can be seen in Chapter 14 (Fig. 14.3).

5.6 Dominance and Separability

5.6.1 Motivation

Let us think of a poset (*X*, IB) with many objects. Often there is an additional information available by which a partitioning of *X* is possible. For example, students in a class may be evaluated by their knowledge in different disciplines. The set of students can be partitioned by the regions from where they come. Is it possible to rank the regions on the basis of the order relations among the students? This question will normally be answered by an appropriate aggregation by which attribute values of students of a certain region are transformed for the corresponding region (by forming means, or medians or adding up, etc.). Here we outline that a procedure is available which does not need to define an aggregation function to perform the transition from the microscale (the students and their evaluations in different disciplines) to a macroscale (regions and their evaluation with respect to different disciplines).

5.6.2 Concept

For any two subsets $X_1, X_2 \subset X/\cong$, $X_1 \cap X_2 = \emptyset$, $\mathrm{Sep}(X_1, X_2, \mathrm{IB})$ may be between 0 and 1. We define

$$\begin{aligned} \mathrm{Dom}(X_1, X_2) &:= |\{(x, y) \in X_1{}^*X_2, x \geq y\}|/(|X_1|^*|X_2|) \\ \mathrm{Dom}(X_2, X_1) &:= |\{(x, y) \in X_1{}^*X_2, x \leq y\}|/(|X_1|^*|X_2|) \end{aligned} \tag{5.17}$$

and

$$\mathrm{Sep}(X_1, X_2) := |U(X_1, X_2)|/(|X_1|^*|X_2|) = |\{(x, y) \in X_1{}^*X_2, x \,||\, y\}|/(|X_1|^*|X_2|)$$

then

$$\begin{aligned} &\mathrm{Dom}(X_1, X_2) + \mathrm{Dom}(X_2, X_1) + \mathrm{Sep}(X_1, X_2) = 1 \\ &\mathrm{Dom}(X_1, X_2) \neq \mathrm{Dom}(X_2, X_1), \mathrm{Dom}(X_i, X_j) \in [0, 1] \end{aligned} \tag{5.18}$$

We speak of X_i dominates X_j to the degree $\mathrm{Dom}(X_i, X_j)$. The dominance relation can be represented as a directed graph (digraph) as follows: (i) each subset X_i is drawn as a vertex labeled with i, (ii) vertices are connected by a directed edge (i, j) if $\mathrm{Dom}(X_i, X_j) > 0$, and (iii) the directed edges are weighted by $\mathrm{Dom}(X_i, X_j)$ and pointing from vertex i to vertex j. The directed and weighted graph – a network – can be transferred into a simple digraph as follows:

> If $\mathrm{Dom}(X_i, X_j) > \varepsilon$, then ($i$, j) are connected by an edge starting from i and pointing to j. If $\mathrm{Dom}(X_i, X_j) \leq \varepsilon$, then there is no connection from vertex i to vertex j. For an example, see Section 5.6.4.

5.6.3 Is the Dominance Relation a Partial Order?

Is the $\mathrm{Dom}(X_1, X_2) > 0$ and $\mathrm{Dom}(X_2, X_3) > 0$ sufficient to call dominance relations among subsets a partial order among subsets? The following example (Fig. 5.15) shows that a dominance relation is not necessarily transitive.

The number of elements in each of the three subsets is $|X_1| = 3$, $|X_2| = 6$, and $|X_3| = 3$.

$\mathrm{Dom}(X_1, X_2) = 9/18$, $\mathrm{Dom}(X_2, X_3) = 9/18$; however, $\mathrm{Dom}(X_1, X_3) = 0$.

Restrepo and Bruggemann (2008) show that, for $\varepsilon \geq 0.5$, the digraph is a partial order.

5.6.4 Illustrative Example

In Fig. 5.16, a Hasse diagram is shown. Furthermore, three sets are defined by encircling objects: $X_1 = \{h, f, b\}, X_2 = \{e, a\}$, and $X_3 = \{d, g, c\}$.

By counting one finds

$$\begin{array}{l} \mathrm{Dom}(X_1, X_2) = 5/6,\ \mathrm{Dom}(X_2, X_1) = 0,\ \mathrm{Sep}(X_1, X_2) = 1/6 \\ \mathrm{Dom}(X_2, X_3) = 0,\ \mathrm{Dom}(X_3, X_2) = 3/6,\ \mathrm{Sep}(X_2, X_3) = 3/6 \\ \mathrm{Dom}(X_1, X_3) = 1/9,\ \mathrm{Dom}(X_3, X_1) = 0,\ \mathrm{Sep}(X_1, X_3) = 8/9 \end{array}$$

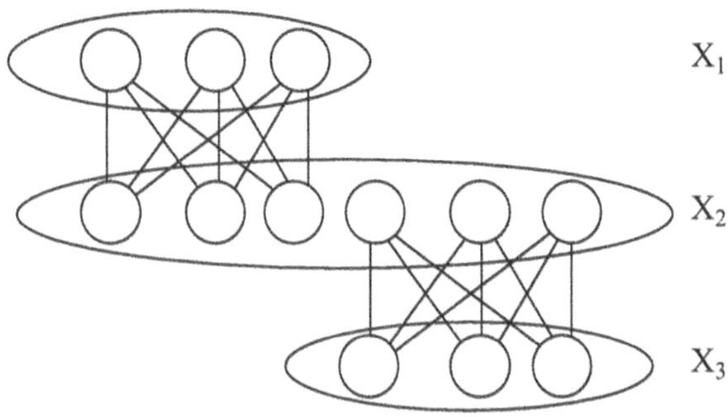

Fig. 5.15 Three subsets X_1, X_2, X_3 mutually disjoint

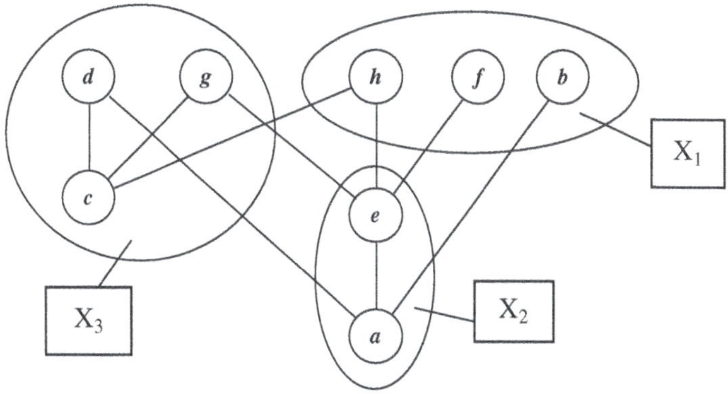

Fig. 5.16 Dominance of subsets of X due to the order relations of their elements

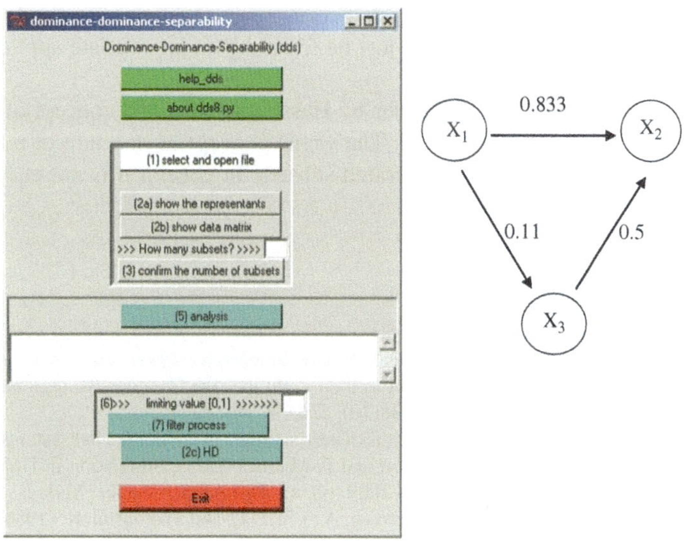

Fig. 5.17 (*LHS*) Graphical user interface of PyHasse module dds8.py and the weighted directed graph (*RHS*) corresponding to Fig. 5.16

We apply the PyHasse program "dds8.py" (see Chapter 17). Figure 5.17 shows its graphical user interface (LHS). After the user input of ε, the program dds8.py provides the corresponding directed graph (RHS).

From the directed graph (also called a dominance diagram), we can derive the dominance sequence: $X_1 > X_3 > X_2$.

The articulation point search or depth-first search for graph theoretical components of the Hasse diagram may be helpful. Whenever promising subsets are found, their separation can be assessed by examining the separability. Once separated subsets are found, we can identify the corresponding smallest "antagonistic indicator base," AIB, capable of explaining their separation. We provide an example in which

|AIB| > 2 has implications on the data matrix. If a partition of the object set X is available by external knowledge, we can calculate not only the separability but also dominance. Instead of searching for order relations referring to objects, we can scale up and search for relations among the subsets of the partition. Introduction of a threshold ε leads to a digraph in which subsets relate to each other. This digraph is a partial order if $\text{Dom}(X_i, X_j) > \varepsilon \geq 0.5$.

5.7 Summary and Commentary

Partial orders can be very complex; therefore we need different tools to perform an adequate analysis. The shape of the Hasse diagrams and the analysis of the incomparabilities per level allow an overview about the data matrix with respect to the order relation it is inducing. It turns out that the concept of level is very useful. Another tool is provided by down sets or up sets because they allow some insights into the data profiles. An "ideal object" may just be found by an appropriate application of Eq. (5.9).

By the visualization of partial order by Hasse diagrams, the concept of a structure of a partial order was motivated. The vague concept of structure of posets can be sharpened by the concept of separated subsets. In general it is not easy to find separated subsets.

References

Bruggemann, R., Pudenz, S., Voigt, K., Kaune, A. and Kreimes, K. (1999). An algebraic/graphical tool to compare ecosystems with respect to their pollution. IV: Comparative regional analysis by Boolean arithmetics. Chemosphere, 38(10), 2263–2279.

Bruggemann, R. and Voigt, K. (2009). Analysis of partial orders in environmental systems applying the new software PyHasse. In W. Jochen and F. Michael (Eds.), Simulation in Umwelt- und Geowissenschaften, Workshop Potsdam 2009 (pp. 43–55). Aachen: Shaker Verlag.

Dutka, B.J., Walsh, K., Kwan, K.K., El Shaarawi, A., Liu, D.L. and Thompson, K. (1986). Priority site selection from degraded areas based on microbial and toxicant screening tests. Water Pollut. Res. J. Can., 21(2), 267–282.

Myers, W.L. and Patil, G.P. (2008). Semi-subordination sequences in multi-measure prioritization problems. Chapter 7. In M. Pavan and R. Todeschini (Eds.), Ranking methods: Theory and applications, Data Handling in Science and Technology (pp. 159–168, Vol. 27). Amsterdam, The Netherlands: Elsevier.

Restrepo, G. and Bruggemann, R. (2008). Dominance and separability in posets, their application to isoelectronic species with equal charge. J. Math. Chem., 44, 577–602.

Simon, U. (2003). Multikriterielle bewertung von wasserwirtschaftlichen Maβnahmen aus gewaesseroekologischer Sicht – Beispiel Berlin. Berlin: Tenea.

Simon, U., Bruggemann, R. and Pudenz, S. (2004a). Aspects of decision support in water management – Example Berlin and Potsdam (Germany) I – Spatially differentiated evaluation. Water Res., 38, 1809–1816.

Simon, U., Bruggemann, R. and Pudenz, S. (2004b). Aspects of decision support in water management – Example Berlin and Potsdam (Germany) II – Improvement of management strategies. Water Res., 38, 4085–4092.

Chapter 6
Hasse Diagrams Based on Transformed Data Matrices

6.1 Motivation

We have seen in Chapter 5 as to why and how the structure of partial order (*X*, IB) can be related to properties of the data matrix. However, partial order with many objects can lead to messy Hasse diagrams with too many lines hiding the structure. What may be the reason for complexity in such diagrams? The number of objects $|X|$ is not necessarily causing messy Hasse diagrams because chains of height $|X|$ or antichains of width $|X|$ certainly allow clear visualizations. There is another reason for complexity: In partial orders, we obtain either $x < y$ or $x \| y$ even if the numerical difference ε between attribute values is small:

1. If $q_1(x) = q_{10}(x) + \varepsilon,\ q_2(x) = q_{20}(x) - \varepsilon,\ \varepsilon > 0$, and $q_1(y) = q_{10}(x),\ q_2(y) = q_{20}(x)$, then $x \| y$, "irrelevant incomparabilities."
2. If $q_1(\mathrm{x}) = q_{10}(x) + \varepsilon,\ q_2(x) = q_{20}(x) + \varepsilon,\ \varepsilon > 0$, and $q_1(y) = q_{10}(x),\ q_2(y) = q_{20}(x)$, then $y < x$, "irrelevant comparabilities."

This ordinal interpretation of the data matrix is at the root of cover relations (see Chapter 2) and lines in the Hasse diagram, although they are representing irrelevant incomparabilities or comparabilities. Irrelevant incomparabilities or comparabilities may better be interpreted as equivalence relation.

The following question arises: How can we manipulate Hasse diagrams to draw useful information, without losing the connection to the original data matrix? Chapter 6 outlines some answers and is organized as follows:

1. complexity ("ordinal modeling") in more detail,
2. discretization procedures,
3. the concept of fuzzy partial order, and
4. the concept of p-algorithm.

R. Brüggemann, G.P. Patil, *Ranking and Prioritization for Multi-indicator Systems*, Environmental and Ecological Statistics 5, DOI 10.1007/978-1-4419-8477-7_6,

6.2 Ordinal Modeling

Complexity of (*X*, IB) can be handled by

1. transformations of the data matrix without aggregations of the attributes (object-related manipulations) and
2. suitable aggregations by which the multitude of phenomena is condensed to an averaged behavior (attribute-related manipulations) (see Chapter 7).

Any kind of transformation which helps us to find out the "ordinal truth" of the data matrix we call "ordinal modeling." Assume a mapping which relates two posets, (*X*, IB), based on raw data matrix, and $(X, \text{IB})_\text{T}$, based on certain transformations. If the map $(X, \text{IB}) \rightarrow (X, \text{IB})_\text{T}$ is order preserving (Chapter 3), then any order relation once found in a messy Hasse diagram will be reproduced in the transformed one. Therefore, we can answer the same questions posed on the original Hasse diagram without having to worry about irrelevant relations.

6.3 Discretization of Attributes, Continuous in Concept

6.3.1 Method

There are two variants of discretization:

1. equidistant discretization (Bruggemann and Bartel, 1999) and
2. equidistributional classification (will not be discussed here).

6.3.1.1 Equidistant Discretization

Performing an equidistant discretization, an interval $I(q_i)$ corresponding to each attribute, i.e., $\min_i$ and $\max_i$, must be found. Often we take $\min_i$ and $\max_i$ from the data matrix:

$$I(q_i) = [\min_x(q_i(x), \max_x(q_i(x))],\ x \in X \tag{6.1}$$

The interval $I(q_i)$ is subdivided in $K(q_i)$ subintervals having the same lengths $I_k(q_i)$, $k = 1, \ldots, K(q_i)$, such that

$$I(q_i) = \bigcup I_k(q_i)$$

with $k = 1, \ldots, K(q_i)$, and

$$I_k(q_i) = \min_i + \frac{\max_i - \min_i}{K(q_i)} \cdot [k - 1, k) \tag{6.2}$$

with $k = 1, \ldots, K(q_i)$.

If $k = K(q_i)$ then the closed interval is to be taken.

If there are no contextual arguments, then it is recommended

$$K(q_1) = K(q_2) = \ldots = K(q_m) = K \tag{6.3}$$

Through selection of $\min_i$, $\max_i$, and $K(q_i)$ $(i = 1, \ldots m)$, a discretization scheme is defined.

By Eq. (6.2) we obtain scores $s_i(x)$ of object x:

$$s_i(x) = k :\Leftrightarrow q_i(x) \in I_k(q_i) \tag{6.4}$$

The collection $s_1(x), s_2(x), \ldots, s_m(x)$ is as usual denoted as $s(x)$. Often the matrix with entries $s_i(x)$ is considered as a "new" data matrix and we write $q_i(x)$ not to overburden the text with new symbols.

6.3.1.2 Discretization is Order Preserving

To prove that the discretization (Eqs. (6.1) and (6.2)) is order preserving, it is sufficient to show that $q(x) < q(y) \Rightarrow s(x) \leq s(y)$.

$q(x) < q(y) \Rightarrow q_i(x) \leq q_i(y) \Rightarrow$ there are some $q_i \in \mathrm{IB}_1$ with $q_i(x) = q_i(y)$ and some $q_j \in \mathrm{IB}_2$ with $q_j(x) < q_j(y)$. Take $q_i \in \mathrm{IB}_1$, then $s_i(x) = s_i(y)$, take $q_j \in \mathrm{IB}_2$, then $s_j(x) \leq s_j(y)$ by Eq. (2.3). Hence $s_i(x) \leq s_i(y)$ with $q_i \in \mathrm{IB}_1 \cup \mathrm{IB}_2$.

What happens in the case of $x \| y$?

Then there are two disjoints IB_1 and IB_2 such that $\mathrm{IB} = \mathrm{IB}_1 \cup \mathrm{IB}_2$:

$q_i \in \mathrm{IB}_1$: $q_i(x) \leq q_i(y)$ with at least one i^* with $q_{i^*}(x) < q_{i^*}(y)$ and
$q_j \in \mathrm{IB}_2$: $q_j(x) \geq q_j(y)$ with at least one j^* with $q_{j^*}(x) > q_{j^*}(y)$.

From $q_i(x) \leq q_i(y)$ and $q_j(x) \geq q_j(y)$, we get the following possibilities (Fig. 6.1). In Fig. 6.1, we see the following:

All combinations including (4): $x \| y$ in $(X, \mathrm{IB}) \rightarrow x \| y$ in $(X, \mathrm{IB})_T$
All combinations consisting solely of (1): $x \| y$ in $(X, \mathrm{IB}) \rightarrow x \cong y$ in $(X, \mathrm{IB})_T$

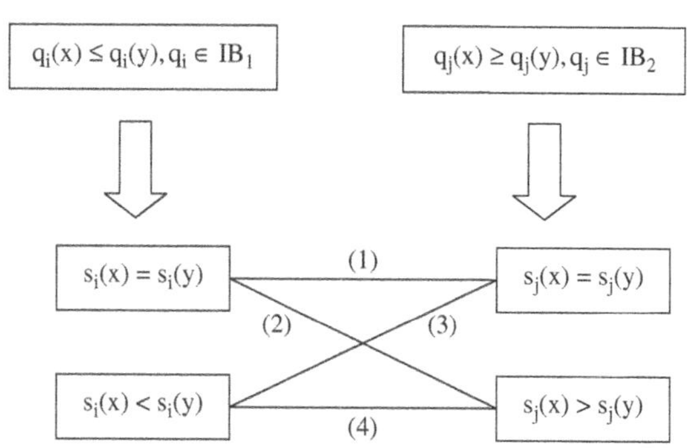

Fig. 6.1 Incomparabilities in (X, IB) and the outcome in $(X, \mathrm{IB})_T$

Combination (2): $x \parallel y$ in $(X, \text{IB}) \rightarrow x > y$ in $(X, \text{IB})_\text{T}$
Combination (3): $x \parallel y$ in $(X, \text{IB}) \rightarrow x < y$ in $(X, \text{IB})_\text{T}$

6.3.2 Advantages and Disadvantages

Advantages:

1. The numerical procedure is easily performed.
2. The method preserves the order of the original poset.

Disadvantages:

1. There is some arbitrariness in selecting the parameters $\max_i$ and $\min_i$ and $K(q_i)$.
2. At the boundaries of the subintervals, irrelevant comparabilities and incomparabilities still remain.
3. Order reversals (see next section).

6.3.3 Order Reversal

Discretizing the attributes, one after another, is order preserving as was discussed in Section 6.3.1.2. Incomparabilities may remain incomparabilities or transform to > or < relations, according to different discretization schemes. We can construct an example where in one discretization scheme, $x <_{(X,\text{IB})\text{T1}} y$, whereas in another discretization scheme, $x >_{(X,\text{IB})\text{T2}} y$. This phenomenon is called an order reversal (Fig. 6.2).

Hence we have to be aware of the order reversals. The only way to check the selected discretization is to compare it with others (Bruggemann and Welzl, 2002).

6.3.4 Discretization and Shape

Discretization often leads to Hasse diagram with a triangular shape (vertex at the bottom) because of a simple combinatorial effect: Consider an indicator vector of only three components, and consider $(1/3)^*S = (1/3)^* \sum q_i(x)$ as a measure for the average values in each level of a Hasse diagram. Then the number of realizations of a given S can be obtained from the formal power series:

$$\prod_{i=1}^{m} (1 + y + y^2 + ... + y^{K(q_i)})$$

The product contains terms like $a_i{}^* y^i$. The number of possible realizations of the sum S can be obtained from the coefficients a_i. It is clear that

	q_1 three classes	q_2 three classes
a	1	2
b	2	1
c	2	2
d	3	2
e	3	3

q_1: original	q_2: original
1	5
6	1
8	7
9	6
12	10

q_1: four classes	q_2: four classes
1	2
2	1
3	3
3	2
4	4

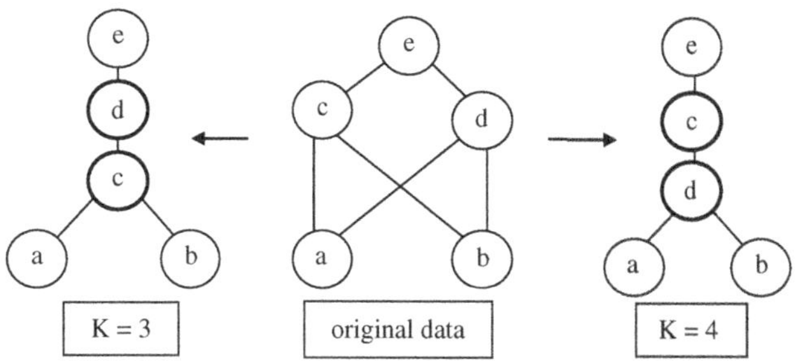

Fig. 6.2 Data matrices are shown at the *top*. For objects c and d, we find c < d or c > d, depending on *K*

- there is only one possible vector for which $S = 0$;
- there is an increasing number of realizations if S is increasing until a middle range of S is reached;
- there is a decreasing number of realizations if S is increasing beyond the middle range; and finally
- there is only one realization if all attributes get their maximum score $K(q_i)$.

Therefore, the shape of a Hasse diagram after discretization is schematically shown in Fig. 6.3.

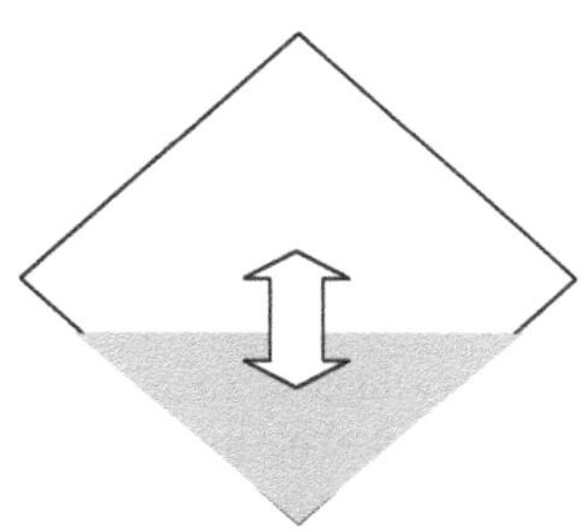

Fig. 6.3 The shape of a *diamond* arises from the number of all possible vectors; the *grey shape* indicates the number of realizations due to a data matrix

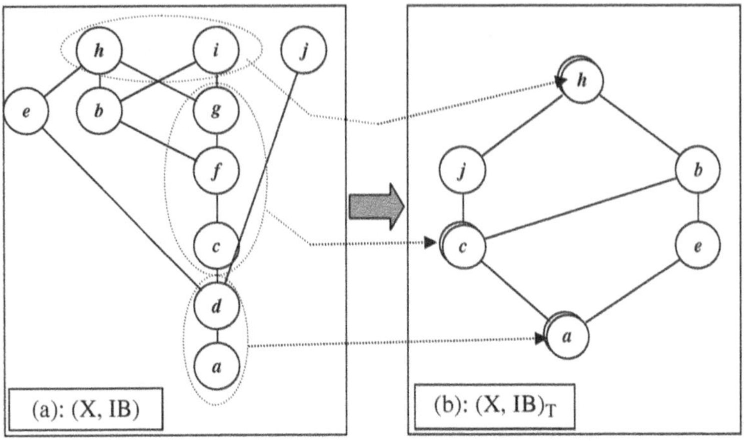

Fig. 6.4 Hasse diagrams based (**a**) on the original data (X, IB) and (**b**) on scores (X, IB)$_{\mathrm{T}}$. Equivalent: {g, f, c}, {h, i}, {a, d}

6.3.5 Illustrative Example

In Fig. 6.4, two Hasse diagrams are depicted, one with the data matrix shown in Table A.1 and the second after discretization of each attribute. The discretization scheme is as follows:

$$K(q_1) = K(q_2) = K(q_3) = K = 3 \text{ (Eq. (6.3))}.$$

$\max_i$ and $\min_i$ are derived from the data matrix according to Eq. (6.1).

Thus, the attributes q_1, q_2, and q_3 get the scores 0, 1, or 2.

Instead of the original values for q_i, an object gets the scores s_i, and from them a Hasse diagram is obtained.

One sees that

- all < relations in (a) are transformed in either < or $\cong$ relations;
- some || relations are transformed to equivalence relations, see $h \,||_{(X,\mathrm{IB})} i$;
- some || relations are transformed to < relations, see objects j and h. (6.5)

6.4 Fuzzy Partial Order

6.4.1 Method

The very idea of fuzzy partial order is to replace the crisp < relation by a fuzzy subsethood. The motivation for that can be demonstrated by Fig. 6.5, where two objects with a mild crisscrossing of their data profiles are shown.

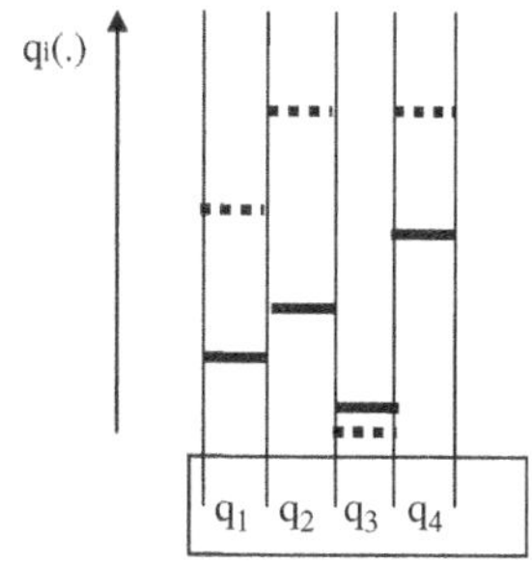

Fig. 6.5 The *bold lines* represent the data profile of object x and the *broken lines* represent that of object y

In Fig. 6.5, object x has a data profile which crisscrosses that of object y. Therefore, the application of the product order (Chapter 2) would lead to $x \| y$. However, evidence shows that object x is "almost" below object y. The only exception is in the attribute q_3. By a fuzzy membership function the wording "almost below" becomes quantified.

6.4.1.1 Kosko Fuzzy Subsethood

Let a, b be two objects characterized by m dimensionless (normalized) attributes, then:

$$\mathrm{SH}(a,b) = \frac{\sum_{i=1}^{m} \min(q_i(a), q_i(b))}{\sum_{i=1}^{m} q_i(a)}, \text{ if } \sum_{i=1}^{m} q_i(a) \neq 0, \text{ else : } \mathrm{SH}(a,b) = 1 \tag{6.6}$$

SH(a,b) is the membership function, describing to which extent object a can be considered as being below object b.

If $a < b$, then $\mathrm{SH}(a,b) = 1$,

if $a \| b$: $0 \leq \mathrm{SH}(b,a) < 1$, both $\mathrm{SH}(a,b)$ and $\mathrm{SH}(b,a) \in [0,1)$. If in Fig. 6.5, object x has the data profile (0.2, 0.3, 0.1, 0.45), whereas object y has (0.5, 0.6, 0.08, 0.6), then $\mathrm{SH}(x,y) = \frac{0.2+0.3+0.08+0.45}{0.2+0.3+0.1+0.45} = 0.98$ and $\mathrm{SH}(y,x) = \frac{0.2+0.3+0.08+0.45}{0.5+0.6+0.08+0.6} = 0.58$.

The subsethood of x relative to y has a large membership, confirming that x is almost below y. It also tells us that y can be considered to be less than x, however to a low degree.

It may be interesting to note that the Kosko measure evaluates incomparable objects x, y by two numbers $\mathrm{SH}(x,y)$ and $\mathrm{SH}(y,x)$. Therefore, it seems to be attractive to establish a relation between SH(.,.) and the mutual probability.

6.4.1.2 Relational Matrix

Application of SH for all object pairs leads to a matrix R (labeled by object identifiers) with entries between 0 and 1. The matrix R cannot be considered as being an expression for partial order. The crucial point is the transitivity. The transitivity axiom as formulated in Chapter 2 refers to crisp relations which can be written as $R(a,b) = 1$ and $R(b,c) = 1$ implies $R(a,c) = 1$. In the setting of fuzziness, three fractional numbers are to be compared and for fuzzy transitivity, it is convenient to require

$$\min(R(a,b),\ R(b,c)) \leq R(a,c) \tag{6.7}$$

The matrix R, obtained from the Kosko measure, i.e., $R(a,b) = \mathrm{SH}(a,b)$, does not necessarily obey Eq. (6.7). Hence an approach is needed to find a transitive closure for R, i.e., to replace some entries in R such that Eq. (6.7) is fulfilled.

6.4.1.3 Transitive Closure

De Baets and De Meyer (2003) suggest an approach that guarantees fuzzy transitivity by replacing as less entries of R as possible. They propose the "matrix method": There the essential step is to calculate $R^{(n)}$ from $R^{(n-1)}$ as follows:

Start: $R^{(1)}(a,b) = \mathrm{SH}(a,b)$

Interation: $R^{(n)}(x,y) = \max[\min(R^{(n-1)}(x,w), R^{(n-1)}(w,y)]$, for all $w \in X$, (n) indicating the nth step in the iteration loop. (6.8)

Stop: When the matrices $R^{(n)}$ and $R^{(n-1)}$ no more differ by a certain threshold ε, the iteration stops, say at R.

6.4.1.4 α Cut

The final matrix R is transitively closed, hence consistent with partial order. It may have at most n^2 different values. For defuzzification of R, it is appropriate to rank order its entries and call them α cuts: $\alpha_1 \leq \alpha_2 \leq \ldots \leq \alpha_{n^2} = 1$, so that we can perform the transformation:

$$R^{\mathrm{crisp}}(x,y) = \begin{cases} 1, & \text{if } R(x,y) \geq \alpha \\ 0, & \text{else} \end{cases} \tag{6.9}$$

Arbitrary choice can be made for the threshold α. Three cases arise in the application of Eq. (6.9):

1. $R^{\mathrm{crisp}}(x,y) = R^{\mathrm{crisp}}(y,x) = 0$: x and y are incomparable
2. $R^{\mathrm{crisp}}(x,y) = 1,\ R^{\mathrm{crisp}}(x,y) = 0$: $x < y$ or $R^{\mathrm{crisp}}(y,x) = 1$: $x > y$
3. $R^{\mathrm{crisp}}(x,y) = R^{\mathrm{crisp}}(y,x) = 1$: $x \cong y$

6.4.1.5 Tolerance

If α has a low value, then almost all entries of R will get a 1, hence there is little differentiation among the objects. If however $\alpha = 1$, then only the entries having value 1 in the original SH matrix (Eq. (6.6)) will be retained, and the order relations of the original data matrix are reproduced. If α is varied, we find the following:

- For $\alpha \in (\alpha_i, \alpha_{i+1})$, the crisp matrix R does not depend on α.
- The α values taken from different intervals of α cuts will induce different crisp matrices R and therefore different equivalence classes and partial orders.

It is convenient to call α a tolerance level.

6.4.1.6 Extraction

The matrix $R^{(\text{crisp})}$ contains not only the order relations but also equivalence relations. In order to obtain a Hasse diagram, equivalent elements must be identified and the order relations of the representative elements extracted.

6.4.2 Advantages and Disadvantages

6.4.2.1 Advantages

The partial orders, indexed by α, are order preserving:

$$(X,\ \mathrm{IB})_{\alpha 1} \subseteq (X,\ \mathrm{IB})_{\alpha 2},\ \ \alpha_1 > \alpha_2 \tag{6.10}$$

(Van de Walle et al., 1995)

Hasse diagrams evolve in a systematic manner, depending on α.

6.4.2.2 Disadvantages

Equation (6.6) implies that a sum is to be performed over different attributes. A sacrilege in the eyes of partial order theory! Furthermore, an objective selection of the α value is difficult. Annoni et al. (2008) propose a measure for selecting a suitable α value.

6.4.3 Illustrative Example

In Table 6.1, the labels of the two matrices are as follows: object a, first row/column; object b, second row/column; object c, third row/column. SH: One can see that $a < b$ and $a < c$. The entries for both b, c and c, b have deviating values from 1, thus documenting that b and c are incomparable. The transitive closure of SH is matrix $R^{(1)}$: For example, R, (c, b) is obtained as follows:

Table 6.1 Illustrative example for fuzzy analysis (performed with PyHasse, see Chapter 17)

	Attributes	
Objects	q_1	q_2
a	0.1	0.2
b	0.6	0.8
c	0.2	0.9

$$\mathrm{SH} = \begin{pmatrix} 1.0 & 1.0 & 1.0 \\ 0.214 & 1.0 & 0.71 \\ 0.27 & 0.91 & 1.0 \end{pmatrix} \qquad R^{(1)} = \begin{pmatrix} 1.0 & 1.0 & 1.0 \\ \mathbf{0.27} & 1.0 & 0.71 \\ 0.27 & 0.91 & 1.0 \end{pmatrix}$$

The attributes q_1 and q_2 are considered dimensionless
The fuzzy relation matrix SH and the transitive closure $R^{(1)}$ are shown

$$\max[\min(0.27, 1), \min(0.91, 1), \min(1.0, 0.91)] = \max[0.27, 0.91, 0.91] = 0.91$$

The matrix method changed one entry: $\mathrm{SH}(b, a) = 0.214$ is replaced by the value 0.273 (indicated by bold literals). There are four different values in the transitive closure, matrix $R^{(1)}$ and correspondingly four different α cuts: 0.273, 0.714, 0.909, and 1.0.

If we started with $\alpha = 0.2$, which is less than the smallest entry of $R^{(1)}$, then $R^{(1)}(x, y) > \alpha$, hence the matrix entries would contain nothing else than 1. Therefore – with that high degree of tolerance – all numerical differences are ignored and consequently all three elements belong to one equivalence class.

Let us select $\alpha = 0.4$: We obtain a crisp matrix "cq" as follows:

$$\mathrm{cq}(\alpha = 0.4) = \begin{matrix} & a\ b\ c \\ a: & \\ b: & \\ c: & \end{matrix} \begin{pmatrix} 1 & 1 & 1 \\ 0 & 1 & 1 \\ 0 & 1 & 1 \end{pmatrix}$$

Objects b and c are considered as equivalent. The extraction leads to a reduced matrix.

Order relations extracted from cq due to α are summarized in the matrix 'order'.

$$\mathrm{order} = \begin{matrix} & a\ b \\ a: & \\ b: & \end{matrix} \begin{pmatrix} 1 & 1 \\ 0 & 1 \end{pmatrix}$$

(order $= \zeta + 1$, 1 being the unit matrix, ζ; see Chapter 3). The corresponding partial order is the second (from the left) Hasse diagram in Fig. 6.6.

We select $\alpha = 0.8$:

$$\mathrm{cq}\,(\alpha = 0.8) = \begin{matrix} & a\ b\ c \\ a: & \\ b: & \\ c: & \end{matrix} \begin{pmatrix} 1 & 1 & 1 \\ 0 & 1 & 0 \\ 0 & 1 & 1 \end{pmatrix}$$

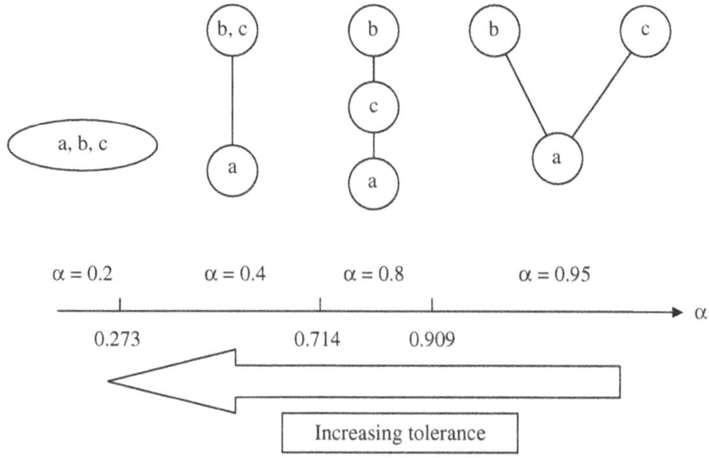

Fig. 6.6 Evolving partial orders depending on α

This matrix indicates that there is no more an equivalence relation but a chain: $a < c < b$ (see also Fig. 6.6).

Finally, if $\alpha = 0.95$, then we obtain

$$\mathrm{cq}\,(\alpha = 0.95) = \begin{matrix} & a\ b\ c \\ a: & \\ b: & \\ c: & \end{matrix}\begin{pmatrix} 1 & 1 & 1 \\ 0 & 1 & 0 \\ 0 & 0 & 1 \end{pmatrix}$$

The matrix cq($\alpha = 0.95$) represents the partial order of the raw data matrix (Fig. 6.6).

6.5 An Algorithm to Focus on Priority Objects

6.5.1 Concept

Often the task of a partial order analysis is directed toward the identification of priority objects. The so-called p-algorithm (Bruggemann et al., 1999) supports this task and consists of two steps:

1. Consider one of the attributes q_i. Select a limiting value q_{i0} such that $P\%$ of objects are excluded, because their q_i values are less than q_{i0}.
2. Perform the transformation:

$$p_i(x) = \begin{cases} q_i(x), \text{ for all } x \in X \text{ for which } q_i(x) \geq q_{i0} \\ -\infty, \text{ else} \end{cases} \tag{6.11}$$

The fraction of $P/100$ of all objects will be excluded by taking an appropriate high value of q_{i0}. We are speaking that these objects are "put into the swamp, SW_i" (with respect to the attribute q_i):

$$SW_i := \{x \in X :\ q_i(x) < q_{i0}\} \tag{6.12}$$

$$SW = \bigcap_{i=1,\dots,m} SW_i$$

The set of remaining objects is as follows:

$$RM = X - \bigcap_{i=1}^{m} SW_i \tag{6.13}$$

6.5.2 Properties of p-Algorithm

6.5.2.1 p-Algorithm is Order Preserving

We have to show that $x \leq y$ in $(X,\ IB) \Rightarrow x \leq y$ in $(X, IB)_T$. Subscript "T" indicates that a transformation due to the p-algorithm is performed.

We think of three cases:

1. There are some q_i with $q_i(x) < q_i(y)$ and $q_i(x)$ gets $-\infty$. Then the $\leq$ relation remains.
2. There are some q_j with $q_j(x) < q_j(y)$ and $q_j(y)$ gets $-\infty$. As $q_j(x)$ is supposed to be less than $q_j(y)$, $q_j(x)$ must also get to $-\infty$. Then the $\leq$ relation remains.
3. There are some q_k with $q_k(x) < q_k(y)$ and both $q_k(x)$ and $q_k(y)$ get to $-\infty$. Then the result depends on the result of the first two cases. Because $x \leq y$ in (X, IB), either $x \cong_{(X,\ IB)T}\ y$ or $x \leq_{(X,\ IB)T}\ y$ will be obtained.

Therefore, the p-algorithm is order preserving.

6.5.2.2 Swamp and Remaining Set

Let us consider the object set X and two attributes.

(i) *Correlation*: If attribute q_2 were correlated with the first one, q_1, then the selection of q_{10} which puts $(P/100)^*\ |X|$ into the swamp with respect to attribute q_1 would do the same for attribute q_2. Hence, in the extreme case of a set of m high-correlated attributes, the same objects would be excluded, and only $(1 - P/100)^*\ |X|$ would remain for a partial order study:

$$SW_1 = SW_2 \text{ and } RM = X - SW_1 = X - SW_2 \tag{6.14}$$

(ii) *Anticorrelation*: Let us now imagine that two attributes q_1 and q_2 are anticorrelated, then q_{10} would send a certain subset of objects in the swamp, and q_{20} would put another different subset of objects into the swamp:

$$\mathrm{RM} = X - \bigcap_{i=1}^{m} \mathrm{SW}_i \qquad |\mathrm{RM}^{\mathrm{ac}}| \leq |\mathrm{RM}^{\mathrm{c}}|,$$

With superscripts ac and c indicating anticorrelation and correlation, respectively (6.15)

Figure 6.7 may help understand the two extreme cases.

Usually there are more than two attributes and their behavior is neither correlated nor anticorrelated. The elements of X which get at the same time $-\infty$ for all attributes are forming one equivalence class, the swamp. All other objects may have some components in their data row, having values $\neq -\infty$. They undergo further partial order analysis.

To assess as to how many objects may be put into the swamp, we estimate the number of elements:

$$|\mathrm{SW}| = (P/100)^{\kappa *}\,|X| \tag{6.16}$$

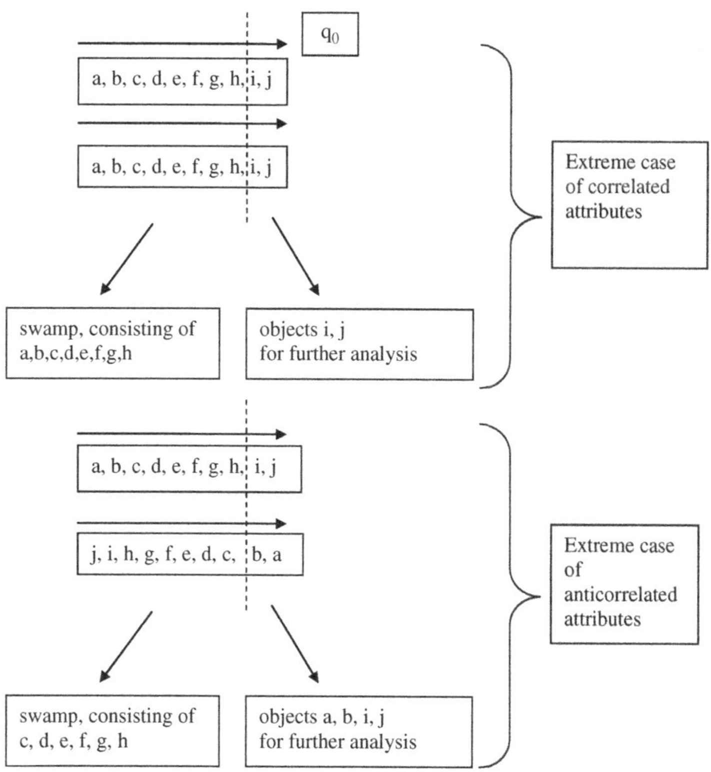

Fig. 6.7 The correlative character of the multi-indicator system determines the number of objects for further analysis

κ is a function of the correlation properties of the attributes.
$\kappa = 1$ for perfectly correlated attributes and $\kappa > 1$ for other cases.

Heuristically, we set $\kappa \in [1, |\text{IB}|]$.

6.5.2.3 Shape

Often Hasse diagrams, resulting from the p-algorithm, get the shape of a triangle, with the vertex at the bottom. Can we give an explanation? Similarly of what was discussed in Section 6.3.4, we find the following (Fig. 6.8).

If we set $q_i(x) \neq -\infty$ formally 1, and $q_i(x) = -\infty$ formally 0, then a sum $S = \Sigma q_i(x)$ measures the average values in each level. The lowest and the highest values of S can be realized by only one vector, namely (0,0,. . .,0) and (1,1,. . .,1). For interim values of S, there are many realizations possible. Hence the shape of Hasse diagrams looks similar to diamonds as shown in Fig. 6.8.

In Fig. 6.8 the shape of a diamond arises because of the combinatorial number of possible realizations of vectors. The grey parts indicate actual realizations due to an empirical data matrix.

Where and why the p-algorithm may be applied:

1. Focus on most important objects ("hot spot detection").
2. By putting many objects into the "swamp," one gets a clearer Hasse diagram.
3. Let (X, IB) be the poset of the original and $(X, \text{IB})_T$ that after performing the p-algorithm. Then the map $(X, \text{IB}) \rightarrow (X, \text{IB})_T$ is order preserving.
4. The data-driven navigation (see below) is facilitated.

6.5.3 Illustrative Example

6.5.3.1 Hasse Diagrams

In Fig. 6.9, a Hasse diagram together with its data matrix is shown.

Performing the transformation of putting 80% of objects into the swamps $\text{SW}_i(i = 1, \ldots, 4)$ results in a highly simplified Hasse diagram (Fig. 6.10).

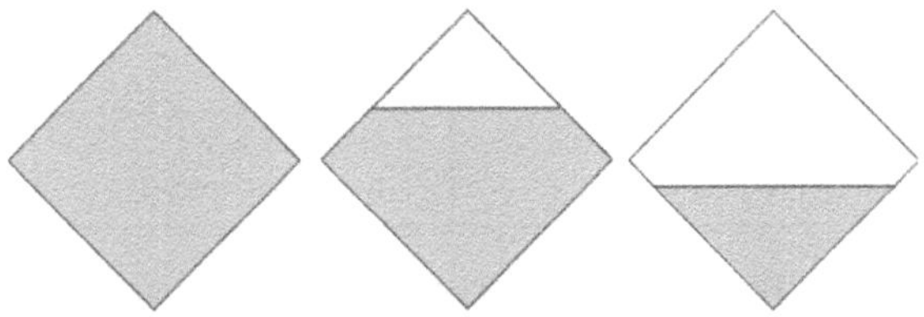

Fig. 6.8 Shapes of Hasse diagrams after p-algorithm

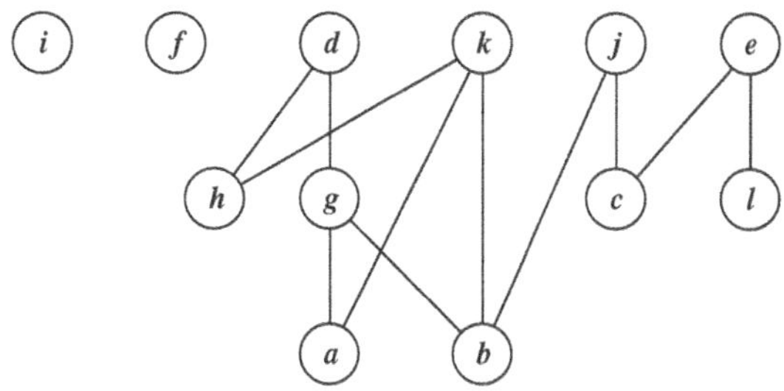

	q_1	q_2	q_3	q_4
a	1	2	4	5
b	2	3	1	6
c	3	6	2	1
d	3	3	7	8
e	8	9	3	4
f	5	2	7	1
g	3	3	5	6
h	2	1	5	8
i	8	2	6	1
j	4	8	3	8

Fig. 6.9 Hasse diagram and its data matrix

Fig. 6.10 Hasse diagram after p-algorithm, with $P = 80\%$. Equivalence class, the swamp: $\{a, b, g\}$

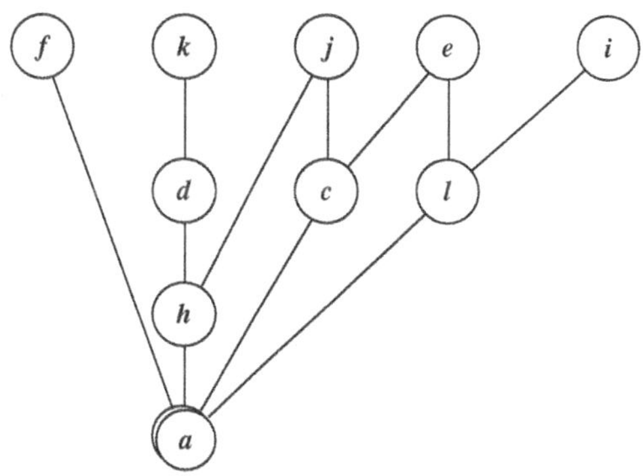

6.5.3.2 Swamp

The swamp has only three objects. If $\kappa = 4$ is applied, then 5 objects are put into the swamp and if $\kappa = 1$, then approximately 10 objects are put into the swamp. Obviously there are attributes which are anticorrelated (Table 6.2).

The range of $\rho_{i,j}$, $i \neq j$, is –0.533 to 0.221 confirming the overall impression of attributes pretty anticorrelated.

6.5.3.3 Navigation

We navigate through the Hasse diagram by means of the tools described in Chapter 5:

- *Object k*: After p-transformation, its profile (see Chapter 3) is $(-\infty, 5, 8, 8)$, hence all objects $\in O(k)$ must have a profile $(-\infty,\ q_2(x) \leq 5,\ q_3(x) \leq 8,\ q_4(x) \leq 8)$.
- *Object j*: After p-transformation, its profile (see Chapter 3) is $(-\infty, 8, -\infty, 8)$, hence all objects $\in O(j)$ must have a profile $(-\infty,\ q_2(x) \leq 8,\ -\infty,\ q_4(x) \leq 8)$.

Table 6.2 Spearman correlation index, ρ

			Correlations			
			q_1	q_2	q_3	q_4
Spearman rho	q_1	Correlation coefficient	1.000	0.147	–0.072	–0.533
		Sig. (two-tailed)		0.650	0.824	0.074
		N	12	12	12	12
	q_2	Correlation coefficient	0.147	1.000	–0.231	0.124
		Sig. (two-tailed)	0.650		0.470	0.702
		N	12	12	12	12
	q_3	Correlation coefficient	–0.072	–0.231	1.000	0.221
		Sig. (two-tailed)	0.824	0.470		0.490
		N	12	12	12	12
	q_4	Correlation coefficient	–0.533	0.124	0.221	1.000
		Sig. (two-tailed)	0.074	0.702	0.490	
		N	12	12	12	12

- *Object e*: After p-transformation, its profile (see Chapter 3) is $(8, 9, -\infty, -\infty)$, hence all objects $\in O(e)$ must have a profile $(q_1(x) \leq 8,\ q_2(x) \leq 9,\ -\infty,\ -\infty)$.
- *Object c*: $c \in O(j) \cap O(e)$; according to Eq. (5.9), the profile of c must be $(-\infty,\ q_2(x) \leq 9,\ \infty,\ -\infty)$.

6.6 Attribute Value Sensitivity

Chapter 6 is devoted to changes of the data matrix. Changing a single entry of the data matrix to get insight into attribute value-related sensitivity may therefore be a relevant section here.

Concerning the attribute value sensitivity, there are two questions:

- What effect does a change in a cell of the data matrix have for the position of the corresponding object in the Hasse diagram?
- What effect will it have on the linear or the weak order?

6.6.1 Basic Idea

We assume that the attributes are discretized to get k different scores (see Section 6.3 for more details). Attribute value sensitivity analyzes the effect of changing the score of a certain attribute by an amount Δ to the partial order in terms of

$|O(x)|$, $|F(x)|$, $|U(x)|$ as well as $|S(x)|$ and $|P(x)|$. We call these quantities "characteristics of the considered object" and denote them as $C(x, \text{IB})$ and if no confusion is possible, we can even denote as C.

If Δ is varying, while $q_i \in \text{IB}$ and $x \in X$ are fixed, then a line graph of C vs Δ is useful (Fig. 6.11).

Depending on the property C, on $x \in X$, and on $q_i \in \text{IB}$, one is observing the thresholds Δ_u and Δ_d with different numerical values. Both thresholds can be considered as inertia of the poset against increasing or decreasing the value of $q_i(x)$.

If Δ is fixed (say at 1), $x \in X$ is selected while browsing through IB, then a representation of the results by a histogram may be useful (Fig. 6.12).

6.6.2 Triangular Representation of Partial Orders

If we want to analyze the effect of Δ on cells of the data matrix and their posetic impact, then we must simultaneously consider $|F(x)|$, $|U(x)|$, and $|O(x)|$ (Chapter 3). These three quantities obey the equation $|F(x)|+|U(x)|+|O(x)| = n+1$ (see Section 3.7). Therefore, any object can be located as a point in an equilateral triangle of altitude $n+1$ with vertices at O, F, and U.

Any line perpendicular to an edge, say FU, and connected with the point x measures the coordinate $|O(x)|$. Hence for an object x in Fig. 6.13, $|U(x)| < |O(x)|$

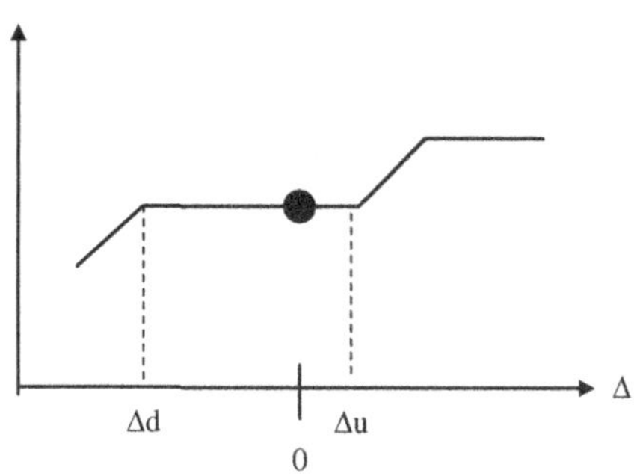

Fig. 6.11 Sketch of $C(x, \text{IB})$ vs Δ; the *black circle* marks the "standard" (see text)

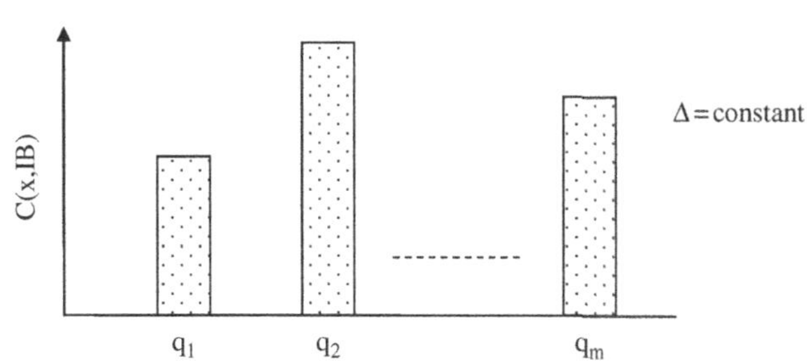

Fig. 6.12 Sketch of $C(x, \text{IB})$ vs $q_i(x)$. Sometimes it is useful to use a stacked bar diagram to see simultaneously more than one property C of the partial order

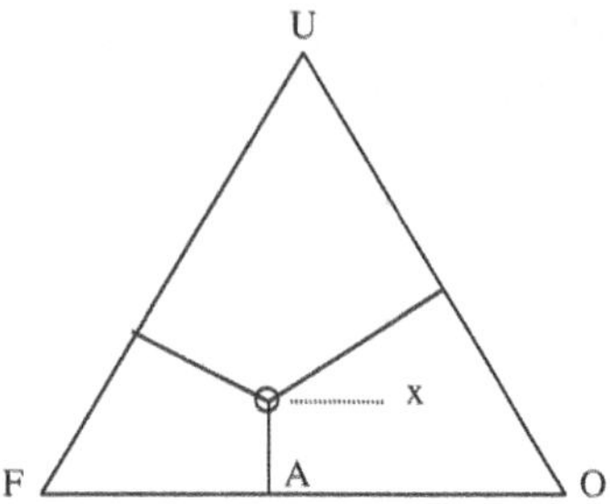

Fig. 6.13 Equilateral triangle (*OFU*) of altitude *n*+1 for presentation of objects with the coordinates *U*, *F*, and *O* (see text)

$< |F(x)|$. If $|U(x)| = 0$, then object *x* is located on the edge *FO*, say at A in which case *FA* is proportional to the rank of *x* from below and *AO* is proportional to the rank of *x* from above. One application of the triangular representation is to see how the coordinates (i.e., $|O(x)|$, $|F(x)|$, and $|U(x)|$) of an object *x* vary when we study the effect of Δ.

6.6.2.1 Example

In Fig. 6.14, a Hasse diagram together with its data matrix is shown.

We first consider the Δ value as fixed and apply to any object and to any attribute and then vary Δ for all attributes but consider only the object *c*.

6.6.2.2 Δ Value Fixed

Let us perform an attribute value sensitivity by keeping $\Delta = 1$. Hence we must observe the responses of *C*(*x*, IB) for every object and every attribute. Therefore, Table 6.3 carries two rows for every object: First row, the simulated attribute values and second row, $|P(x)|$, $|S(x)|$, $|U(x)|$ (abbr., *PSU*) for each object and each attribute.

Simulated value in bold letters. *PSU* results: italic (bold letters if there is a change relative to the standard)

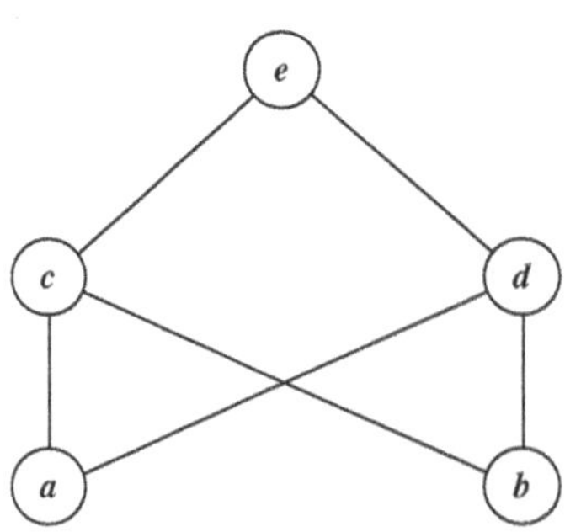

	q_1	q_2	q_3
a	1	2	3
b	2	1	4
c	3	3	6
d	3	4	5
e	4	5	6

Fig. 6.14 $X = \{a, b, c, d, e\}$, $\text{IB} = \{q_1, q_2, q_3\}$, visualization of (*X*, IB)

Table 6.3 Attribute value sensitivity for the example

	Standard: $q_1(x)$ $q_2(x)$ $q_3(x)$	Simulation concerning q_1	Simulation concerning q_2	Simulation concerning q_3
a: data	1 2 3	2 2 3	1 3 3	1 2 4
a: PSU	*3, 0, 1*	*3, 0, 1*	*3, 0, 1*	*3, 0, 1*
b: data	2 1 4	3 1 4	2 2 4	2 1 5
b: PSU	*3, 0, 1*	*3, 0, 1*	*3,* ***1****, 0*	*3, 0, 1*
c: data	3 3 6	4 3 6	3 4 6	3 3 7
c: PSU	*1, 2, 1*	*1, 2, 1*	*1,* ***3, 0***	***0****, 2,* ***2***
d: data	3 4 5	4 4 5	3 5 5	3 4 6
d: PSU	*1, 2, 1*	*1, 2, 1*	*1, 2, 1*	*1,* ***3, 0***

Remarks:

- Objects *a* and *b*, *c* and *d* are order theoretically symmetric, hence their triple $(|P(x)|, |S(x)|, |U(x)|)$ is the same in the standard case. However, if the simulation is carried on, then they behave differently as the attribute value sensitivity is dependent on the data matrix.
- Object *e* is a greatest element. Any Δ added to its $q_i(e)$ values will not change the position.

As indicators for the changes in the poset, we select $|S(x)|$ and $|U(x)|$, and Fig. 6.15 shows the bar diagram.

Figure 6.16 shows the triangular representation of the complete object set and shows how object *c* varies with adding Δ to its attribute value.

In Fig. 6.16, the point *C*0 is the object *c* with the original attribute values. The other points correspond to the sensitivity simulation. Point *C*1 results from $\Delta=1$ added to $q_1(c)$ and the consequences in term of the *O*, *F*, *U* coordinates, similarly

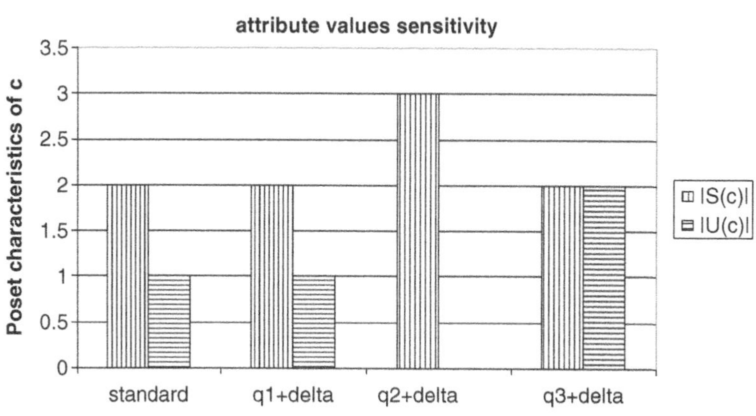

Fig. 6.15 Attribute value sensitivity, $\Delta=1$, comparison through different q_i

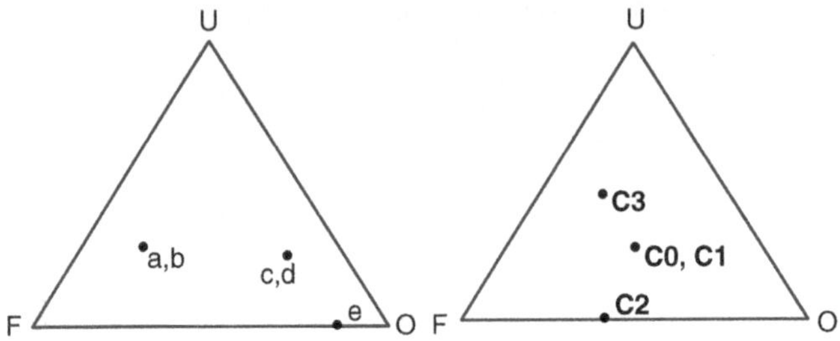

Fig. 6.16 *OFU* triangles. All objects of Fig. 6.12 (*LHS*). Simulation concerning object *c* (*RHS*) (see the text)

*C*2 is obtained for the case where Δ is added to q_2, and *C*3 is obtained for the case where Δ is added to $q_3(c)$.

One can see that attribute q_3 is crucial for object *c* because it increases $|U(c)|$ while keeping *F* and *O* almost constant. A perturbation of the value $q_1(c)$ by adding $\Delta=1$ does not change at all the posetic configuration of *c*, whereas addition of Δ to $q_2(c)$ reduces the incomparabilities of *c* to 0. The location of *C*2 at edge *FO* shows that *C*2 must have slightly more predecessors than successors; correspondingly the rank from the bottom will be less than the rank from the top.

6.6.2.3 Δ Value Varied

We can also perform a study where the attribute is fixed and we vary Δ. How will $|P(x)|$, $|S(x)|$, $|U(x)|$ change? In Fig. 6.17, we select $|U(x)|$ vs Δ for q_1, q_2, and q_3.

Even if $|P(x)|$, $|S(x)|$, $|U(x)|$ do not change, as it is the case for $q_2(c) + \Delta$ with $\Delta = 3$ and 4, the Hasse diagram may change. Changes of $q_i(c)$ may let

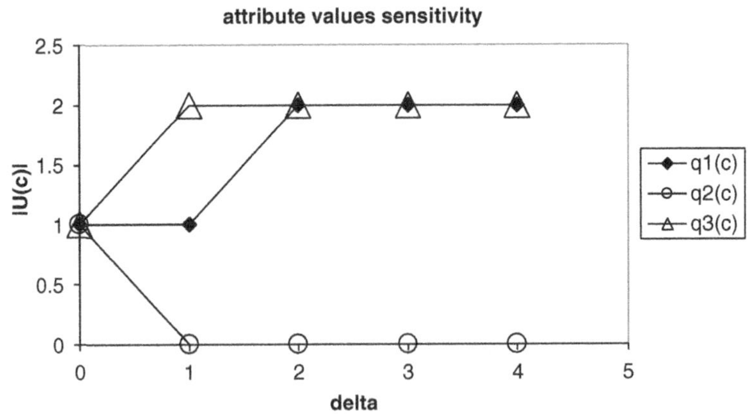

Fig. 6.17 Attribute value sensitivity Δ varies

$|P(c)|$, $|S(c)|$, $|U(c)|$ invariant but may change $|P(x)|$, $|S(x)|$, $|U(x)|$, $x \neq c$. In the example above, only increasing values of Δ are studied. Hence, only the threshold values of Δ_u can be identified. They are $q_1 = 1$, $q_2 = 0$, and $q_3 = 0$. In case studies, we will toggle between $|U(x)|$ or $|S(x)|$ as indicating quantity.

6.7 Summary and Commentary

The starting point is how we get a clear Hasse diagram without getting lost in irrelevant comparabilities and incomparabilities. We think of corresponding techniques as ordinal modeling, being aware that ordinal analysis does not in general need that sharpness in data as required by many statistical exploration and inference techniques.

We described (i) discretization of any single attribute, (ii) fuzzy analysis, (iii) p-algorithm, and (iv) attribute value sensitivity. In Table 6.4, we compare the three methods (i)–(iii) of simplifying the partial order.

Applications of all three methods are found in many case studies in the second part of the monograph.

Attribute value sensitivity helps with decision on which indicator the management should focus to improve their positional ranking. A new concept, the variance analysis-based sensitivity of partial orders applied on chemical risk assessment, can be found in Annoni et al. (2012) (subm.).

Table 6.4 Comparison of discretization, fuzzy analysis, and p-algorithm

	Advantage	Disadvantage	Remark
(i) Discretization	Strong simplification Order preserving	Order reversal Subjectivity in selecting $K(q_i)$, $\min_i$, and $\max_i$	Checks by varying $K(q_i)$, $\min_i$, and $\max_i$ are recommended
(ii) Fuzzy analysis	Well-elaborated theoretical background Simplifications in a systematic manner Order preserving	Attributes are numerically combined according to the Kosko measure	There is an implicit approximation because of the need to find a transitive closure
(iii) p-algorithm	Strong simplification Tools of Chapter 5 are most suitable for the resulting Hasse diagrams Order preserving	By focusing on priority objects, there is some loss of information. The definition of q_{i0} bears some subjectivity	Checks by varying q_{i0} are recommended

References

Annoni, P., Fattore, M. and Bruggemann, R. (2008). Analyzing the structure of poverty by fuzzy partial order. In J. Owsinski and R. Bruggemann (Eds.), Multicriteria ordering and ranking: Partial orders, ambiguities and applied issues (pp. 107–124). Warsaw: Systems Research Institute Polish Academy of Sciences.

Annoni, P., Fattore, M. and Bruggemann, R. (2012). A multi-criteria fuzzy approach for analyzing poverty structure. Statistica & Applicazioni, accepted.

Bruggemann, R. and Bartel, H. (1999). A theoretical concept to rank environmentally significant chemicals. J. Chem. Inf. Comput. Sci., 39(2), 211–217.

Bruggemann, R., Bucherl, C., Pudenz, S. and Steinberg, C. (1999). Application of the concept of partial order on comparative evaluation of environmental chemicals. Acta Hydrochim. Hydrobiol., 27(3), 170–178.

Bruggemann, R. and Welzl, G. (2002). Order theory meets statistics – Hasse diagram technique. In K. Voigt and G. Welzl (Eds.), Order theoretical tools in environmental sciences – order theory (Hasse diagram technique) meets multivariate statistics (pp. 9–39). Aachen: Shaker-Verlag.

De Baets, B. and De Meyer, H. (2003). On the existence and construction of T-transitive closures. Inf. Sci. 152, 167–179.

Van de Walle, B., De Baets, B. and Kersebaum, K.C. (1995). Fuzzy multi-criteria analysis of cutting techniques in a nuclear dismantling project. Fuzzy Sets Syst., 74, 115–126.

Chapter 7
Reducing the Number of Incomparabilities

7.1 Introduction

In Chapter 6, we have shown as to how we can obtain simpler Hasse diagrams from messy ones. We transformed the data matrix so that incomparabilities or comparabilities disappear because objects become equivalent.

This chapter discusses as to how we can enrich the partial order by numerically combining the attributes. Why do we want to enrich partial orders? Because too many incomparabilities hamper the insight into the ranking positions of the objects.

In this chapter, we will (i) revisit the concept of an index, (ii) introduce the concept of mmm order (min, median, and max), and (iii) formulate the concept of stepwise aggregation.

We will discuss how far tools of partial order can help to get insights into the consequences of uncertainties in weights to composite indicators.

7.2 Weighted Sums

7.2.1 Index

One of the simplest approaches is the weighted sum of attributes, which we call an index (for convenience, we use the symbol Γ, and we will use the term "index" (or "composite indicator") exclusively for weighted sums of the attributes):

$$\Gamma(x) = \sum g_i{}^* q_i(x) \tag{7.1a}$$

$$1 = \sum g_i, \quad 1 \geq g_i \geq 0 \tag{7.1b}$$

- The g_i values are the weights and do not depend on the specific object. Equations (7.1b) are the boundary conditions for selecting the weights. If the weights are not derived from the data matrix, they reflect expert opinion about the degree of mutual substitution of the attributes (Munda, 2008). In a monograph of the OECD (2008), methods to obtain weights are compiled.

R. Brüggemann, G.P. Patil, *Ranking and Prioritization for Multi-indicator Systems*, Environmental and Ecological Statistics 5, DOI 10.1007/978-1-4419-8477-7_7,

Γ is a continuous and positive monotone function; it induces an order O_Γ and we write $h_\Gamma(x)$ or $h_{\text{Index}}(x)$ to denote the height (rank) values of x. Also, we say that O_Γ is consistent with (X, IB) to indicate that the map $(X, \text{IB}) \to O_\Gamma$ is order preserving.

Equation (7.1a) provokes some caveats:

1. Order theoretical applications need that a linear or a weak order with respect to any single indicator is definable. Combination of attributes by a weighted sum (or any other positive monotone function), however, implies an appropriate scaling level.
2. Attributes must be normalized.
3. Expert weights may be subject to controversy.
4. A weighted sum representing an index is an averaging over the indicator values. According to Munda (2008), this is equivalent to a high compensation: By a weighted average, low values of some attributes (implying a low rank) can be compensated by large values of some attributes to get nevertheless a good ranking position.

As the weights are of much concern, we need some more formulations:

- We call a set of weights for m attributes a weight vector, obeying the boundary conditions (7.1b).
- Weights are often associated with importance of the attributes. As Munda (2008) shows, this is only in a very restricted sense correct. Scaling levels and ranges of the indicator can influence the numerical values of the weights.
- We will speak of weights in the sense of influence: If the attributes are columnwise normalized, the weights express how much influence a variation of the numerical value of attributes has on the index.

7.2.2 Superindicators

If the calculation of a weighted sum $\sum_{q_i \in \text{IB}'} g_i \cdot q_i(x)$, with $\text{IB}' \subset \text{IB}$ does not include all attributes, then we speak of a "superindicator" (or super-attribute) and together with the non-used attributes $q_i \in \text{IB} - \text{IB}'$ or other superindicators a new data matrix can be built.

For example, starting with five attributes ($\text{IB}_0 = \{q_1, q_2, q_3, q_4, q_5\}$), we get a partial order $X_0 = (X, \text{IB}_0)$. Forming a superindicator Γ of the first three attributes, we obtain a new information base $\{\Gamma, q_4, q_5\}$ and a new partial order $X_1 = (X, \{\Gamma, q_4, q_5\})$. We observe that the map $X_0 \to X_1$ is order preserving, because any comparability found in X_0 is retained in X_1, whereas some incomparabilities in X_0 are transformed into comparabilities in X_1. Because we refer to the same object set X, we get an enrichment of the partial order: A diagram may be helpful (Fig. 7.1).

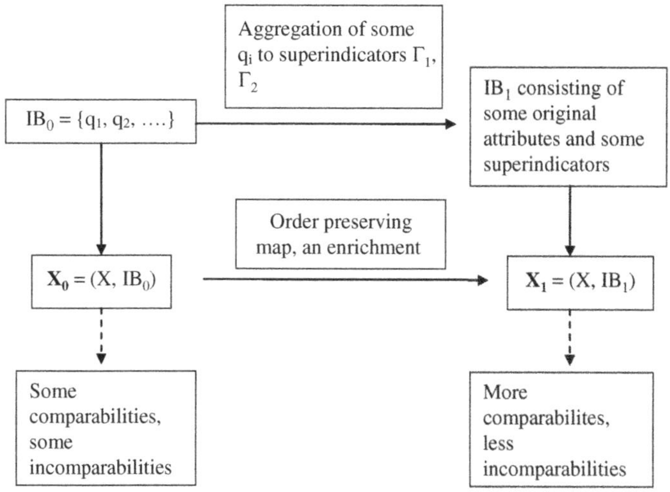

Fig. 7.1 Enrichment of partial order by stepwise aggregation

The stepwise aggregation will be useful if

- there is an unambiguous preference among some attributes so that they can be condensed to a superindicator, thus eliminating the incomparabilities arising from them, and
- an already existing indicator hierarchy is defined by the experts of a study: Aggregation is understood as a coarsening process, whereas disaggregation corresponds to a detailing of the evaluation analysis (see Fig. 7.2). Examples can be

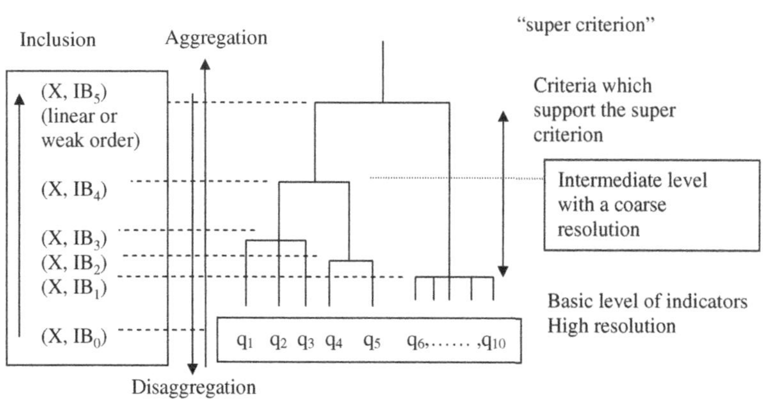

Fig. 7.2 Hierarchy in evaluation. The series (X, IB_i), $i = 0, \ldots, 5$, indicates that different partial orders are obtained during aggregation (see text)

found for the bridge (Chapter 13), the watershed (Chapter 14), or the EPI study (Chapter 15).

Figure 7.2 exemplifies the following:

1. Indicators of $IB_0 = \{q_1, \ldots, q_{10}\}$ describe the objects. They are the basic indicators of the problem. The resulting partial order (X, IB_0) may have many incomparabilities.
2. The basic indicators $q_6 - q_{10}$ are forming the superindicator Γ_1, because they may describe contextually a common aspect. We need four weights (normalization assumed). The information base is $IB_1 = \{q_1, q_2, q_3, q_4, q_5, \Gamma_1\}$ and the partial order (X, IB_1) is an enrichment of (X, IB_0). We write $(X, IB_0) \subseteq (X, IB_1)$.
3. The next step is to generate a superindicator Γ_2 from q_4 and q_5. We need one weight. After these first two steps, we have a new information base $IB_2 = \{\Gamma_1, \Gamma_2, q_1, q_2, q_3\}$ and consequently a new partial order (X, IB_2), i.e., $(X, IB_1) \subseteq (X, IB_2)$.
4. By aggregation of q_1, q_2, and q_3 to Γ_3 for which we need two weights, we obtain (X, IB_3), $(X, IB_2) \subseteq (X, IB_3)$. Now, the set of basic attributes is exhausted and we continue the aggregation with Γ_1, Γ_2, and Γ_3 as candidates.
5. We aggregate Γ_2 and Γ_3 to get Γ_{23}. $IB_4 = \{\Gamma_{23}, \Gamma_1\}$ and the partial order is (X, IB_4), i.e., $(X, IB_3) \subseteq (X, IB_4)$.
6. The last step finally is to obtain only one function, and for the objects, a linear or a weak order can be found $(X, IB_5) = O_\Gamma$, $O_\Gamma \supseteq (X, IB_4)$.
7. With the steps 1 – 6, we get a chain in the inclusion order of posets.

7.2.3 Illustrative Example for an Index Calculation

In Fig. 7.3, a Hasse diagram together with its data matrix is shown.

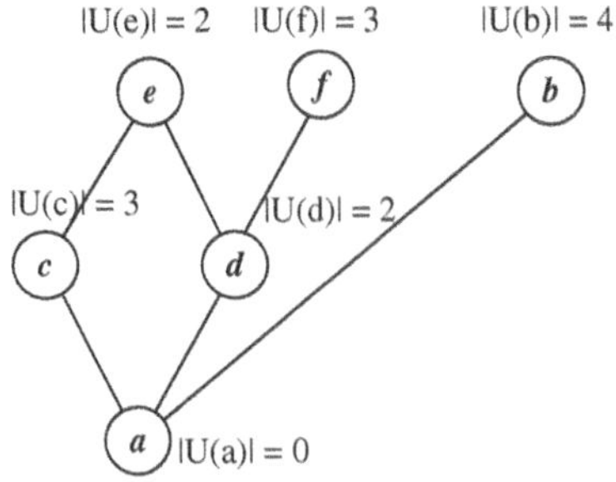

	q_1	q_2
a	1	1
b	10.2	1
c	2	3.3
d	4.2	2.6
e	6	7.4
f	7.3	2.8

Fig. 7.3 Hasse diagram of six objects. $|U(x)|$ is additionally indicated for every object

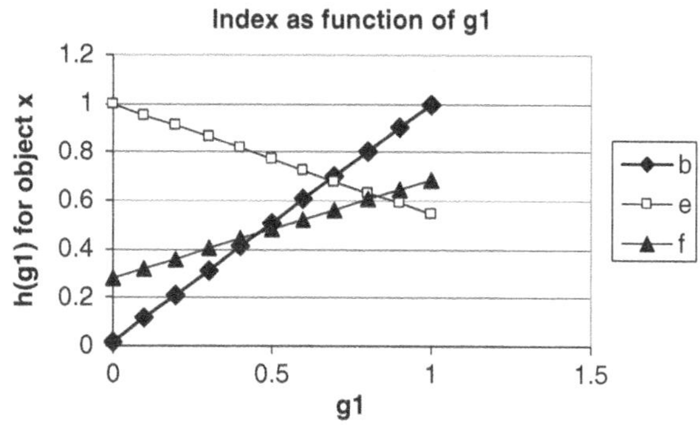

Fig. 7.4 Variation of height $h_\Gamma(x, g_1)$, $x = b, e, f$ (Fig. 7.3)

Now let us calculate an index from two attributes, normalized to [0,1]. The height h_Γ of an object $x \in X$ as a function of weights (here of g_1) we call "$h_\Gamma(x, g)$ function" and it is shown in Fig. 7.4.

Among the three objects e, f, and b, object b has the largest number of incomparable objects ($|U(b)| = 4$) and has the largest slope (taken as absolute value). The results of Chapter 3 tell us that the maximal height interval depends on $|U(x)|$. An object x with large difference in (normalized) attribute values $q_i(x)$ and $q_j(x)$ tends to get large $|U(x)|$ values and is sensitive to a variation in weights. Furthermore, crossing of two $h_\Gamma(x, g)$ functions is possible only for incomparable objects, because comparable objects, say $x \leq y$, will maintain that relation for all values of the weights. Thus in Fig. 7.4 on the one hand, the line for object d should be located below that of object e, but on the other hand, the line for object d would cross the lines of objects f, b, and c (not shown).

7.2.4 Representability Problem

Imagine that an index is to be constructed and you have a partial order, (X, IB), based on your data matrix at hand. We know that any index is consistent with the partial order. Furthermore we know that all linear extensions are by definition consistent with the partial order. Is it possible that every linear extension is realizable as a result of an appropriately selected set of weights to obtain the composite indicator? We call this problem the "representability problem" (see Patil, 2005).

Let us consider the set of all orders O_Γ obtained with admissible weights (Eq. (7.1b)). If this set of all orders O_Γ contains less orders than does the set of linear extensions, then we can conclude that the partial order is more general than the index. We will show by a counterexample that there is no O_Γ which reproduces all linear extensions of (X, IB). In Fig. 7.5, a Hasse diagram together with the data matrix is shown.

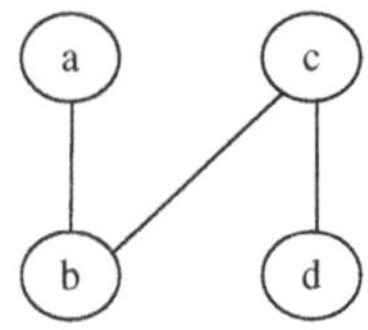

Object	q_1	q_2
a	0.333	1
b	0	0.333
c	1	0.666
d	0.666	0

Fig. 7.5 Hasse diagram (data see *RHS*)

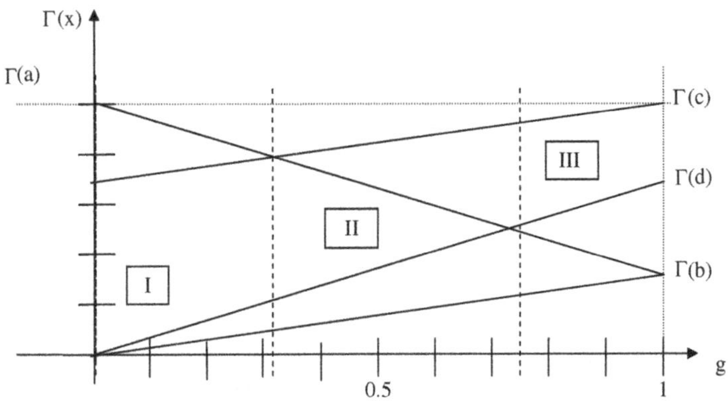

Fig. 7.6 The system of four functions $\Gamma(x)$, $x \in \{a, b, c, d\}$. The allowed range for g is divided (by *broken lines*) into three sections (I, II, and III) (see text)

The aggregation function is an index as a weighted sum of q_1 and q_2: $\Gamma(x) = g^* q_1(x) + (1 - g)^* q_2(x)$. Figure 7.6 displays the index as a function of g for all four objects.

In each section (I, II, or III), one linear order, induced by Γ, is found. Taking $g = 0$ or $g = 1$ gives two weak orders ($g = 0$: $d \cong b < c < a$; $g = 1$: $a \cong b < d < c$). The linear extension (d, b, a, c) of (X, IB) cannot be represented by O_Γ. Thus we see that there are only three linear orders derived from Γ, whereas there are five linear extensions of the partial order of Fig. 7.5. Therefore, not every linear extension is realizable by an index. (7.2)

7.2.5 *Simultaneous Variation of Several Weights (Monte Carlo Simulation)*

It is difficult to overview the role of weights when there are more than one weight. A Monte Carlo simulation (PyHasse) can be performed and the resulting distribution of heights can be obtained (Fig. 7.7 and its data matrix).

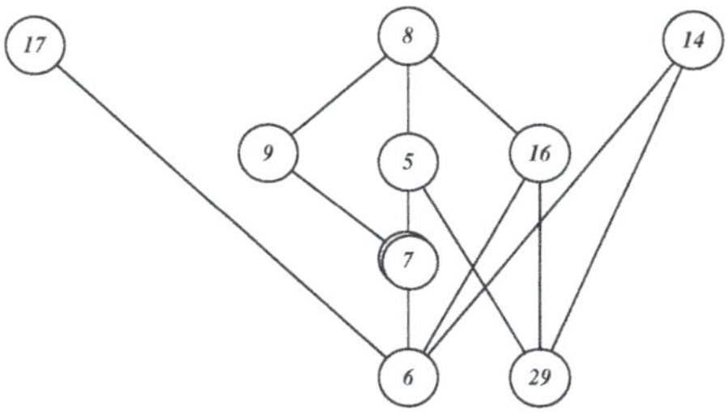

Id	q1	q2	q3
6	11	0.2	31
8	20	0.4	55
7	14	0.3	41
17	13	0.3	63
9	17	0.3	45
16	13	0.4	51
22	14	0.3	41
14	12	0.6	41
5	14	0.4	45
29	9	0.4	29

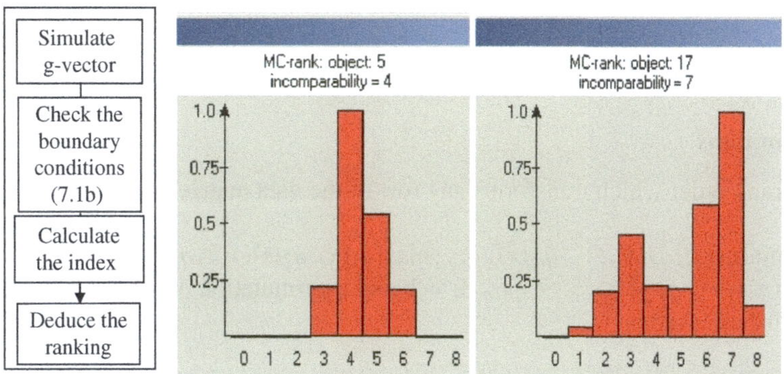

Fig. 7.7 Monte Carlo simulation (see text)

In Fig. 7.7, at the top, the Hasse diagram of 10 objects (object 22 $\cong$ object 7) and its data matrix are shown, whereas at the bottom, the principle of MC simulation and the MC simulations of the weights are shown.

In detail the Monte Carlo simulation is performed as follows:

1. For any weight, take a value $\in [0,1]$ at random.
2. Form the sum $\sum g_i$ and test whether the sum is equal to 1. If not, divide each weight by the sum.
3. Calculate the index from this weight vector according to (7.1a).
4. Repeat the calculation with a new choice of randomly selected weights.

For an application on chemicals, see Carlsen and Bruggemann (2009).

We see that the height distribution of object 5 ($|U(5)| = 4$ (LHS)) is much more concentrated than that of object 17 ($|U(17)| = 7$ (RHS)).

7.3 The Min-, Median-, Max- (mmm) Order

7.3.1 Prerequisites

Often a data matrix consists of so many attributes that at least for a first screening, the individual meaning of each attribute is of minor importance. This is the case if, for instance, surface waters are characterized by concentrations of many chemicals or if child well-being is described by a variety of attributes.

If we replace the attribute set of a data matrix $\{q_1, \ldots, q_m\}$ by {min, max} or {min, median, max} for each object (mapping M), then the attributes will need to have a common scale or dimension, or need to be dimensionless. Therefore it is recommended to normalize them (columnwise).

7.3.2 Partial Order, Rank Order, and m^r Order

7.3.2.1 Definitions

We apply a rank order which transforms any row of the data matrix as follows:

$$(\min(q_1(x), q_2(x), \ldots, q_m(x)), \ldots, \max(q_1(x), q_2(x), \ldots, q_m(x))) \\ = (q_{\sigma(1)} \leq q_{\sigma(2)} \leq \ldots \leq q_{\sigma(m)}),\ \sigma \text{ being a permutation of the attribute's index} \quad (7.3)$$

We perform two simplifications: We replace the rank order by (a) (min(x), median(x), max(x)) and call the resulting partial order the m^3 order. (7.4)

and

(b) (min(x), max(x)), calling that order the m^2 order. (7.5)

Equation (7.5) may furthermore be interpreted as follows: There is a class of students and instead of an evaluation based on their skill for every discipline, we are looking at the worst and the best performance.

7.3.2.2 Properties of $m^r (r = 2 \text{ or } 3)$ Order

It is easy to show

$$q(x) \leq q(y) \Rightarrow m^r(x) \leq m^r(y) \quad (7.6)$$

Hence the mapping M is order preserving.

The reverse implication does not hold in general, as the following simple counter example shows: $x \rightarrow (2, 0, 3, 4)$ and $y \rightarrow (1, 2, 3, 5)$. Then $m^2(x) = (0, 4)$ and $m^2(y) = (1, 5)$. Although $m^2(x) \leq m^2(y)$, we find that $x \parallel y$. Furthermore it is obvious that

$$m^2(x) \parallel m^2(y) \Rightarrow q(x) \parallel q(y) \quad (7.7)$$

from which the results follow for m^3.

Incomparable pairs $m^2(x) \parallel m^2(y)$ can be ordered by ordinary interval subset relations.

A proper inclusion $\subset_p$ is $[\min(x), \max(x)] \subset [\min(y), \max(y)]$, with $\min(x) \neq \min(y)$ and $\max(x) \neq \max(y)$.

(a) $[\min(x), \max(x)] \subset_P [\min(y), \max(y)] \Rightarrow x \parallel y$ in the m^2 order. (7.8)

(b) $[\min(x), \max(x)] \subset [\min(y), \max(y)]$, with $\min(x) = \min(y)$ or (exclusive) $\max(x) = \max(y)$; improper inclusion implies $x < y$ in the m^2 order. (7.9)

(c) $[\min(x), \max(x)] \subset [\min(y), \max(y) \Rightarrow \Delta h_\Gamma^{\max}(x) \leq \Delta h_\Gamma^{\max}(y)$. (7.10)

Equation (7.10) is best understandable by taking the example of students in a class. If the worst skill of student y is worse than that of student x and the best skill of student y is better than that of student x, then the disparity in the disciplines of student y is much larger than that of student x. Hence an aggregation to get a total score for student y depends more on the weight one gives the single disciplines than that for student x.

In Fig. 7.8 we summarize some important facts of this section.

7.3.2.3 Illustrative Example

A simple example will now support this theoretical aspect (Table 7.1 and Fig. 7.9).

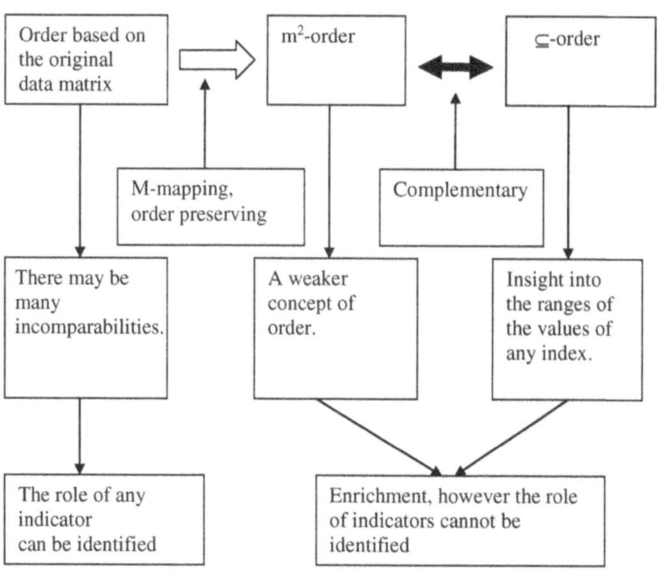

Fig. 7.8 Summary among the three possible orders (usual product order m^r and inclusion order)

Table 7.1 Illustrative example explaining the interplay between inclusion and m^2 orders

	q_1	q_2	q_3	Min	Max
a	0	2	3	0	3
b	2	3	5	2	5
c	3	4	3	3	4
d	1	6	1	1	6
e	4	2	7	2	7

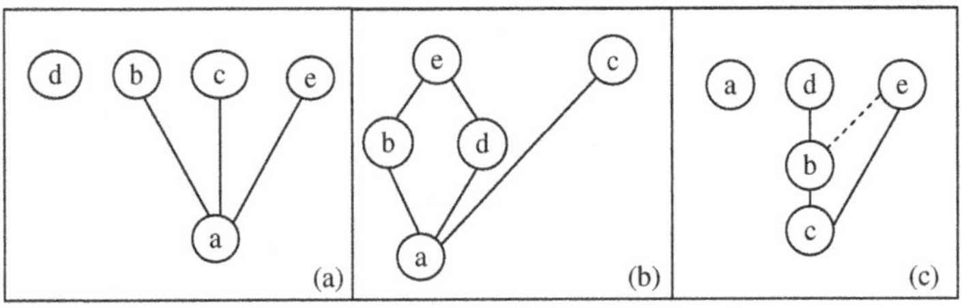

Fig. 7.9 Hasse diagrams based on different orders (see text)

In Fig. 7.9, the three orders are displayed.

Figure 7.9 shows the following: (a) the Hasse diagram of the order relations induced by the three attributes q_1, q_2, and q_3; (b) Hasse diagram based on the m^2 order; and (c) the Hasse diagram based on the inclusion of intervals (Eqs. (7.11) and (7.12)). The improper inclusion is presented as broken line. In detail, Figure 7.9 demonstrates that any incomparability in the inclusion order represents an order relation in the m^2 order. The improper inclusion [min(b), max(b)] $\subset$ [min(e), max(e)], with min(b) = min(e) is realized as $b < e$ in the m^2 order. Finally [min(c), max(c)] $= [3, 4]$ and [min(e), max(e)] $= [2, 7]$. Hence in m^2, $e \parallel c$, whereas in the inclusion order $c < e$.

7.4 METEOR

The concept of METEOR (method of evaluation by order theory) was developed in order to allow a step-by-step aggregation as described in Section 7.2 (see Simon et al., 2005, 2006; Bruggemann et al., 2008). The main ideas are as follows:

1. avoiding to know all weights at once and
2. ability to analyze the role of weights by identifying so-called stability fields and "hot spots" in the weight space.

7.4.1 Iterative Aggregation

Whenever an index has to be set up, the very starting point is the definition of the index framework (OECD, 2008). The framework usually starts with a set of indicators. If the set of indicators is large due to the complexity of the objects to be ranked, then it is convenient to aggregate them as per commonalities. The interim aggregations are called pillars. An application of an iterative aggregation is to compute each pillar and then to apply partial order on them. This has the key advantage to retain the structure of the composite indicator, i.e., its aim, while avoiding aggregation at the pillar level. Keeping pillars separated is important because most often policy makers are interested on the pillar level. Avoiding aggregation across pillars allows for staying away from compensatory effects.

Hence an evaluation may start with basic attributes and then proceed by aggregating some attributes to describe the phenomenon corresponding to its pillars. This process may be iterated, and we get some kind of attribute hierarchy: As each subsequently performed aggregation is order preserving, an enrichment of the partial orders until finally a linear order is obtained (see Fig. 7.2). We demonstrate the iteration by an illustrative example (Figs. 7.10 and 7.11).

The aggregation scheme is as follows:

- We combine q_1 with q_2 with weights $g_1 = 0.4$ and $g_2 = 0.6$, hence a super-attribute $q12 = g_1{}^*q_1 + g_2{}^*q_2$ is obtained, $\mathrm{IB}_1 = \{q12,\ q_3,\ q_4\}$.
- A parallel aggregation is $q34 = 0.5^*q_3 + 0.5^*q_4$, $\mathrm{IB}_2 = \{q_1,\ q_2,\ q34\}$.
- The super-attributes can be simultaneously considered, i.e., $\mathrm{IB}_3 = \{q12,\ q34\}$.
- The final subsequent aggregation based on $q12$ and $q34$ is $q1234 = 0.666^*q12 + 0.333^*q34$. Here $\mathrm{IB}_4 = \{q1234\}$.

See Fig. 7.11 for the partial order among $(X, \{q12, q_3, q_4\})$, $(X, \{q34, q_1, q_2\})$, $(X, \{q12, q34\})$, and $(X, \{q1234\})$.

The partial orders arising from different aggregation schemes are themselves partially ordered (by inclusion of the sets of ordered pairs $(x, y) \in X^2$ (see Chapter 2)).

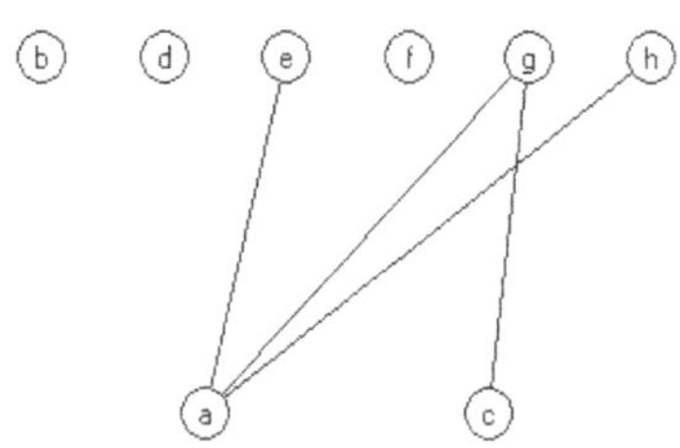

	q_1	q_2	q_3	q_4
a	0	0.166	0.286	0
b	0.5	0.166	0	0
c	0.166	0.333	0.143	0.286
d	0.5	0	0.143	0.571
e	0	1	0.857	0.143
f	1	0	1	0
g	0.166	0.5	1	1
h	0.2	0.166	0.571	0.714

Fig. 7.10 Hasse diagram (X, IB), $\mathrm{IB} = \{q_1,\ q_2,\ q_3,\ q_4\}$ and its data matrix of normalized attributes

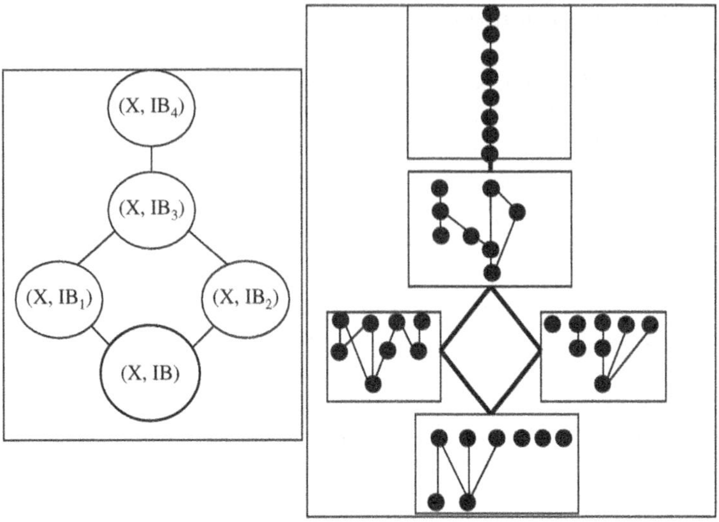

Fig. 7.11 Partial order on partial orders due to the enrichment while aggregating attributes (we neglect the labeling for the sake of clarity)

7.4.2 Comparability Acquisition Profile

7.4.2.1 Idea

Here we introduce a quality measure for stepwise aggregation (see Patil, 2005): The idea is that if there is no evidence which helps us to prefer one weight vector and one sequence of stepwise aggregation (called a "weighting scheme"), then that weighting scheme should be favored whose comparability acquisition profile (CAP) is the better one (see below).

7.4.2.2 Method

It is clear that a positive monotonous transformation applied to correctly oriented data preserves the order relation. At every step of the aggregation, the data matrix produced by the indicators and superindicators results in a new poset. In order to characterize the aggregation strategy, we use the total number of comparabilities V:

$$V = |\{(x, y) \in (X, \mathrm{IB})\}|\,, x \neq y \tag{7.11}$$

V is the number of pairs of objects which are comparable. We have seen that the aggregation of two indicators in one aggregation step cannot decrease V, since aggregation is order preserving. To compare two different weighting schemes, we cumulate the number of comparabilities after each step of aggregation for a particular weighting scheme. We start with the initial data matrix, which we call the 0th step. Specifically, we can compare weighting schemes w_1 and w_2, and look at their CAP at each aggregation step.

Weighting scheme w_1 is preferred to w_2 if $V(i, w_1) \geq V(i, w_2)$ for every $0 \leq i \leq m - 1$, where $V(i, w)$ is the number of

$$\text{comparabilities of the data matrix using the weighting scheme } w \tag{7.12}$$

at the ith step of the aggregation, and m is the number of indicators in the original data matrix.

We will apply CAP to real-life examples in application chapters and give here an illustrative example.

7.4.2.3 Illustrative Example

We assume that an index is defined as follows (see Table 7.2):

$$\Gamma = (1/6)^*(q_1 + q_2 + q_3 + q_4 + q_5 + q_6),\ g_i = 1/6,\ \text{for } i = 1, \ldots, 6$$

We define different weighting schemes:

Weighting scheme w_1: Take the weights $g_i = 1/6$ and start with q_1 until all attributes are included.

Weighting scheme w_2: Take the weights $g_i = 1/6$ and start with q_6 until last step q_1 is aggregated.

Weighting scheme w_3: Take the weights $g_i = 1/6$. That aggregation will be selected which has the lowest value in the Spearman correlation among either

- attributes
- attributes and already aggregated attributes (super-attributes) and
- super-attributes.

Table 7.2 Data matrix for the illustrative example demonstrating CAP (normalized attributes)

	q_1	q_2	q_3	q_4	q_5	q_6
a	0.1	0.4	0.2	0.5	0.6	0.4
b	0.4	0.5	0.1	0.7	0.6	0.5
c	0.3	0.9	0.7	0.8	0.7	0.6
d	0.2	0	1	0.2	0	1
e	0.7	0.4	0.3	0.6	1	0.6
f	0.9	0.3	0.3	0.7	0.6	0.5
g	0	0.7	0.5	1	0.2	0.7
h	1	0.6	0.9	0	0.4	0
i	0.5	1	0.2	0.4	0.8	0.8
j	0.2	0.1	0	0.3	0.9	0.9

The Hasse diagram of the 10 objects is shown in Fig. 7.12.

The resulting CAP (Fig. 7.13) shows that the three weighting schemes are incomparable. There is no best strategy.

The automatic, i.e., Spearman-driven aggregation, leads to the following sequence (only the actual aggregated attributes are shown):

$$(q_3, q_4) \rightarrow (q_3, q_5)(q_1, q_6) \rightarrow (q_3, q_4, q_5)(q_1, q_6) \rightarrow (q_3, q_4, q_5)(q_1, q_2, q_6) \rightarrow (q_1, q_2, q_3, q_4, q_5, q_6)$$

Although the Spearman-driven scheme w_3 has in the latter steps the steepest increase, the first aggregation step is worse than that for aggregation scheme w_1. The unexpected effect that w_3 lets the number of comparisons constant, even if anti-correlated attributes are aggregated, can be explained when the correlation matrix is examined (Table 7.3).

The pair of attributes with the lowest correlation is q_3, q_5. Their aggregation will average out large disparities in the data values. However, there is still a pair of attributes, namely q_1 and q_6 with a high degree of anticorrelation. Therefore the number of comparabilities can only weakly increase after the single aggregation step of q_3 and q_5.

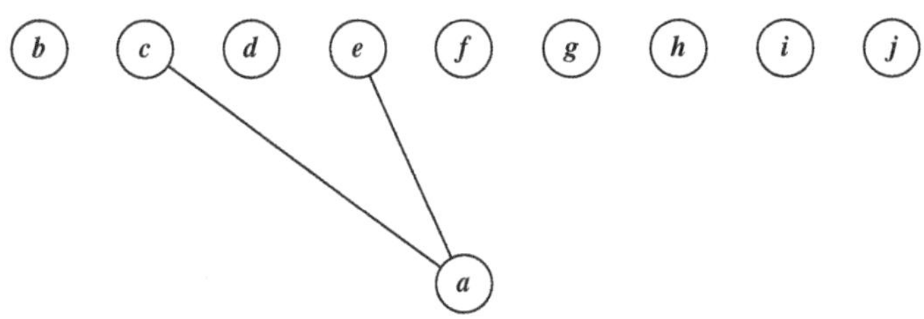

Fig. 7.12 A certainly not complex Hasse diagram

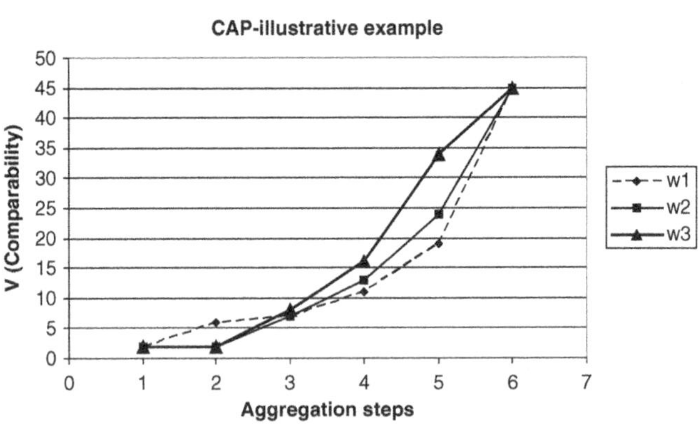

Fig. 7.13 CAP, following the alternatives of weighting schemes, based on PyHasse

Table 7.3 Spearman correlation matrix of the attributes of Table 7.2

			q_1	q_2	q_3	q_4	q_5	q_6
Spearman rho	q_1	Correlation coefficient	1	0.11	0.122	–0.262	0.252	–0.428
		Sig (two-tailed)		0.763	0.736	0.464	0.482	0.217
		N	10	10	10	10	10	10
	q_2	Correlation coefficient	0.11	1	0.055	0.372	0.111	–0.205
		Sig (two-tailed)	0.763		0.88	0.29	0.761	0.57
		N	10	10	10	10	10	10
	q_3	Correlation coefficient	0.122	0.055	1	–0.095	–0.599	0
		Sig (two-tailed)	0.763	0.88		0.794	0.067	1
		N	10	10	10	10	10	10
	q_4	Correlation coefficient	–0.262	0.372	–0.095	1	0.055	–0.092
		Sig (two-tailed)	0.464	0.29	0.794		0.879	0.801
		N	10	10	10	10	10	10
	q_5	Correlation coefficient	0.252	0.111	–0.599	0.055	1	0.099
		Sig (two-tailed)	0.482	0.761	0.067	0.879		0.786
		N	10	10	10	10	10	10
	q_6	Correlation coefficient	–0.428	–0.205		–0.092	0.099	1
		Sig (two-tailed)	0.217	0.57	1	0.801	0.786	
		N	10	10	10	10	10	10

7.4.3 Stability Fields and Hot Spots in the Space of Weights

7.4.3.1 Method

Let us take two attributes called q_1 and q_2. The super-attribute $q12(g) = g^* q_1 + (1-g)^* q_2$ is considered as a linear function of $g \in [0, 1]$. Accordingly we write $q12(g,\ a)$ to indicate the value of $q12$ for weight g and object a. Let $(a, b) \in U_{X/\cong} = \{(x, y),\ (x, y),\ \text{a pair of representants}, x \| y\}$ (Section 4.3). Then there exists one and only one crucial weight g_c such that $q12(g_c,\ a) = q12(g_c,\ b)$. If we consider all pairs of $U_{X/\cong}$, a rectangular scheme is useful, where rows and columns are labeled by the objects. Any cell gets one and only one crucial weight value. Because X is a finite object set, there is a finite number of different g_c values, say n_c. We order these from the smallest to the largest and call the resulting order the crucial weight sequence.

We introduce a map G:

G: $[0, 1] \in \mathrm{IR} \to X \times X$
$G\ g_c \to E(g_c)$, the set of object pairs for which $q12(g_c, x) = q12(g_c, y)$.

To each g_c of the crucial weight sequence belongs a set of object pairs $E(g_c)$ for which the $q12(g_c)$ values are the same. The pairs $(g_c, |E(g_c)|)$ allow the following interpretation: Any crucial weight indicates where a selection of weight has an impact on the ranking by a composite indicator and by $|E(g_c)|$ as to how severe this impact will be. Pairs belonging to $E(g_c)$ undergo an order reversal if the weight g is varied from a value less than g_c to a value larger than g_c. We prove that between two successive crucial weights, say $g_{c,i}$ and $g_{c,i+1}$, constituting the interval $I_g = (g_{c,i}, g_{c,i+1})$, the ranking due to $q12$ does not depend on the value of $g \in I_g$.

The proof will be performed by contradiction.

Assume that $g_1, g_2 \in I_g$ exist such that two different linear orders due to $q12$ are induced. Then there must be a pair $(x, y) \in U_{X/\cong}$ such that at g_1, $x <_{q12(g1)} y$ and at g_2, $x >_{q12(g2)} y$. Hence there exists $g_c \in (\min(g_1, g_2), \max(g_1, g_2)) \subset I_g$ for which $q12(x, g_c) = q12(y, g_c)$ in contradiction to the exhaustive count of the crucial weights, which leads to n_c values.

The pairs $(g_c, |E(g_c)|)$ allow a visualization in the following manner (Fig. 7.14).

Between two successive crucial weights, there is one and only one linear order when we speak of a "stability field." If a composite indicator is to be constructed aiming at a ranking, the exact value of a weight may not be known. If, however, the study of weights produces a value near g_c, then a slight numerical change will change the ranking result of the composite indicator and the impact will be large if $|E(g_c)|$ is large. Hence pairs $(g_c, |E(g_c)|)$ with large $|E(g_c)|$ are "hot spots" in the space of weights.

7.4.3.2 Illustrative Example

We select the example shown in Fig. 7.7. In our example, the first two attributes of the data matrix are aggregated to get $q12$. We construct a presentation of the $(g_c, |E(g_c)|)$ pairs like in Fig. 7.14 to see where the weights are sensitive for the ranking due to the composite indicator. The result is shown in Fig. 7.15, applying the software PyHasse (see Chapter 17). In any stability field one finds one linear order. There are nine crucial weights. From these, seven have $|E(g_c)| = 1$ and two have $|E(g_c)| = 3$.

If the weights are varied, then each crossing of a g_c position will change the linear order by reverting the rank positions of any two objects. Especially at two positions, three pairs of objects will undergo an inversion, hence much care is needed

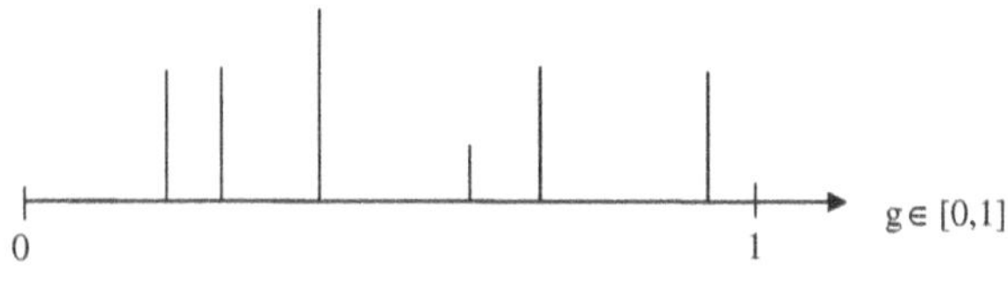

Fig. 7.14 Along the g-axis the sequence of crucial weights is located and to every position, belongs $|E(g_c)|$

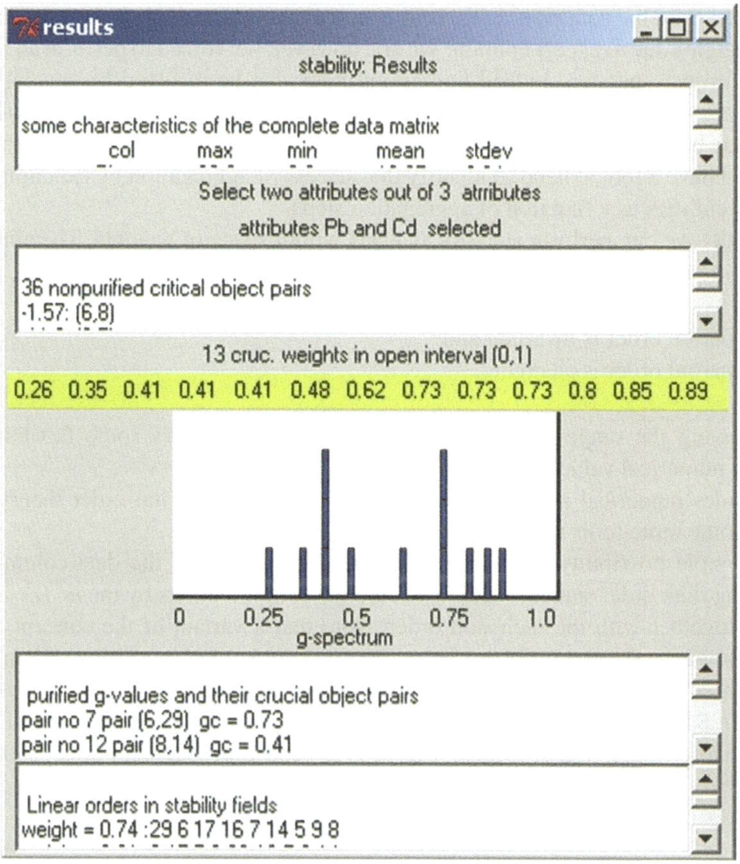

Fig. 7.15 Stability plot (PyHasse)

if weights are supposed to be in the neighborhood of such "hot spots." We will reexamine the stability field in the chapter dealing with the analysis of watersheds (Chapter 14). For more details, see Bruggemann et al. (2008), Restrepo et al. (2008), and Voigt and Bruggemann (2008).

7.5 Summary and Commentary

We started with the question of how we can reduce the number of incomparabilities? In Chapter 7, attributes, i.e., the columns of a data matrix, are aggregated through weighted sums and thus the number of incomparabilities can be reduced.

In many ranking studies, the strategy is to develop a data matrix with detailed information about the objects by including many attributes. The question about who or what is at the top and about who or what is at the bottom, cannot directly be extracted from the data matrix. Therefore, in most of the cases, an index was derived with weights due to expert opinion. We are, however, not forced to perform an aggregation in just one step. Indeed finding an index can be resolved by several steps where any step leads to partial order, which is an enriched one. Therefore the process may be stopped when the partial order renders enough information. With CAP we even have a tool at hand to identify the success of aggregation by examining the comparabilities as a function of aggregation steps.

Finally we can perform stability analysis within space of weights. The aim is to identify those ranges in the space of weights, where

a. the partial order is invariant and
b. the partial order is changing.

Knowing the range of invariance of partial orders allows some flexibility in finding numerical values of weights.

Besides numerical aggregation (eventually stepwise), partial order theory provides some more tools to help the expert.

A simple possibility is to forget the individual labels of the data columns by applying rank order statistics and to discuss the simplifications by the m^r ($r = 2, 3$) order, together with the inclusion order. Note that a variant of the concept of m^2 (or m^3) order was used by Myers et al. (2006) as rank range run (RRR). Compared with Hasse diagrams, RRR gives an impression of the object set X even if $|X|$ is very large. In RRR the individual labeling of the data matrix columns is lost as in some other methods. See in that context Yager (1993) and Carlsson and Fuller (2002) for their OWA operators (ordered weighted averaging operators).

References

Bruggemann, R., Restrepo, G. and Voigt, K. (2008). Towards a new and advanced partial order program: PyHasse. In J. Owsinski and R. Bruggemann (Eds.), Multicriteria ordering and ranking: Partial orders, ambiguities and applied issues (pp. 11–33). Warsaw: Systems Research Institute Polish Academy of Sciences.

Carlsen, L. and Bruggemann, R. (2009). Partial order ranking as a tool in environmental impact assessment. PAH and PCB pollution of the river main as an illustrative example. In G.T. Halley and Y.T. Fridian (Eds.), Environmental impact assessment (pp. 335–354). Hauppauge, NY: Nova Science Publishers.

Carlsson, C. and Fuller, R. (2002). Fuzzy reasoning in decision making and optimization. Heidelberg: Physica-Verlag.

Munda, G. (2008). Social multi-criteria evaluation for a sustainable economy (pp. 1–210). Berlin: Springer.

Myers, W.L., Patil, G.P. and Cai, Y. (2006). Exploring patterns of habitat diversity across landscapes using partial ordering. In R. Bruggemann and L. Carlsen (Eds.), Partial order in environmental sciences and chemistry (pp. 309–325). Berlin: Springer.

OECD (Nardo, M., et al.). (2008). Handbook on constructing composite indicators – methodology and user guide (pp. 1–158). Ispra: OECD.

Patil, G.P. (2005). Cross-disciplinary class room notes. Center for Statistical Ecology and Environmental Statistics, Penn State University.

Restrepo, G., Bruggemann, R., Weckert, M., Gerstmann, S. and Frank, H. (2008). Ranking patterns, an application to refrigerants. Match – Commun. Math. Comput. Chem., 59, 555–584.

Simon, U., Brüggemann, R., Behrendt, H., Shulenberger, E. and Pudenz, S. (2006). METEOR: A step-by-step procedure to explore effects of indicator aggregation in multi criteria decision aiding – Application to water management in Berlin, Germany. Acta Hydrochim. Hydrobiol., 34, 126–136.

Simon, U., Bruggemann, R., Mey, S. and Pudenz, S. (2005). METEOR – Application of a decision support tool based on discrete mathematics. Match – Commun. Math. Comput. Chem., 54(3), 623–642.

Voigt, K. and Bruggemann, R. (2008). Ranking of pharmaceuticals detected in the environment: Aggregation and weighting procedures. Comb. Chem. High Throughput Screen., 11, 770–782.

Yager, R.R. (1993). Families of OWA operators. Fuzzy Sets Syst., 59, 125–148.

Chapter 8
Formal Concept Analysis

8.1 Motivation

So far the core of all considerations was the partial order and its visualization by a Hasse diagram. On the one hand, the system of lines allowed us to identify comparabilities and on the other hand, it also revealed the status of objects relative to the others. In some cases, the Hasse diagram had a structure so that it was possible to explain as to why a certain relative position was obtained for an object. The concept of antagonistic indicators helped in clarifying the reasons for certain positions. The Hasse diagram is a graph focusing on the objects and their mutual relations. It will be extremely helpful, if we can construct a directed graph, where at the same time the constellation of the relevant attribute values responsible for the position of the object is exhibited. As we have seen in Chapters 6 and 7, we may perform ordinal modeling by focusing on object-related or attribute-related manipulations. In the theory of "formal concept analysis," mutual relationship of the position of an object with the values of its attributes inducing its position is depicted into one single diagram (Davey and Priestley, 1990; Ganter and Wille, 1986; Wolff, 1993; Gugisch, 2001; Carpineto and Romano, 1994; Annoni and Bruggemann, 2008, 2009; Bartel and Nofz, 1997; Bartel, 1997; Kerber, 2006).

8.2 The Concept

8.2.1 Intuitive Introduction

The term "concept" is a central, technical term and has its origin in philosophy. The idea is to characterize a subset of objects uniquely by a subset of properties[1] and a subset of properties is uniquely characterized by a subset of objects. Let us consider

[1] An object has a property or not. Although we can describe the presence or the absence of a property by a binary attribute, we are using the concept "property" for the sake of the simplicity of the text.

R. Brüggemann, G.P. Patil, *Ranking and Prioritization for Multi-indicator Systems*, Environmental and Ecological Statistics 5, DOI 10.1007/978-1-4419-8477-7_8,

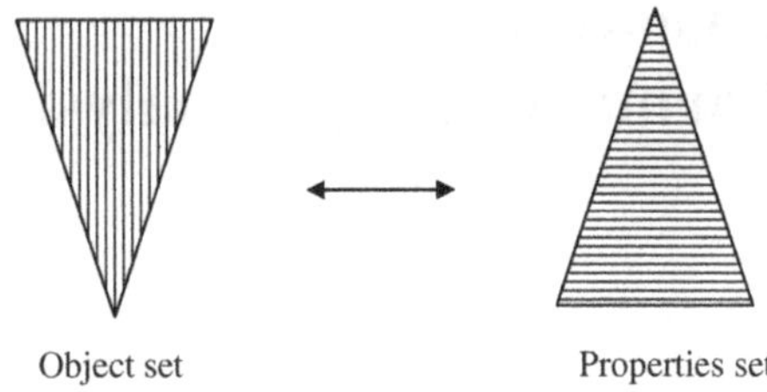

Fig. 8.1 The larger the set of properties to be fulfilled by objects, the smaller the object set fulfilling them

a set of objects having some properties in common. If an additional property is considered, not all of the objects may have this additional property. Hence, increasing the set of properties and requiring that objects at the same time have the corresponding properties must consequently decrease the set of objects. Conversely, increasing the object set by requiring that properties be simultaneously fulfilled can be done only by reducing the number of properties, i.e., by relaxing the conditions which are to be fulfilled. Figure 8.1 shows this schematically.

Let us take a class of students. The property "being member of the class" is common to all students of the class. The set of students is reduced by the additional requirement of being good in mathematics. An additional requirement of having good knowledge in chemistry reduces the set further.

8.2.2 A Formalized Relation Between Object Subsets and Property Subsets

We will here give only a schematic description of the most important steps.

Consider a data matrix with objects denoted as x and properties as q.

1. Define a relation I, (xIq) expressing that x "has" the property q. The set of properties is called IB.
2. Derive a table with the objects as rows and the properties as columns and insert 1 if (xIq). This table is called a context table.
3. Think of a new matrix where the rows are elements of the power set of X and the columns are elements of the power set of IB ("power set" matrix).
4. Define the derivation of a subset $X' \subseteq X$ as that set of properties $\mathrm{IB}' \subseteq \mathrm{IB}$ where for all $x \in X'$, (xIq), $q \in \mathrm{IB}'$ holds.
5. Define a derivation of a subset $\mathrm{IB}' \subseteq \mathrm{IB}$ as that set of objects X" where for all $q \in \mathrm{IB}'$, (xIq) holds.
6. Checkmark those cells of the power set matrix for which the derivation of X' is a set $\mathrm{IB}^{(+)}$ and the derivation of $\mathrm{IB}^{(+)}$ is X'. Such subsets of X and IB are called "Galois connected:"

$$\text{derivation of } X' = \mathrm{IB}^{(+)} \text{and derivation of } \mathrm{IB}^{(+)} = X' \tag{8.1}$$

We will use the symbol d for derivation and write $d(X')$.

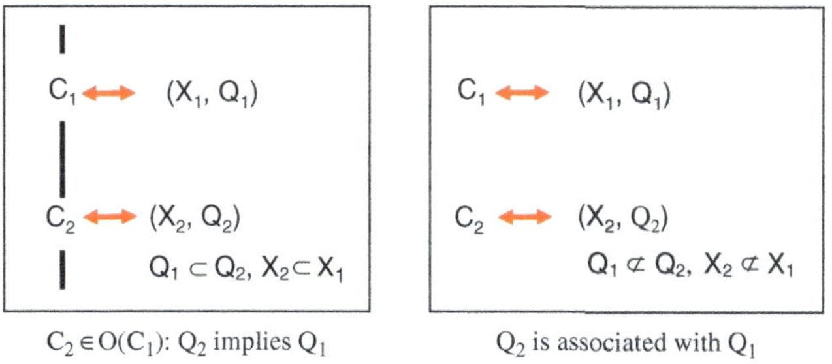

Fig. 8.2 Formal concept analysis, leading to implications and associations

7. Consider the checkmarked cell as new object (called concept), corresponding to a certain object subset and a certain attribute subset.
8. Draw a Hasse diagram of the concepts, with the inclusion relation among the object subsets. Increase object subsets by walking from the bottom to the top of the diagram.
9. Label the concepts by their attribute and object subsets.
10. Reduce the labels by keeping only the smallest possible subsets. The full information can then be reconstructed by union operations, following the lines of the graph.
11. Check for object set inclusion relations to deduce associations and implications among the attributes. Let X_2 be the set of objects for which the premise holds and X_1 the objects for which the conclusion is fulfilled. Then, the extent of association EoA: $= |X_2 \cap X_1| \,/\, |X_2|$.
12. Software is provided by Yevtushenko (2000): Conexp1.3.

A figure may be helpful to understand step 11 (Fig. 8.2).

In the following, we will illustrate some steps.

8.3 Context

8.3.1 Context Table

Let us imagine three objects *a*, *b*, and c and three properties q_1, q_2, and q_3. Then an entry 1 in Table 8.1, the context table, means that $d(\{x_j\}) = \{q_i\}$ and $x_i \in d(\{q_j\})$.

From Table 8.1, we conclude the following:

Table 8.1 Assignment of properties with objects and vice versa (context table)

	q_1	q_2	q_3
a	1	1	0
b	1	0	0
c	1	1	1

- Object a has the properties q_1 and q_2, $d(\{a\}) = \{q_1, q_2\}$.
- Object b has the property q_1.
- Object c has the properties q_1, q_2, and q_3.
- Property q_1 is a property in common for a, b, and c, $d(\{q_1\}) = \{a,\ b,\ c\}$.
- Property q_2 is a property in common for a and c.
- Property q_3 is a property of c alone.

8.3.2 Application of the Derivation

Let us perform some examples of how to use the "derivation." When we start with the example above, the object set as well as the attribute set has three elements. Hence there are eight subsets possible for the objects and eight for the properties. Generally the number of concepts $\leq |\text{Pow}(X)| * |\text{Pow(IB)}| = 2^{|X|*}2^{|\text{IB}|}$.

Clearly, in reality we will only get some few concepts because of the condition (8.1): Only those pairs are concepts whose object subsets (extents) and property subsets (intents) are Galois connected.

Object subsets:

$$d(\text{Ø}_X) = \{q_1,\ q_2,\ q_3\}(\text{Ø}_X\text{: empty object subset}) \tag{O.1}$$

$$d(\{a\}) = \{q_1,\ q_2\} \tag{O.2}$$

$$d(\{b\}) = \{q_1\} \tag{O.3}$$

$$d(\{c\}) = \{q_1,\ q_2,\ q_3\} \tag{O.4}$$

$$d(\{a, b\}) = \{q_1\} \tag{O.5}$$

$$d(\{a,\ c\}) = \{q_1,\ q_2\} \tag{O.6}$$

$$d(\{b,\ c\}) = \{q_1\} \tag{O.7}$$

$$d(\{a,\ b,\ c\}) = \{q_1\} \tag{O.8}$$

Property subsets:

$$d(\text{Ø}_Q) = \{a,\ b,\ c\}(\text{Ø}_Q\text{: empty property subset}) \tag{P.1}$$

$$d(\{q_1\}) = \{a,\ b,\ c\} \tag{P.2}$$

$$d(\{q_2\}) = \{a,\ c\} \tag{P.3}$$

$$d(\{q_3\}) = \{c\} \tag{P.4}$$

$$d(\{q_1,\ q_2\}) = \{a,\ c\} \tag{P.5}$$

$$d(\{q_1,\ q_3\}) = \{c\} \tag{P.6}$$

$$d(\{q_2, q_3\}) = \{c\} \tag{P.7}$$

$$d(\{q_1, q_2, q_3\}) = \{c\} \tag{P.8}$$

8.3.3 Concepts

We check (P.1)–(P.8) by looking at the corresponding subsets in (O.1)–(O.8) and examine whether and where the constraint Eq. (8.1) is fulfilled.

(P.1) is not Galois connected with (O.8) because $d(\emptyset_Q) = \{a,\ b,\ c\}$, however, $d(\{a,\ b,\ c\}) = \{q_1\}$.
(P.2) is Galois connected with (O.8), thus we find one concept, which we write as a pair: Concept $1 = [\{a,\ b,\ c\},\ \{q_1\}]$.
(P.3) is not Galois connected with (O.6), because $d\{q_2\} = \{a,\ c\}$, however, $d\{a,\ c\}$ is not $\{q_2\}$.
(P.4) is not Galois connected with (O.4).
(P.5) is Galois connected with (O.6), thus a second concept is found: Concept $2 = [\{a, c\},\ \{q_1,\ q_2\}]$.
(P.6) is not Galois connected with (O.4).
(P.7) is not Galois connected with (O.4).
(P.8) is Galois connected with (O.4), thus a third concept is found: Concept $3 = [\{c\}, \{q_1, q_2, q_3\}]$.

8.4 Order Relation Among Concepts

8.4.1 Inclusion Relation

We can in a natural way order the concepts by applying the set-theoretical inclusion operation: Apply the inclusion relation on either the extents or the intents. By the constraint Eq. (8.1), a superset–set inclusion relation interpreted as greater than relation among the object subsets $X_1 \supset X_2$ is uniquely accompanied by a subset–set inclusion relation interpreted as a less than relation of the attribute sets $Q_1 \subset Q_2$. We construct the Hasse diagram of the concepts by applying the inclusion of object subsets as order relation. Hence, the complete object set is on the top, whereas the complete attribute set is at the bottom of the diagram. There is only one top and only one bottom element. In our example, Table 8.1, we obtain a chain, consisting of the three concepts we have found (Fig. 8.3 (LHS)).

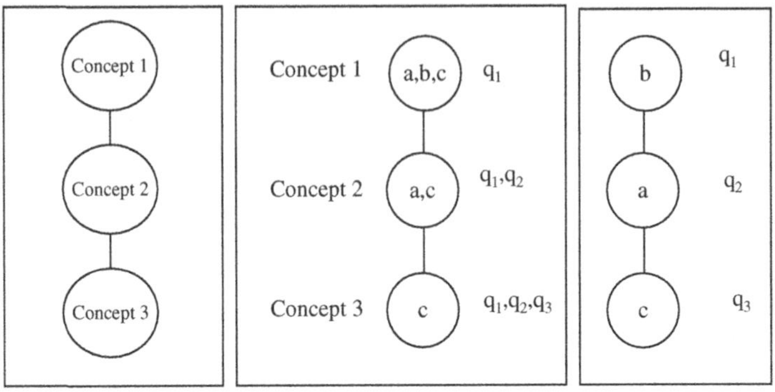

Fig. 8.3 Evolution of a concept lattice based on the context table (Table 8.1)

In Fig. 8.3, instead of the name "Concept," we write its extent within and its intent outside the circle (Fig. 8.3 (middle), Fig. 8.3 (left), see below).

8.4.2 Lattice

Generally, lattices of concepts not only are chains but also can be more complicated partial orders. However, as a lattice (see Birkhoff, 1984; Ganter and Wille, 1996; Grätzer, 1998), the Hasse diagram of concepts fulfills more axioms than partial order, namely the following: (i) one and only one greatest element, (ii) one and only one least element, and (iii) only one component, i.e., in terms of ordinal graph, any concept is connected by a sequence of edges with any other. The additional axioms exclude Hasse diagrams which look like those shown in Fig. 8.4.

Because of the inclusion relation as order relation, we can also draw the Hasse diagram of the concepts of Table 8.1 as shown in Fig. 8.3 (RHS). Going upward, we are gathering objects. The lowest concept had c, so the next concept (Concept 2) has the label a for the object set. Hence the extent of Concept 2 is $\{a, c\}$. The top concept (Concept 1) has the label b, therefore the subset is $\{a, b, c\}$, being the object set. Going downward, we are gathering properties, starting from the top: Concept 1: $\{q_1\}$, Concept 2 has the property set $\{q_1, q_2\}$, and Concept 3 has all three properties. Once again, one can see how Fig. 8.2 is realized. Enrichment of the object set is accompanied by reduction of the set of properties and enrichment of the set of properties is followed by a reduction of the set of objects. More technically,

Fig. 8.4 Some forbidden structures if the visualization of a partial order should represent a lattice

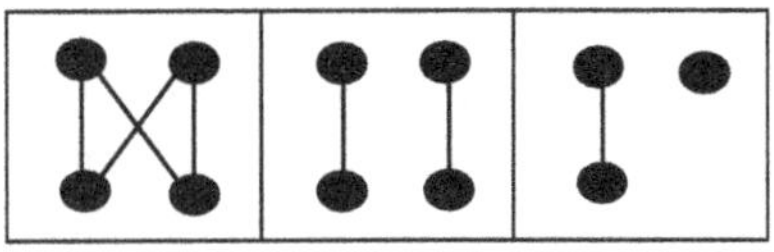

increasing the extent of a concept implies decreasing intent (the more the objects we like to include, the less the number of properties they obey). Increasing the intents implies decreasing the extents (the more the properties we want to be present for the objects, the less the objects will fulfill them).

8.4.2.1 Illustrative Example Concerning Formal Concept Lattices

A slight modification of the context leads to a more interesting lattice (Table 8.2).

From Table 8.2 we obtain six concepts, applying the same process as for Table 8.1:

Concept 1: $[\{a,\ b,\ c\}, \emptyset_{\mathrm{IB}}]$
Concept 2: $[\{a,\ b\},\ \{q_1\}]$
Concept 3: $[\{a,\ c\},\ \{q_2\}]$
Concept 4: $[\{a\},\ \{q_1,\ q_2\}]$
Concept 5: $[\{c\},\ \{q_2,\ q_3\}]$
Concept 6: $[\emptyset_X,\ \{q_1,\ q_2,\ q_3\}]$

The Hasse diagram made of the concepts (abbrev. C_1, C_2, ...) can be seen in Fig. 8.5:

(a) Examples of walking upward:
Starting from C_5 and C_4, the unique covering vertex is C_3
Starting from C_3 and C_2, the unique covering vertex is C_2

Table 8.2 Context table

	q_1	q_2	q_3
a	1	1	0
b	1	0	0
c	0	1	1

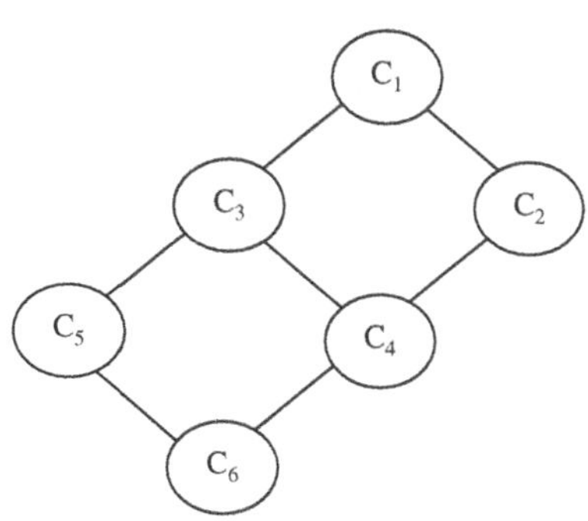

Fig. 8.5 Concept lattice based on Table 8.2

(b) Examples of walking downward:
Starting from C_3 and C_2, the unique vertex covered by C_3 and C_2 is C_4
Starting from C_5 and C_4, the unique vertex covered by C_5 and C_4 is C_6

Walking upward, the resulting object set of the covering concept is always the union of the object subsets belonging to the vertices from where we started.

Walking downward, the resulting attribute set of the covered vertex is always the union of the attribute subsets belonging to the vertices from where we started.

In Fig. 8.6a, we use the extended labeling, similar to Fig. 8.3 (middle). In Fig. 8.6b, we use the reduced labeling, helping to increase the clarity of the graph applied (like in Fig. 8.3 (RHS), which makes use of the laws of a lattice.

As for Hasse diagrams, there are different graphical representations. We use the Conexp1.3 software of Yevtushenko (2000). The context displayed in Table 8.2 is drawn as follows (Fig. 8.7).

In Fig. 8.7, the filled upper semicircle indicates that there is a property attached to the corresponding concept, whereas the filled lower semicircle indicates an object attached to the corresponding concept. Furthermore, we see six concepts and the

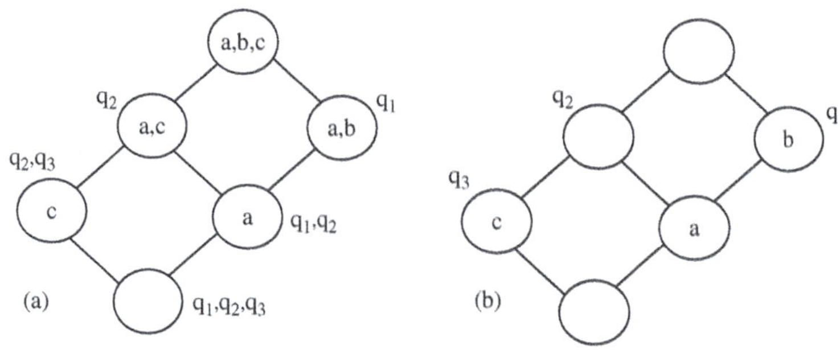

Fig. 8.6 Labeling: (**a**) extended labeling, (**b**) reduced labeling

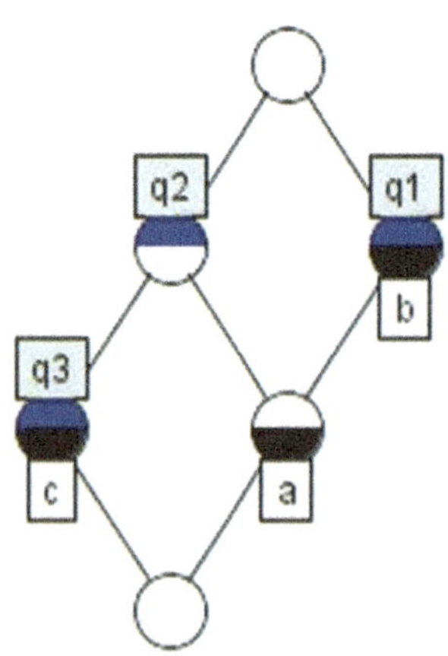

Fig. 8.7 Representation of the context of Table 8.2 by the software Conexp1.3

full information with respect to the extent and the intent of every concept can be easily reconstructed: If C_1 is the concept covered by $C_2, C_3, \ldots$, then C_1 inherits the properties of $C_2, C_3, \ldots$. Further, if C_1 covers $C_2, C_3, \ldots$, then $C_2, C_3, \ldots$ inherit the objects of C_1.

8.5 Implications

The lattice of concepts is based on the inclusion relations of the extents (or the intents) as Fig. 8.2 shows. For example, the label q_2 in Fig. 8.7 means that q_2 is a property of all extents of those concepts which are elements of $O(C_2)$, i.e., $\{c\}$,$\{a\}$, and $\{c,a\}$. If another attribute label which selects smaller object subsets can be found, then obviously this property implies the first one. In the example of Fig. 8.7, $d(\{q_3\}) \subset d(\{q_2\})$ with $d(\{q_3\}) = \{c\}$ and $d(\{q_2\}) = \{a, c\}$. Hence q_3 implies q_2 or, having a look at the context table, if $q_3 = 1$, then $q_2 = 1$.

Determining such implications by hand is difficult. Fortunately, implications are automatically generated by Conexp1_3 software (called there "association rules" because not always EoA = 100). Thus, the formal concept analysis does not only help in identifying the reasons for a certain location of an object within its Hasse diagram but also provide us with a system of automatically generated implications (Ganter, 1987). See Annoni and Bruggemann (2009) for a recent application in sociology. Clearly, these implications or associations are related to the data matrix and should therefore be considered as hypothesis generators.

We will apply this facility later in the application part of this monograph.

8.6 Multivalued Contexts

Up to now, we discussed the dichotomic case: Having or not having a property. In statistical analysis, this restriction to mono-valued contexts would make the formal concept analysis almost useless. However, we can consider any value of a certain attribute as if it is a mono-valued property. Most generally, we replace the m columns of m binary attributes by $m \times n$ columns which correspond to n different values of any attribute of any object. For example, if q_1 gets the values 1.0, 1.4, and 7.9, then we consider

- q_1 with the value ≥ 1.0 as one property,
- q_1 with the value ≥ 1.4 as another one, and finally
- q_1 with the value ≥ 7.9 as the third property.

Instead of one column for q_1, we get now three columns in the context table for q_1.

8.6.1 Scaling Model

The important point to consider now is the logical interaction of the three properties of q_1. Does a high value of q_1 imply the lower ones or should this value be considered like a nominal value, a label. For example, if a student in a class has learnt five subdisciplines of chemistry, then she/he also knows any subset of these five disciplines. Number 5 implies that 4, 3, 2, 1 are also true. If, however, the student has learnt just the fifth discipline, she/he does not necessarily know the others. Scaling models analyze these kinds of questions (Ganter and Wille, 1996). In general, we assume that the simplest case is present: A high value in an attribute implies the presence of smaller ones. Thus, an object having the value of q_1 of 7.9 also has the lower values, i.e., the context table for that object would get three 1 s, namely 1 for q_1 with the value 1.4 and one for q_1 with the value 1.0. In general, sensitivity studies are recommended when there is no clear evidence for the scaling model.

An example may help to see how the construction of multivalued context works.

8.6.2 Illustrative Examples Concerning Multivalued Contexts

In Fig. 8.8, the concept lattices based on Table 8.3 (LHS) and of Table 8.4 (RHS) are shown, once interpreted as ordinal and once as nominal evaluation of data.

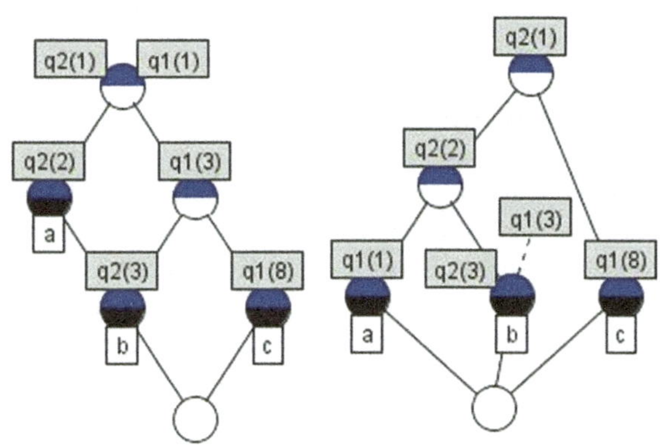

Fig. 8.8 (*LHS*) Concept lattice based on context of Table 8.3; (*RHS*) concept lattice based on context of Table 8.4 where the attribute values of q_1 are interpreted as nominal (see text)

Table 8.3 Small data matrix as an example (LHS). Context derived from the q_1 and q_2 columns. The columns of the context are headed by $\geq q_i$ to indicate the ordinal scaling model

	q_1	q_2	$\geq q_1 = 1$	$\geq q_1 = 3$	$\geq q_1 = 8$	$\geq q_2 = 1$	$\geq q_2 = 2$	$\geq q_2 = 3$
a	1	2	1	0	0	1	1	0
b	3	3	1	1	0	1	1	1
c	8	1	1	1	1	1	0	0

Table 8.4 Formal concept analysis of attributes, mixed in their scaling level. Context derived from the data of Table 8.3

	$q_1 = 1$	$q_1 = 3$	$q_1 = 8$	$\geq q_2 = 1$	$\geq q_2 = 2$	$\geq q_2 = 3$
a	1	0	0	1	1	0
b	0	1	0	1	1	1
c	0	0	1	1	0	0

From Fig. 8.8, we can see that for a, b, c, only the values $q_1 = 1$ and $q_2 = 1$ are found simultaneously, indicated in the graph by $q_1(1)$ and $q_2(1)$. The object subsets of the concept (top vertex in Fig. 8.8 (LHS)) are the same for $q_1(1)$ and $q_2(1)$. Therefore, we find the implication $q_1(1) \Leftrightarrow q_2(1)$ which can be easily verified by looking at Table 8.3. The object subset $\{a, b\}$ "has" $q_1(1)$ and $q_2(2)$ and $q_2(1)$. As a 1 in the cell of the context Table 8.4 indicates $q_2 \geq 2$ is true, it is also true that $q_2 \geq 1$. Hence there is a 1 too and $q_2(1)$ is in the graph located above $q_2(2)$. This is a trivial case of an implication, which arises just from our ordinal scaling of q_2.

Let us consider the values of q_1 as a nominal label, whereas q_2 is still interpreted as ordinal scaled (Table 8.4).

As can be seen in Fig. 8.8 (RHS), the first attribute is labeling the objects a, b, and c.

8.7 Why Objects Have a Certain Position

8.7.1 Overview

As example, we select the Lake Ontario data (see Chapter 5). Also see Annoni and Bruggemann (2008). Figure 8.9 shows the Hasse diagram of the formal concept lattice with 20 sediment sites and with five multivalued attributes FC, CH, CP, MT, and GT, describing the degradation status of sediments in hygienic, health, and ecotoxicological aspects. In Fig. 8.9, we see that the concept lattice is pretty small as there are not as many Galois connections as can be expected, taking the members of the power set of X and IB into consideration. The concept lattice allows us to identify the Hasse diagram of the objects because the sampling sites are located in the reverse orientation (compare Fig. 5.7). The reverse orientation becomes clear if we take into consideration that we want to have the full object set at the top of the diagram (corresponding to the scheme in Fig. 8.1). There are no attribute values which simultaneously are valid for all sites. Going downward, more and more attributes represent less and less objects. Therefore, the objects with high values of their attributes in Fig. 8.9 are here near the bottom of the diagram.

Annoni and Bruggemann (2008) point out that the formal concept lattice allows us a symmetric view. We can either examine the attributes and their values to see which objects belong to them, or we can look at objects and see which attributes, with which values, characterize them.

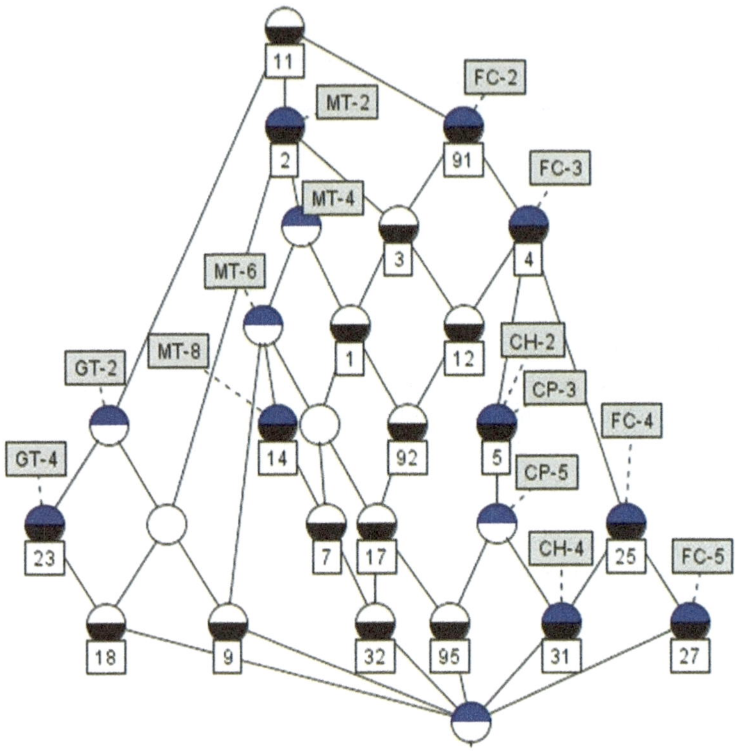

Fig. 8.9 Formal concept lattice of Lake Ontario. The *number labels* refer to sediment sites; the labels like CP-5 describe the attribute CP, which has value 5

We apply the following scheme:

1. Examine one attribute with its values and see what the objects are.
2. Examine several attributes and see what we can say about the objects.
3. Examine one object and see what the attributes and their values are.
4. Examine several objects and see what happens.
5. Finally, examine association rules.

8.7.2 Attributes

(1) Which objects obey CP-5?

- *First step*: Identify the corresponding concept, C.
- *Second step*: Look to its down set $O(C)$.
- *Third step*: Gather all objects which belong to $x \in O(C)$.

We find that the object set {31, 95} has CP-5 and therefore due to our scaling model, all values of CP ≤ 5.

(2) Which objects obey MT-2 and simultaneously FC-2?

- *First step*: Identify the infimum of the concepts bearing MT-2 and FC-2, which we call C_{inf}.
- *Second step*: Look to the down set $O(C_{\text{inf}})$.
- *Third step*: Gather all objects which belong to $x \in O(C_{\text{inf}})$. They all have simultaneously the properties MT-2 and FC-2.
- The two attributes MT and FC with value 2 are located near the top of the lattice. Hence without taking a closer look at the diagram, we can expect that these two characterizations, namely MT-2 and FC-2, will be valid for almost all objects. The only exception is site 11, which is at the top. MT-2 and FC-2 are labels at different vertices, therefore there will be some objects, which belong only to one of these attribute values (Fig. 8.10).

In Fig. 8.10, two intersecting subsets are visualized to show how to find objects with common attribute values and those with exclusively one of the two attribute values. The set for which both MT-2 and FT-2 is valid is in the down set of C_{inf}. Hence it is easy to identify those objects which fulfill only one of the two properties. They must be reachable downward either from MT-2 or exclusively from FC-2. Sites 91, 4, 5, 31, 25, and 27 have the property FC-2, but certainly not the property MT-2 (see scheme Fig. 8.10).

In order to avoid awkward descriptions, we will express "concept labeled by MT-2" as MT-2. Tracing the Hasse diagram downward, we can, for instance, reach MT-4. We see that fewer objects are in the down set. For example, sites 2 and 3 have MT-2 but not MT-4.

Which sediment samples have some genotoxicity potential (attribute GT)?

We start at GT-2. All objects in the down set are of interest. We find sites 23, 18, and 9. Are there sites which at the same time have no acute toxicity? Hereto we examine as to how far below the objects 23, 18, and 9 are in the down set of MT-2. Indeed we find two sites out of the three, which have at the same time an acute toxicity potential, namely 9 and 18.

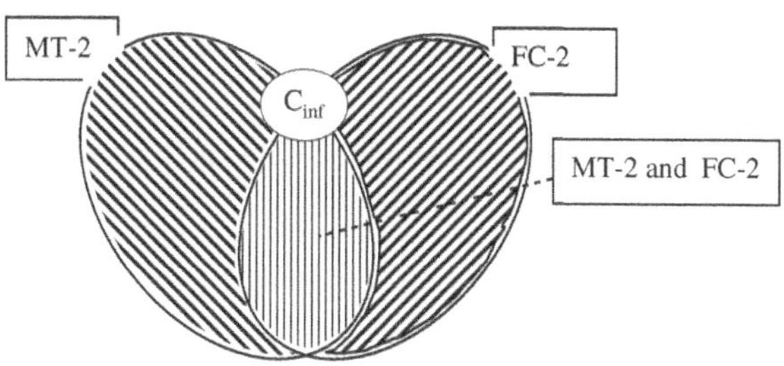

Fig. 8.10 Schematic view on MT-2 and FC-2

8.7.2.1 Redundancy of Attributes

The attributes FC, CH, and CP describe fairly well the same kind of problems, namely hygienic problems due to fecals. We may ask whether it was meaningful to add all three properties to the test battery of Dutka et al. (1986). Indeed, low levels like FC-2 include all objects which have higher values in CH and CP. However, site 27, for instance, has the maximum value of FC, but neither CP nor CH is of concern for this site. Whether or not there is redundancy, say in q_i and q_j, can be examined by determining the symmetric difference set (see Chapter 4) $O(q_i)\ \Delta\ O(q_j)$. The larger the symmetric difference is, the less redundant q_i and q_j are. Note that we use an abbreviated notation: $O(q_i)$ stands for the down set of the concept having as label q_i.

8.7.3 Objects

(3) Characterization of objects
Which values of which attributes may be characteristic of objects?

- The site 18 has a high value in GT but a low value in MT.
- Site 9 has a weak genotoxicity potential (GT-2), however, a rather high acute toxicity (MT-6). Both sites 18 and 9 are not of concern with respect to the group FC, CH, and CP.
- Site 32 belongs to O(MT-8) but has only a medium value of FC (FC-3).
- Sites 4, 5, 25, 31, and 27 have no genotoxicity, no acute toxicity but different variants of hygienic loadings.

(4) Characterization of object subsets
Following Chapter 5, we may ask as to how far we can identify reasons for the separation of object subsets. An example may clarify this point: In Fig. 8.9, we see that

$X_1 = \{7,\ 14,\ 32\}$ and $X_2 = \{9,\ 18,\ 23\}$ are separated subsets.

The supremum of X_2 is the concept, labeled with GT-2; site 9 has the MT value 6 (MT-6). In terms of the formal concept analysis, no other property {FC-2, FC-3, ...}, {CH-2, CH-4, ...}, {CP-3, CP-5} is common for X_2. The supremum of X_1 is the concept, labeled with MT-8. Site 7 has property FC-2 and site 32 has FC-3. Hence the separation of these two subsets is explained as follows:

X_1: FC ≤ 3, CP = CH = 0, GT = 0, MT > 6
X_2: FC < 2, CP = CH = 0, $2 \leq$ GT ≤ 4, $0 \leq$ MT ≤ 6.

(5) Implications II
We already discussed implications and associations, related to a mono-valued context. In multivalued contexts, we can analogously derive them, because an attribute with different values is considered like two different properties in the mono-valued case (see Annoni and Bruggemann (2008) and a recent example, concerning the pollution by rocket fuels and their degradation products, in Carlsen (2009)).

One example may be sufficient.

CP-3 implies FC-3 and CH-2. How can we see this in the diagram?

O(CP-3) $\subset$ O(CH-2) $\cup$ O(FC-3), i.e., all concepts in O(CP-3) are also reachable downward from either CH-2 or FC-3.

Let us apply the extent of association, EoA: We call PR (premise) to be the set of objects of the premise and CON (conclusion) to be the set of objects of the conclusion. Let us examine |PR $\cap$ CON|/|PR|. We obtain a EoA = 1 if PR $\subset$ CON, otherwise a fraction of 1 tells us that there are some (few) exceptions. See Chapter 15 for an application of the associations and implications.

8.8 Summary and Commentary

Formal concept analysis (FCA) is a powerful mathematical tool to analyze data matrices. By different scaling models (we are using mainly the ordinal scaling), it is possible to analyze a wide span of different cases. For example, FCA provides a tool, where nominal and ordinal data can be handled simultaneously.

There are some hurdles at this time, however, that are difficult to overcome at least with the available software:

- The need of scaling. FCA requires a context and a decision about how to handle continuous variables in concept. HDT can handle such variables without pre-processing.
- The concept lattice can be huge, even with few objects and few attributes. If there are n objects and if there is a context with m properties (either derived from multivalued attributes or from mono-valued properties), then there are 2^n and 2^m subsets and the maximal number of concepts will be $2^{(n+m)}$. The constraint (Eq. (8.1)) filters out the pairs with no correct matchings. Nevertheless, there are difficulties in disclosing the whole lattice.

Table 8.5 Comparison of formal concept analysis (FCA) with partial order analysis (PoA) as done in Chapters 2–7

	Advantages	Disadvantages
PoA	Direct use of the original data matrix is possible	The partial order of the original data matrix can be messy or uninformative
FCA	Symmetric view on objects and attributes. Derivation of implications	A transformation is necessary to obtain the context table. The lattice diagrams can be huge as at maximum they could contain 2^m*2^n concepts, m being the number of attributes and n that of objects

The recommendation is that we select suitable object subsets to utilize the power of FCA and analyze the positions of the objects at least in these smaller concept lattices. The FCA and the visualization it provides can be very helpful.

Finally, implications will help focus on the attributes themselves. This may not offer direct help but allows us to put our fingers on measurement problems and even on the selection of attributes to quantify the criteria.

What is the use of finding an implication and analyzing the formal concept lattice? If the implication is known a priori, it can be easily checked by the context table. However, if the implication is not known, then the formal concept analysis is an elegant way to obtain it. In Table 8.5, we summarize advantages and disadvantages of formal concept analysis in comparison with the partial order analysis we discussed in the former chapters.

References

Annoni, P. and Bruggemann, R. (2008). The dualistic approach of FCA: A further insight into Ontario Lake sediments. Chemosphere, 70, 2025–2031.

Annoni, P. and Bruggemann, R. (2009). Exploring partial order of European countries. Soc. Indic. Res., 92, 471–487.

Bartel, H. (1997). Ein neuer Ansatz zur formalbegriffsanalytischen Objektklassifikation und seine Anwendung auf aromatische heterocyclische Verbindungen. Match – Commun. Math. Comput. Chem., 36, 185–215.

Bartel, H. and Nofz, M. (1997). Exploration of NMR data of glasses by means of formal concept analysis. Chemom. Intell. Lab. Syst., 36, 53–63.

Birkhoff, G. (1984). Lattice theory (Vol. XXV). Providence, RI: American Mathematical Society.

Carlsen, L. (2009). The interplay between QSAR/QSPR studies and partial order ranking and formal concept analyses. Int. J. Mol. Sci., 10(4), 1628–1657.

Carpineto, C. and Romano, G. (2004). Concept data analysis. Chichester: Wiley.

Davey, B.A. and Priestley, H.A. (1990). Introduction to lattices and order. Cambridge: Cambridge University Press.

Dutka, B.J., Walsh, K., Kwan, K.K., El Shaarawi, A., Liu, D.L. and Thompson, K. (1986). Priority site selection from degraded areas based on microbial and toxicant screening tests. Water Pollut. Res. J. Can., 21(2), 267–282.

Ganter, B. (1987). Algorithmen zur formalen begriffsanalyse. In B. Ganter, R. Wille, and K.E. Wolff (Eds.), Beiträge zur Begriffsanalyse (pp. 241–254). Mannheim: BI Wissenschaftsverlag.

Ganter, B. and Wille, R. (1986). Implikationen und Abhängigkeiten zwischen Merkmalen. In: P.O. Degens, H.-J. Hermes, and O. Opitz (Eds.), Die Klassifikation und ihr Umfeld (pp. 171–185). Frankfurt: Indeks-Verlag.

Ganter, B. and Wille, R. (1996). Formale begriffsanalyse mathematische grundlagen (pp. 1–286). Berlin: Springer.

Grätzer, G. (1998). General lattice theory. Basel: Birkhäuser Verlag.

Gugisch, R. (2001). Many-valued context analysis using descriptions. In H. Delugach and G. Stumme (Eds.), ICCS 2001, bd LNAI 2120 (pp. 157–168). Heidelberg: Springer.

Kerber, A. (2006). Contexts, concepts, implications and hypotheses. In R. Bruggemann and L. Carlsen (Eds.), Partial order in environmental sciences and chemistry (pp. 355–365). Berlin: Springer.

Wolff, K.E. (1993). A first course in formal concept analysis. How to understand line diagrams. In F. Faulbaum (Ed.), SoftStat'93: Advances in statistical software 4 (pp. 429–438). Stuttgart: Lucius & Lucius.

Yevtushenko, S.A. (2000). System of data analysis 'concept explorer'. Proceedings of the 7th National Conference on Artificial Intelligence, Russia, K II-2000, K-II, pp. 127–134.

Yevtushenko, S. Software ConExp. http://sourceforge.net/projects/conexp

Chapter 9
Methods to Obtain Linear or Weak Order by Means of Partial Order

9.1 Tasks

In Chapter 3, we have seen how averaged heights of objects hav(x) can be calculated. Thus partial order provides a method to obtain a linear order without the need of making additional assumptions like weights for indicators. The main computational problem, however, is the huge number of linear extensions, which sometimes makes the calculation of averaged heights and from them the linear order difficult. This chapter discusses different procedures to rank objects.

9.2 Levels

In Section 2.5 and in Chapter 5, we introduced the concept of levels.

Levels are a means to derive from posets a weak order, because objects x can be ordered due to their level number lev(x). Let us introduce the equivalence relation

$$\begin{aligned} &\mathfrak{R}: x, y \in X \\ &x\, \mathfrak{R}\, y :\Leftrightarrow \text{lev}(x) = \text{lev}(y) \end{aligned} \tag{9.1}$$

Typically, the equivalence classes due to $\mathfrak{R}$ are large.

Therefore, the disadvantage of ordering by lev is that there are many ties. The advantage however is its simplicity.

9.3 Local Partial Order Model

9.3.1 Idea

The idea behind the "local partial order model" (LPOM) is to select an object x and to characterize its order theoretical environment, i.e., to look at $O(x)$, $F(x)$, and $U(x)$. Because we focus on one single object, for which we want to estimate its averaged height hav (sometimes also called Rkav), we call the method local partial order

R. Brüggemann, G.P. Patil, *Ranking and Prioritization for Multi-indicator Systems*, Environmental and Ecological Statistics 5, DOI 10.1007/978-1-4419-8477-7_9,

model. As we have to do with partial order, the environment cannot be understood only by considering the objects covering x and the objects covered by x, but also objects incomparable to x. The principal down set $O(x)$, the principal up set $F(x)$, and the set of incomparables $U(x)$ need to be considered as determining quantities to estimate hav(x).

9.3.2 Several Local Partial Order Models

There are different local partial order models depending on how the elements of $U(x)$ are (graph theoretically) related to x (see three examples in Fig. 9.1).

In the Hasse diagram A, we get six linear extensions, in which four include y at a position below x. Hence, the averaged height of x hav(x) $= (4{*}5 + 2{*}4)/6 = 4.67$ (Eq. (9.2), see below).

In the Hasse diagram B, we get three linear extensions, because of the reduced number of positions that y can take. From these, there is only one position which increased the height of x in the corresponding linear extension. The averaged height of x, hav(x) $= (1{*}5{+}2{*}4)/3 = 4.333$. One can see that if one ignores the connection (in an ordinary graph theoretical sense) y has with x, an erroneous result will be obtained.

In Hasse diagram C, ignoring y for a moment, there are three possibilities to locate the element a. Depending on the position the element a gets, the influence of y will be more or less pronounced. If element a gets the lowest position, then the result is 4.6, which is close to the value obtained from Hasse diagram A (y as isolated element). If, however, element a gets the position such that it is covered by x, then the result is 4.33 (like in Hasse diagram B).

9.3.3 LPOM

Therefore, the simplest and unique way is to consider all elements of $U(x)$ as isolated. The corresponding local partial order model is called LPOM. The height of

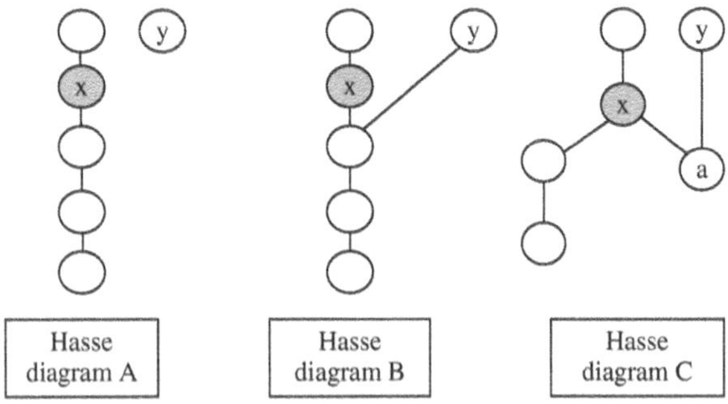

Fig. 9.1 Three Hasse diagrams with $|O_i(x)| = |O_j(x)|$, $|F_i(x)| = |F_j(x)|$, $U_i(x) = U_j(x)$. $i, j =$ A, B, C, $i \neq j$

x must then be a function of $|O(x)|$, $|F(x)|$, and $|U(x)|$ alone. For more involved approximations, see Bruggemann et al. (2004, 2005) and Bruggemann and Patil (2010).

The steps of calculation within LPOM are the following:

1. Select an element x.
2. Find $U(x)$.
3. Consider all elements of $U(x)$ as isolated.
4. All elements of successors of x are arranged into a chain (compare Chapter 3).
5. All elements of predecessors of x are arranged into a chain (compare Chapter 3).
6. Hence a chain results with the following order: elements of $S(x) < x < P(x)$ which we call the $S - x - P$ chain (see Chapter 3).
7. Determine the averaged height of x by inserting the whole set $U(x)$ into one of the positions of the $S - x - P$ chain.

Step 7: Insertion of $U(x)$ into the predecessors of x, i.e., in $P(x)$, would not change the height of x. Insertion of $U(x)$ into the chain made of $S(x)$ will change the height, namely from $|O(x)|$ to $|O(x)| + |U(x)|$. To simplify the notation, we simply write O for $|O(x)|$, F for $|F(x)|$, and U for $|U(x)|$. For the set $U(x)$, there are O positions available which enhance the height of x and F positions which let the height of x invariant. In total, there are $O + F$ positions, i.e., there are $O + F$ linear extensions if $U(x)$ is considered as one object. Therefore

$$\text{hav}(x) = \frac{O}{O+F} \cdot (O+U) + \frac{F}{O+F} \cdot O \tag{9.2}$$

As $O + F$ is the total number of locations where U elements can be positioned, the fractions $\text{pr} <:= O/(O+F)$ and $\text{pr} >:= F/(O+F)$ can be considered as probabilities for object x getting height $O + U$ or getting height O.

For spreadsheet calculations, Eq. (9.2) can be rearranged, taking into account that $|X| = n = O + F + U - 1$:

$$\text{hav}(x) = O^{*}(n+1)/(n+1-U) \tag{9.3}$$

Both Eqs. (9.2) and (9.3) are at first to be considered as a result of an approximation, because the assumption to put $U(x)$ as a whole (i.e., as if it is one object but adds to the height of x by U units) is not justified. In reality, all the elements of $U(x)$ are to be distributed independently over the $S - x - P$ chain. This assumption has been justified (Bruggemann et al., 2004). Several examples appear later in this monograph.

9.4 Bubley Dyer Algorithm

The Bubley Dyer algorithm generates a sample set of linear extensions from which properties like averaged ranks can be obtained. This algorithm is a Monte Carlo Markov chain procedure (MCMC) and the best way to demonstrate it is to show a flow chart (Fig. 9.2, after Denoeux et al., 2005). Bubley and Dyer (1997, 1999) show that a uniform and stationary distribution for linear extensions can be obtained and they estimate that the time needed (under certain conditions) goes with $|X|^4$. The Bubley Dyer algorithm is realized in PyHasse as well as in VB-RAPID (see Chapter 17). The Bubley Dyer algorithm needs a linear extension before it can do its iterations. We call this linear extension a "starter." In PyHasse, the starter is obtained from the levels of the partial order. We begin with the top level and put the elements

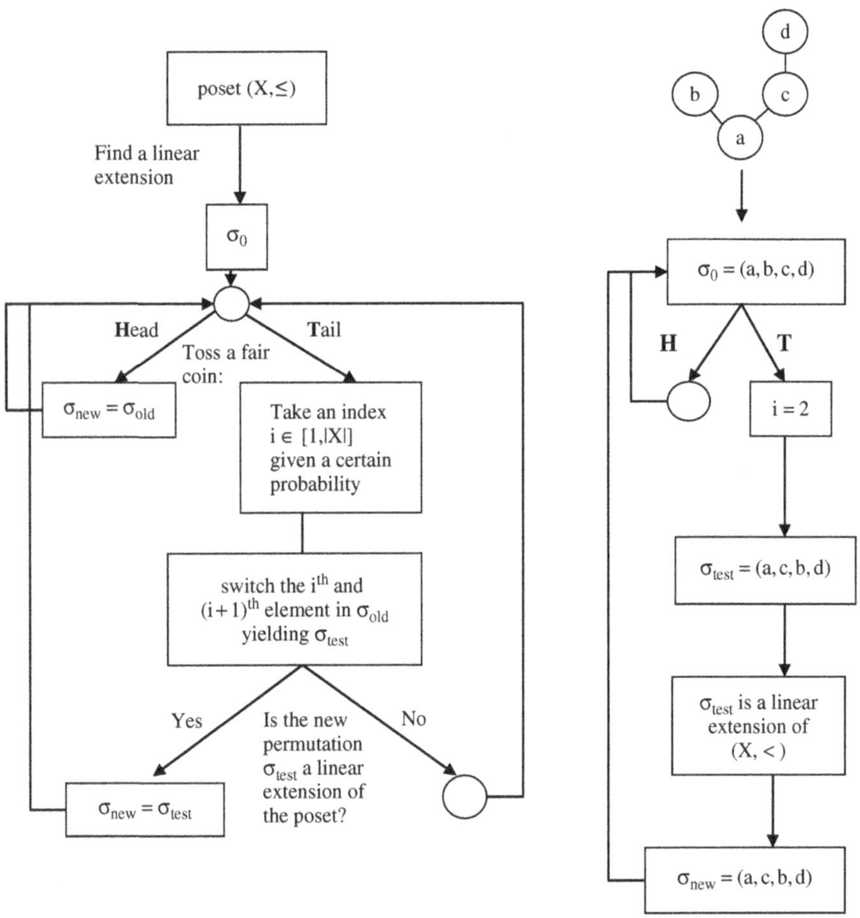

Fig. 9.2 Flow chart for the Bubley Dyer algorithm. *RHS*: A parallel example. See also Denoeux et al. (2005)

of the top level arbitrarily in the upmost positions of the linear extension, then the next level follows analogously, until the bottom level is reached. Any permutation must be checked for its compatibility with the partial order. When the new permutation cannot be considered as a linear extension of the poset, then the next run starts.

9.5 Cumulative Rank Frequency Method

9.5.1 Method

Patil and Taillie (2004) suggest another method to find a linear or a weak order, which they call the cumulative rank frequency (CRF) method. Consider a set of linear extensions LE and Σ prob($h_{\mathrm{le}(i)}(x) \le h$), with le($i$) $\in$ LE and $x \in X/\cong$.[1] The sum is taken over all heights $\le h$. If h is getting the values $[1, \ldots, |X/\cong|]$, we obtain a cumulative rank frequency $\mathrm{CRF}_x(h)$, which is a discrete function of h.

We define

$$x \le y :\Leftrightarrow \mathrm{CRF}_x(h) \ge \mathrm{CRF}_y(h), \text{ for all } h = 1, \ldots, |X/\cong| \tag{9.4}$$

The opposite orientation on the RHS of Eq. (9.4) can be easily understood: Take a least element (see Chapter 2), then its probability = 1 for all h. Take a greatest element, then

$$\mathrm{prob}(h_{\mathrm{le}(i)}(x)) = \begin{cases} 0, & \text{for all } h < |X/\cong| \\ 1, & \text{for } h = |X/\cong| \end{cases}$$

and due to $\mathrm{CRF}_x(h)$, the greatest element would be less than the least element.

Taking $\mathrm{CRF}_x(1)$, $\mathrm{CRF}_x(2), \ldots, \mathrm{CRF}_x(|X/\cong|)$ as new data row for the elements $x \in X$, we get a new matrix whose order relation can be checked, applying Eq. (9.4). Now CRF can be applied once again until the final order relation due to Eq. (9.4) is a linear or a weak one.

Figure 9.3 summarizes the CRF method. The conceptual advantage of the CRF method to obtain the linear or the weak order is that it avoids the interim step of calculating the averaged heights.

9.5.2 Illustrative Example

Consider a data matrix with four objects $\{a, b, c, d\}$, and its Hasse diagram shown in Fig. 9.4 (LHS) and the linear extensions shown in Fig. 9.4 (RHS).

In Table 9.1 the frequencies of $(h_{\mathrm{le}(i)}(x) \le h)$ are counted.

Applying Eq. (9.4), we see that a linear order is obtained: $c < a < d < b$.

In other partial orders, iterations may be necessary (see Patil and Taillie, 2004).

---

[1]Note that according to Chapter 2, we identify the quotient set with the set of representative elements.

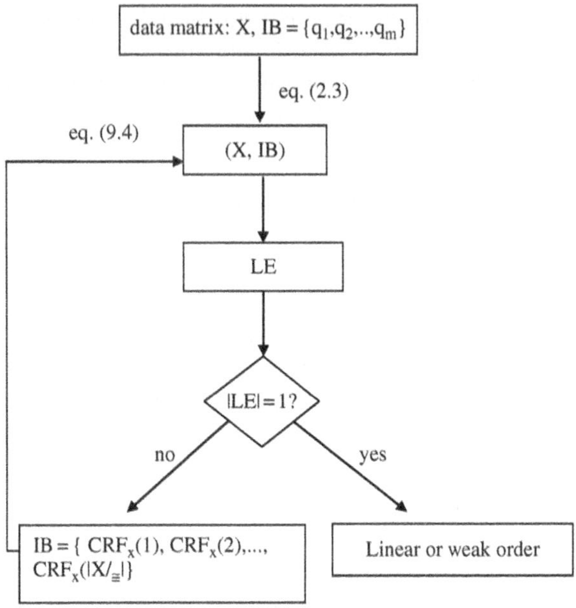

Fig. 9.3 Flowchart of the CRF method

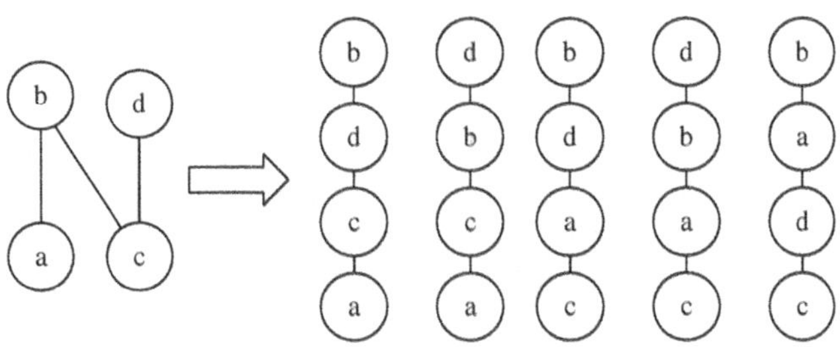

Fig. 9.4 Illustrative example: Hasse diagram and its linear extensions

Table 9.1 Frequencies of $(h_{\mathrm{le}(i)}(x) \leq h)$, cumulative frequencies (last four columns)

	$h=1$	$h=2$	$h=3$	$h=4$	$h\leq 1$	$h\leq 2$	$h\leq 3$	$h\leq 4$
a	2	2	1	0	2	4	5	5
b	0	0	2	3	0	0	2	5
c	3	2	0	0	3	5	5	5
d	0	1	2	2	0	1	3	5

9.6 Averaged Heights (Ranks) Derived from the Lattice of Down Sets

9.6.1 Motivation

The computational problem in calculating the averaged heights sometimes arises from the huge number of linear extensions. Storing and managing all these LT sequences should be avoided. The idea can be sketched as follows (Fig. 9.5).

The network shown in Fig. 9.5 has 12 vertices. If any walk from B to T would represent a linear extension, then we obtain 14 linear extensions. This observation implies that we would need to store only 12 vertices and their cover relations but obtain the larger variety of 14 linear extensions by finding all paths and by calculation of the needed quantities on the fly.

9.6.2 Generalization of Down Sets and Finding All Down Sets of a Poset

We generalize the down sets.

Let $Y \subset X$. Then Y is a down set of (X, IB) if $x \in Y$ and $z \leq x$ implies $z \in Y$.

To find all down sets of a poset (X, IB), we perform the following steps (Davey and Priestley, 1990):

1. Identify all principal down sets $O(x)$.
2. Generate a list of antichains.
3. Let AC(i) be the ith antichain, then any ordered set

$$Z(i) = \bigcup_{x \in \mathrm{AC}(i)} O(x)$$

is a down set.

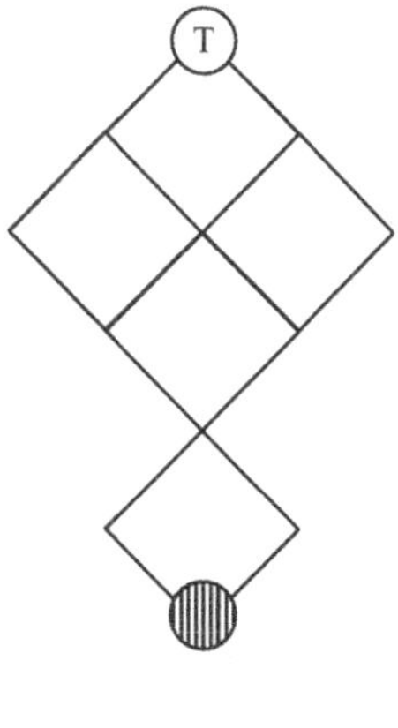

Fig. 9.5 The "Manhattan-like" network represents a digraph which exclusively can be discovered by walks either from the bottom B (*circle hatched*) to the top T (*circle*) or the other way round (see text)

4. Include if necessary the empty set.
5. Include if necessary the poset (X, IB) as a down set.

9.6.2.1 Illustrative Example

Let us take a simple poset, e.g., a fence $F(4)$ (see Chapter 3), and perform the five steps (Fig. 9.6).

The set of all down sets is denoted by J, hence for the fence $F(4)$ we get

$$J(F(4)) = \{\varnothing, \{a\}, \{c\}, \{a, c\}, \{c, d\}, \{a, b, c\}, \{a, c, d\}, \{a, b, c, d\}\}$$

The sets of $J(F(4))$ can be partially ordered by applying the set-theoretical inclusion (Fig. 9.7).

There are many important theorems and statements to be made for the partially ordered down sets. Here we refer only to those which we need for the next steps:

1. The partial order of down sets (ordered by inclusion) is a lattice (see Chapter 8).
2. For any covering vertex v' covering v, the associated down set of v' differs from that of v by one and only $x \in$ (X, IB). Hence the edges of the lattice can be uniquely labeled by x.
3. A path from the bottom of the lattice to the top can be characterized by the edges and their labels which are met.
4. The sequence of edge labels is just a linear extension of (X, IB).

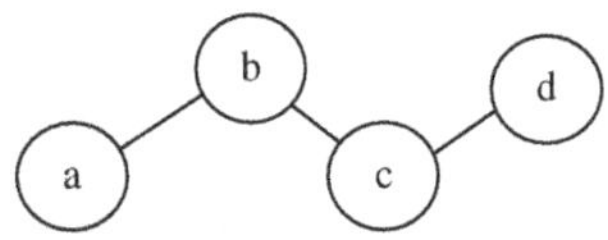

1. Principal down sets:
   O(a) = a
   O(b) = a,b,c
   O(c) = c
   O(d) = c,d
2. Antichains:
   AC(1) = a,c
   AC(2) = a,d
   AC(3) = b,d
3. Perform unions of the down sets:
   O(a) ∪ O(c) = a,c
   O(a) ∪ O(d) = a,c,d
   O(b) ∪ O(d) = a,b,c,d
4. Include ∅
5. O(b) ∪ O(d) = (X, ≤)

Fig. 9.6 Generating all down sets of the fence $F(4)$

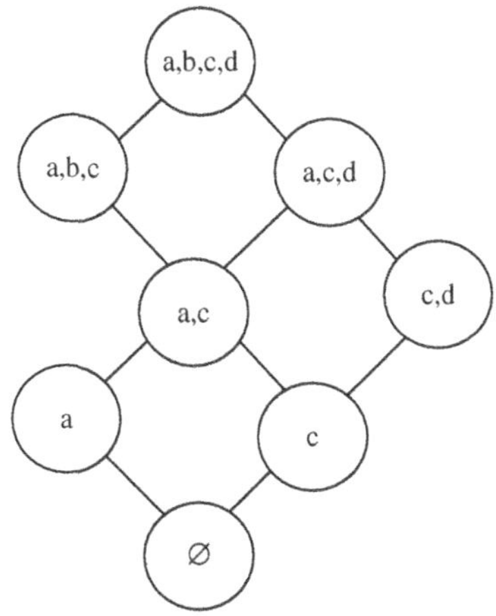

Fig. 9.7 $J(F(4))$, the partial order of down sets of the fence $F(4)$, ordered by inclusion

Following De Loof et al. (2006, 2008), Wienand (2005), and Morton et al. (2006, 2009) the four points are the basis for an alternate computational approach to calculate the averaged heights.

9.7 Mutual Probabilities

9.7.1 Tasks

Suppose that the decision maker is not interested in getting a rank for all objects but wishes to know as to whether one object is better than the other. In the setting of partial order, this question becomes: What is the probability of an element x to be ranked higher than element y? We interpret this as a question for a local analysis of the partial order, because the focus is on two elements only. However, in doing so, we should be aware that each new object changes the value of the mutual probability, probm.

9.7.2 General Outline

The mutual probability probm($x > y$) (see Chapter 3, Eq. (3.4)) can be easily calculated if the set of linear extensions is at hand. Because then one simply has to count the number of linear extensions in which object x has a height above y and divide by the number of linear extensions, LT.

Once again, behind this simple situation can arise a nontrivial computational difficulty. The number of linear extensions gets so large even for empirical posets of moderate size that it is not possible to obtain the set of linear extensions and then perform the needed counts.

The following strategy provides guidance:

- Derive empirical formulas based on easily accessible quantities like $O(x)$, $F(x)$, and $U(x)$.
- Show that the empirical formula works well for a certain training set of posets and pairs (x, y) in it.

9.7.3 Heuristic Approach

As was discussed in Section 9.3, the probability for merging $U(x)$ into an $S - x - P$ chain can be approximately described by the number of accessible locations below and above x. If there are two elements $x \| y$, then in a rough approximation, probm $(y > x)$ will depend on the quotient $Q(x) = F(x)/O(x)$ and $Q(y) = F(y)/O(y)$. If $Q(x) > (y)$, then there are less locations for y to be located below x, hence the probability of $y > x$ will increase with $Q(x)$ and based on similar arguments decrease with $Q(y)$. Therefore, one may write probm$(y > x) \sim Q(x)/Q(y)$. As probm$(x > y)$ must get such a form that probm$(x > y)$ + probm$(y > x) = 1$, the functional form

$$\text{probm}(y > x) = Q(x)/(Q(x) + Q(y)) \tag{9.5}$$

is the simplest possible variant.

9.7.4 Applicability of Equation (9.5)

Equation (9.5) is derived in a pretty heuristic manner. The leading parameters are $F(x)$, $F(y)$, $O(x)$, and $O(y)$. However, Eq. (9.5) may not be quite applicable for an estimation of probm$(x > y)$, $x \| y$, when the content of down sets and up sets is not sufficient to characterize the poset. See, for example, Fig. 9.8.

Furthermore, the approximation of the mutual probability by LPOM may become worse as more incomparable elements are present.

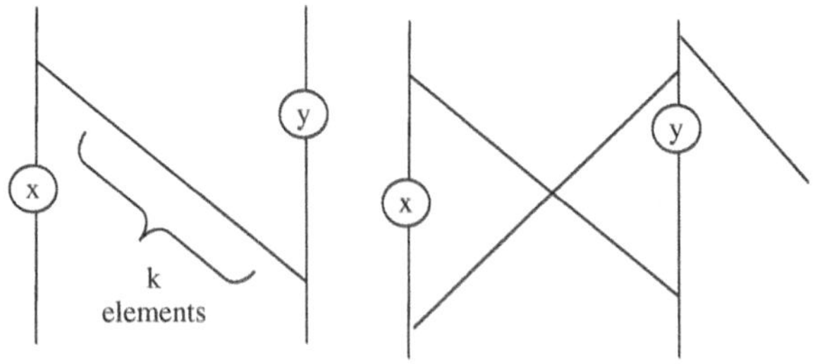

Fig. 9.8 Two examples of partial order, where the description of probm by $F(x)$, $O(x)$, and $F(y)$, $O(y)$ alone may be inappropriate. The *lines* not including x or y are thought of as having at least one element

9.8 Two Illustrative Examples

9.8.1 Revisiting Example of Chapter 7

We are interested in the heights for all objects (Fig. 7.7, Table App2). This is equivalent to seeking the overall ranks according to an unknown attribute. For the convenience of the reader, the Hasse diagram is shown in Fig. 9.9.

To obtain the averaged heights of the objects, we have to perform the steps described in Section 9.3 and demonstrate them for some objects.

Object 5: $S - x - P = 29, 6, 7, 5, 8$; $U(5) = \{9, 14, 16, 17\}$, object 6: $S - x - P = 6, 17, 7, 9, 5, 16, 8, 14$; $U(6) = \{29\}$, object 7: $S - x - P = 6, 7, 5, 9, 8$; $U(7) = \{14, 16, 17, 29\}$, object 8: $S - x - P = 6, 29, 7, 5, 16, 9, 8$; $U(8) = \{14, 17\}$, object 17: $S - x - P = 6,\ 17$; $U(17 = X - \{6, 17\}$.

The results are summarized in Table 9.2.

In Fig. 9.10, the values delta = hav(LPOM) – hav(exact) are shown as a histogram.

There is a bias as LPOM is overestimating the exact values and there are two outliers, namely the objects 17 and 14. For these objects, advanced local partial

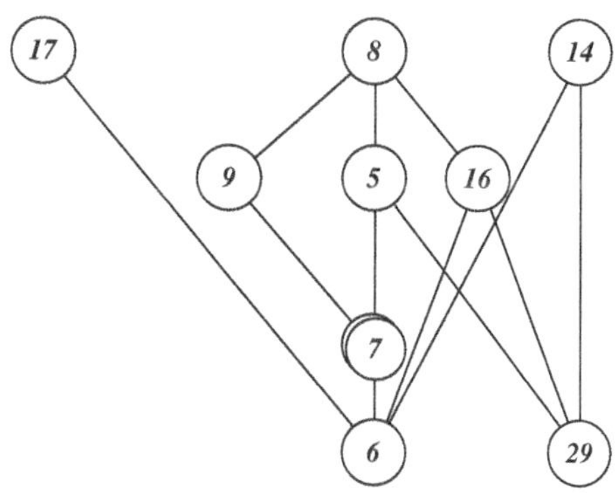

Fig. 9.9 Three attributes. $X = \{5, 6, 7, 8, 9, 14, 16, 17, 29\}$, object 7 is equivalent to 22

Table 9.2 Calculation of averaged heights by LPOM models, last column (exact averaged heights)

Object	$S - x - P$	$U(x)$	hav(LPOM(0))	hav(exact)
5	29, 6, 7, 5, 8	9, 14, 16, 17	6.67	6.16
6	6, 17, 9, 5, 16, 8, 14	29	1.11	1.33
7	6, 7, 5, 9, 8	14, 16, 17, 29	3.33	3.25
8	6, 29, 7, 5, 16, 9, 8	14, 17	8.75	8.67
9	6, 7, 9, 8	5, 6, 14, 17, 29	6	5.96
16	29, 6, 16, 8	5, 7, 9, 14, 17	6	5.58
14	29, 6, 14	5, 7, 8, 9, 16, 17	7.5	6.24
17	6, 17	X-{6, 17}	6.67	5.66
29	29, 5, 16, 14, 8	5, 7, 9, 17	2	2.16

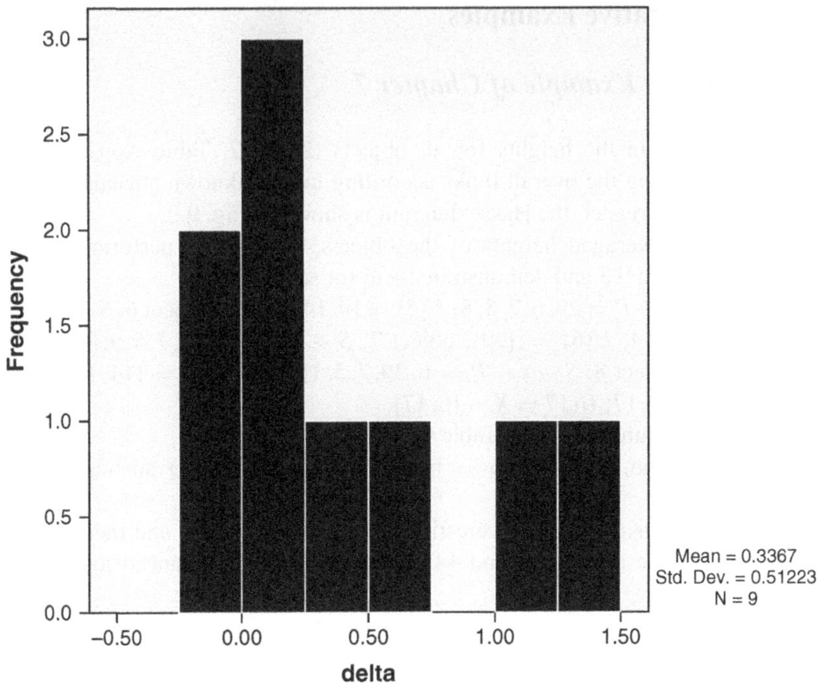

Fig. 9.10 Histogram of the delta values

order models like those published in Bruggemann et al. (2005) and Bruggemann and Carlsen (2011) have far better performance.

Nevertheless, the general statistical quality of LPOM is not so bad: The Pearson correlation is 0.955 and is highly significant.

9.8.2 Example Human Environment Interface Index

For details of the HEI, see Patil (2000), Patil and Taillie (2004), and Singh (2008).

As we are convinced that the local partial order model is a helpful tool, we take a second example, where we want to apply almost all concepts of Chapter 9. We select the partial order of European countries.

For the following determination of the levels, compare Fig. 9.11.

9.8.2.1 Level

There are 10 levels because lg = 9 or the height = 10. Some of them are rendered now:

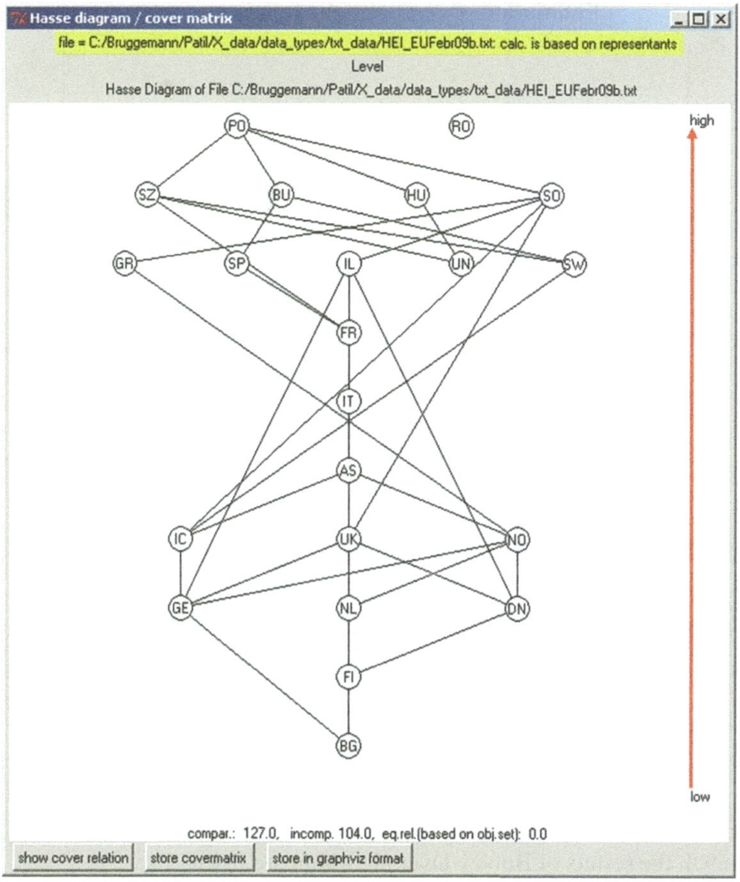

Fig. 9.11 Hasse diagram of European Countries (PyHasse)

The first level, $\text{level}_1 = \{\text{BG}\}$; the second level, $\text{level}_2 = \{\text{FI}\}$; the third level, $\text{level}_3 = \{\text{GE, NL, DN}\}$; the eighth level, $\text{level}_8 = \{\text{GR, SP, IL, UN, SW}\}$; and the tenth level, $\text{level}_{10} = \{\text{PO, RO}\}$.

As discussed above, one can use the level number as a crude parameter-free estimation of a weak order. Indeed the correlation (Pearson) of the results due to Bubley Dyer (see below) with the level number is 0.865.

In Fig. 9.12, the scatter plot of Bubley Dyer averaged heights vs level number is shown.

As expected, strong deviations appear when objects are located in the same level, because then n equivalent elements of one level often have different numbers of successors. The number of successors, however, is decisive for the final averaged height, as one can see from the equations in Section 9.3.3.

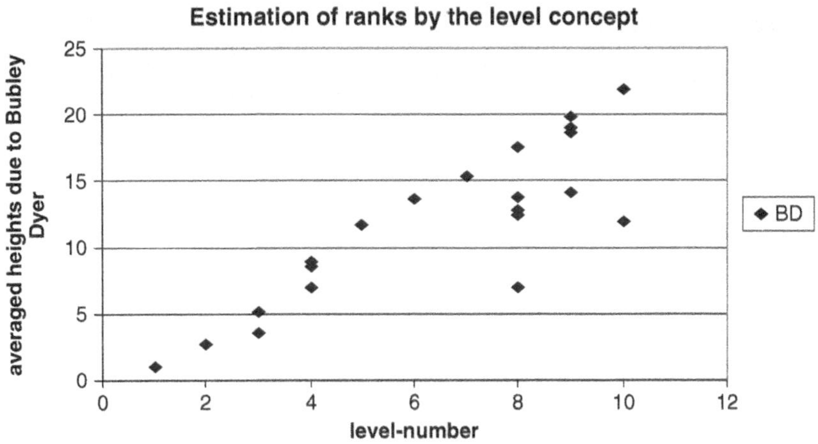

Fig. 9.12 Averaged heights due to the Bubley Dyer algorithm vs level number

9.8.2.2 LPOM(0)

The outcomes of LPOM are shown in Table 9.3.

From Table 9.3 the following weak order is obtained:

PO > SZ ~ BU > SO > SP > GR > FR > IL > IT > AS > HU ~ SW ~ RO > UK > NO > IC > UN > DN ~ NL > FI ~ GE > BG.

9.8.2.3 Bubley Dyer

In Table 9.4, the results of Bubley Dyer algorithm are listed.

Table 9.3 Results of LPOM for 22 countries belonging to EU (HEI study)[a]

No.	Rkav	pr<	pr>	No	Rkav	pr<	pr>
GR	16.1	0.7	0.3	NL	4.313	0.188	0.813
IT	14.375	0.625	0.375	UK	9.2	0.4	0.6
PO	21.955	0.955	0.045	BU	20.125	0.875	0.125
SP	18.4	0.8	0.2	HU	11.5	0.5	0.5
AS	12.938	0.563	0.438	UN	4.6	0.2	0.8
GE	2.706	0.118	0.882	SO	19.462	0.846	0.154
SZ	20.125	0.875	0.125	DN	4.313	0.188	0.813
BG	1.15	0.05	0.95	FI	2.706	0.118	0.882
FR	15.813	0.688	0.313	NO	8.625	0.375	0.625
IC	5.308	0.231	0.769	SW	11.5	0.5	0.5
IL	15.333	0.667	0.333	RO	11.5	0.5	0.5

[a]First column: Identifier of the country. Second column: averaged height (Rkav). Third and fourth columns: Probability of $U(x)$ to be below or above x.

Table 9.4 Bubley Dyer algorithm applied to countries of EU (HEI study)

Nation	Rkav	Nation	Rkav	Nation	Rkav	Nation	Rkav
GR	13.83	SZ	19.04	UK	8.99	FI	2.75
IT	13.67	BG	1.14	BU	19.86	NO	8.65
PO	21.96	FR	15.44	HU	14.23	SW	12.82
SP	17.61	IC	7.03	UN	7.05	RO	12.01
AS	11.82	IL	12.44	SO	18.67		
GE	3.65	NL	5.21	DN	5.18		

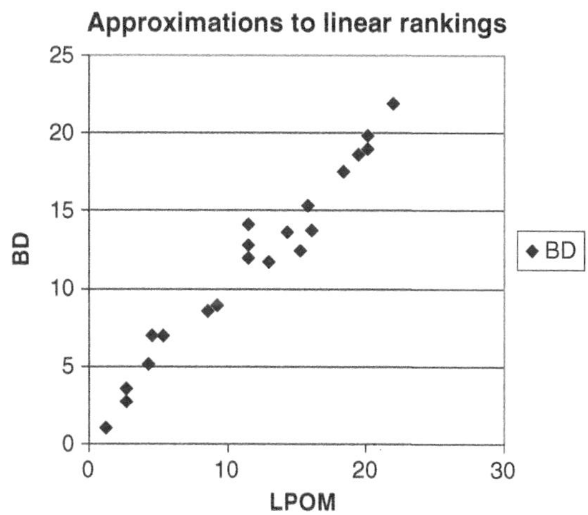

Fig. 9.13 Bubley Dyer algorithm (BD) vs local partial order model (LPOM)

From Table 9.4, we obtain the linear order:

PO > BU > SZ > SO > SP > FR > HU > GR > IT > SW > IL > RO > AS > UK > NO > UN > IC > NL > DN > GE > FI > BG

The LPOM yields astonishingly good results: The (Pearson) correlation coefficient = 0.981 (see also Fig. 9.13 for a scatter plot).

Clearly, as one can see from the weak order and the linear order due to BD, there are broken equivalences and also some inversions. For instance:

LPOM: GR > FR > ... > HU, whereas BD: Fr > HU > GR.

9.8.2.4 Method of the Down Set Lattice

In contrast to the Bubley Dyer algorithm, the lattice method provides exact averaged ranks. Figure 9.14 shows the comparison of (a) lattice method vs LPOM and (b) lattice method vs results of the Bubley Dyer algorithm.

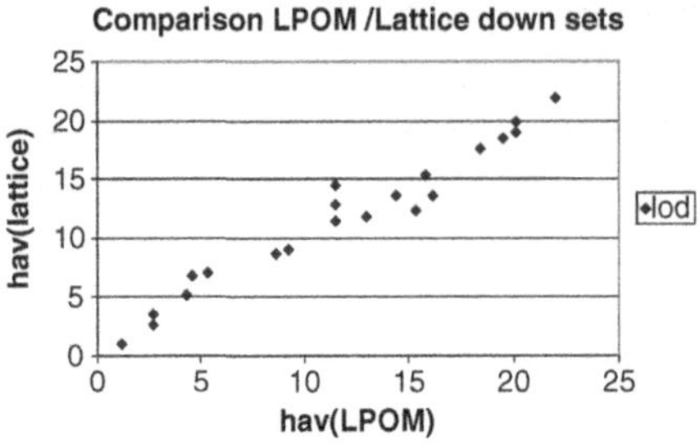

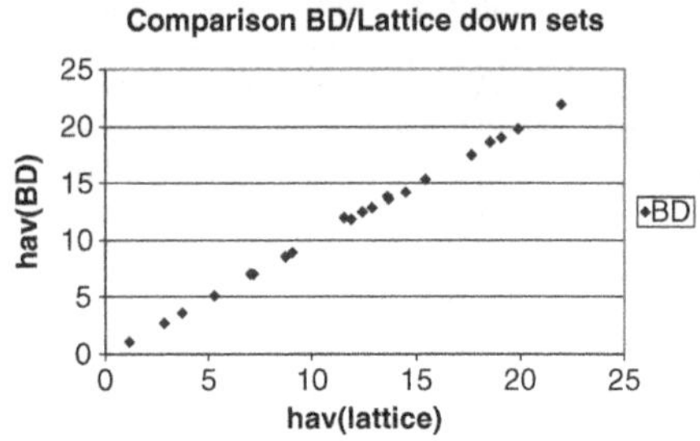

Fig. 9.14 (*LHS*) Comparison of LPOM and (*RHS*) comparison of Bubley Dyer algorithm with exact averaged ranks due to the lattice method (abscissa)

As expected the LPOM method will have some discrepancies to the exact values, whereas Bubley Dyer and the lattice method coincide very good. Hence we can give an advice when to use each of the three methods:

- *LPOM*: It provides quick overview and easy trace back of factors relevant for a certain height. There is no restriction in the number of objects.
- *Lattice method*: When the number of objects is less than 50, then this method provides exact ranks and is recommended.
- *Bubley Dyer algorithm*: This algorithm gets results in an acceptable time even if the number of objects exceeds 50.

9.8.2.5 Mutual Probability

It is only meaningful to calculate the mutual probability for incomparable elements. A stakeholder in Germany may be interested in knowing how probable Germany (GE) is superior to Netherlands (NL).

The heights of GE and NL in either LPOM or BD clearly differ. We find NL > GE.

In Table 9.5, we find following information for GE and NL.

Just by examining the data of Table 9.5, we see that NL has both fewer predecessors and more successors compared to GE. Hence the rough empirical equation (9.5) will favor NL over GE. In Fig. 9.15, the PyHasse user interface is shown, where the information gathered in Table 9.5 is used to obtain averaged ranks and the mutual probability of any two incomparable objects.

Table 9.5 Order theoretical characteristics of GE and NL

	Successors	Predecessors	Incomparable elements
GE	1	14	6
NL	2	12	7

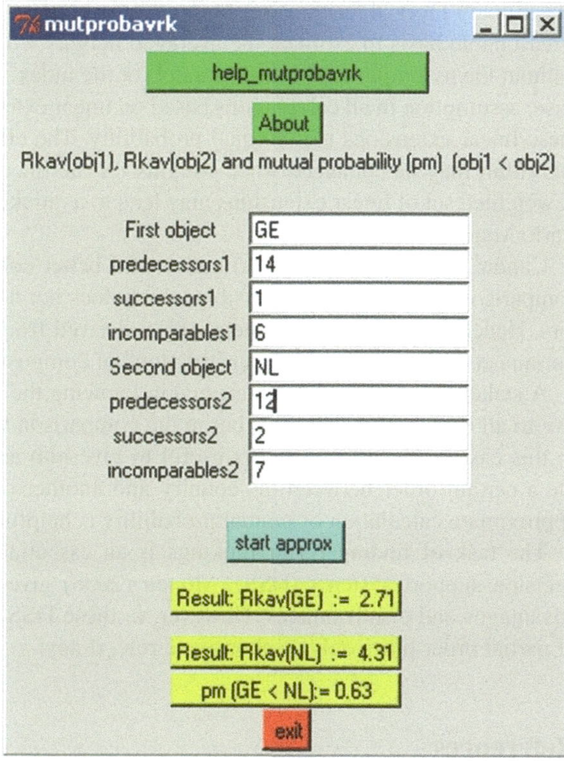

Fig. 9.15 Graphical user interface of the module "mutprobavrk.py"

The answer is that it is more probable that GE is dominated by NL in a linear order, as was expected by the height calculation.

9.9 Summary and Commentary

The concept of levels is rather simple and allows a quick access to ranking of objects.

The LPOM model is recommended for estimation of the canonical order within a preliminary study because of its simplicity and unambiguity with respect to what is to be selected as $S - x - P$ chain. The approximation error of LPOM is a function of the number of incomparable elements for each selected object, because any incomparable element which is not isolated will contribute to an error. We recommend this method for a first screening. Recently, a very interesting approach is provided by De Loof et al. (2006, 2008). Instead of constructing linear extension from the poset and deriving averaged heights and other properties from them, the less complex set of down sets and their lattice is the basis of the algorithm. Once the lattice is found, several quantities of interest can be derived from paths within the lattice.

The Bubley Dyer algorithm is a Monte Carlo Markov chain approach. It provides a reasonable basis to estimate the averaged heights without the use of weights and without the assumption of a linear model for the index. Note however that there is a basic assumption in all calculations based on linear extensions. It is assumed that all these linear extensions are of equal probability. The efficiency of the Bubley Dyer algorithm may be enhanced when weights for the linear extensions are developed. A weighted set of linear extensions may lead to a quicker convergence of the Monte Carlo Markov chain approach.

Canonical orders can serve to understand better composite indicator because a comparison with an order is possible which does not need the weighting of indicators. Hence partial order and linear orders derived from them may helpful in what Saisana et al. (2011) call a "deconstruction" of composite indicators.

A stakeholder may not be interested in knowing the position of his country relative to all of the other countries but in the comparison with only one other country. In this case, a "local" concept is useful to give him an initial idea of how probable a certain order between his country and another one is. For this purpose, the approximate calculation of mutual probability is helpful.

The task of finding linear rankings is an essential part of many well-known decision support systems (DSS). Munda (2008) gives a good overview of their advantages and disadvantages. However, in these DSS, the mathematical structure of partial order plays only a subordinate role, if any.

References

Bruggemann, R. and Carlsen, L. (2011). An improved estimation of averaged ranks of partial orders. Match Commun. Math. Comput. Chem., 65, 383–414.

Bruggemann, R. and Patil, G.P. (2010). Multicriteria prioritization and partial order in environmental sciences. Environ. Ecol. Stat., 17, 383–410.

Bruggemann, R., Simon, U. and Mey, S. (2005). Estimation of averaged ranks by extended local partial order models. Match – Commun. Math. Comput. Chem., 54(3), 489–518.

Bruggemann, R., Sørensen, P.B., Lerche, D. and Carlsen, L. (2004). Estimation of averaged ranks by a local partial order model. J. Chem. Inf. Comput. Sci., 44, 618–625.

Bubley, R. and Dyer, M. (1997). Faster random generation of linear extensions no. http://delivery.acm.org/10.1145/320000/314730/p350-bubley.pdf. School of Computer Studies. University of Leeds, Leeds, UK.

Bubley, R. and Dyer, M. (1999). Faster random generation of linear extensions. Discr. Math., 201, 81–88.

Davey, B.A. and Priestley, H.A. (1990). Introduction to lattices and order. Cambridge: Cambridge University Press.

De Loof, K., De Baets, B., De Meyer, H. and Bruggemann, R. (2008). A hitchhiker's guide to poset ranking. Comb. Chem. High Throughput Screen., 11, 734–744.

De Loof, K., De Meyer, H. and De Baets, B. (2006). Exploiting the lattice of ideals representation of a poset. Fundam Informaticae, 71, 309–321.

Denoeux, T., Masson, M. and Hébert, P. (2005). Nonparametric rank-based statistics and significance tests for fuzzy data. Fuzzy Sets Syst., 153, 1–28.

Morton, J., Pachter, L., Shiu, A., Sturmfels, B. and Wienand, O. (2006). Geometry of rank tests (pp. 1–9). http://arvix.org/abs/math/0605173.

Morton, J., Pachter, L., Shiu, A., Sturmfels, B. and Wienand, O. (2009). Convex rank tests and semigraphoids. SIAM J. Discr. Math. 23, 1117–1134.

Munda, G. (2008). Social multi-criteria evaluation for a sustainable economy (pp. 1–210). Berlin: Springer.
Patil, G.P. (2000). UNEP workshop on human environment interface index. UNEP, Washington, DC.
Patil, G.P. and Taillie, C. (2004). Multiple indicators, partially ordered sets, and linear extensions: Multi-criterion ranking and prioritization. Environ. Ecol. Stat., 11, 199–228.
Saisana, M., Annoni, P., Bruggemann, R., Munda, G., Nardo, M., Saltelli, A. and Tarantola, S. (2011). Pitfalls in deconstructing composite indicators. Publication planned.
Singh, A. (2008). UNEP workshop on human environment interface index. Nairobi, Kenya.
Wienand, O. (2005). http://bio.math.berkeley.edu/ranktests/lcell/index.html.

Chapter 10
Comparison of Partial, Linear, and Weak Orders

10.1 Introduction

There are two reasons to compare different orders:

1. From (X, IB), a linear or weak order, called O_{poset}, can be derived, applying methods rendered in Chapter 9. By calculation of an index (Chapter 7), another linear or weak order can be obtained, which we call O_{Γ}. As there are the same set of indicators, IB, and the same set of objects, X, O_{poset}, and O_{Γ} should ideally be coincident. As can be suspected, this is not necessarily the case and we need measures to quantify the degree of coincidence between O_{poset} and O_{Γ}.
2. There are different indicator sets IB_1, IB_2 inducing partial orders (X, IB_1) and (X, IB_2). Will any comparability $x < y$ in one order be reproduced in another? If not, how can we compare these two partial orders?

In the following, we discuss five concepts which may be useful for comparisons.

10.2 Representation of O_{poset} and O_{Γ} by a Hasse Diagram

10.2.1 Method

Both orders O_{poset} and O_{Index} will be considered as indicators I_{poset} and I_{Γ}, with which we can order the objects. From I_{poset} and $\underline{I}_{\Gamma}$, a new partial order $(X, \{I_{\text{poset}}, I_{\Gamma}\})$ can be found.

A Hasse diagram of $(X, \{I_{\text{poset}}, I_{\Gamma}\})$ may show us the following:

1. Chains of $(X, \{I_{\text{poset}}, I_{\Gamma}\})$: Subsets of objects with coincident mutual orders.
2. Antichains of $(X, \{I_{\text{poset}}, I_{\Gamma}\})$: Pairs of objects for which object rank inversions are found.

R. Brüggemann, G.P. Patil, *Ranking and Prioritization for Multi-indicator Systems*, Environmental and Ecological Statistics 5, DOI 10.1007/978-1-4419-8477-7_10,

3. A linear order (see Chapter 2): The two orders O_{poset} and O_Γ coincide completely. The number of incomparabilities U will be 0.
4. A complete antichain: O_{poset} is the dual (Chapter 3) of O_Γ. $U = n^*(n-1)/2$, with n being the number of objects.

Therefore, the degree of coincidence d_{coin1} can be quantified by the following equation:

$$d_{\text{coin1}} := 1 - \frac{\mid U(X, \{I_{\text{poset}}, I_\Gamma\}) \mid}{\binom{n}{2}} \tag{10.1a}$$

Instead of counting pairwise incomparability (Eq. (1.10)), we can measure the degree of coincidence by the extent of pairwise incomparability. We sum objectwise the absolute difference between ranks of each object due to I_{poset} and I_Γ and normalize this sum by its maximum attainable value of $1 + 2 + \ldots + n - 1 = n^*(n-1)/2 = \binom{n}{2}$. Thus we obtain another coincidence measure d_{coin2}:

$$d_{\text{coin2}} := 1 - \frac{\sum\limits_{x \in X} \mid \text{rank}(x, I_{\text{poset}}) - \text{rank}(x, I_\Gamma) \mid}{\binom{n}{2}} \tag{10.1b}$$

10.2.2 Illustrative Example

Figure 10.1 shows the Hasse diagram of 10 objects, three attributes, and the data matrix.

The order O_{poset} is obtained from the set of linear extensions and from them the averaged height, hav.

The order O_Γ is obtained by assuming the weight vector (0.5, 0.3, 0.2).

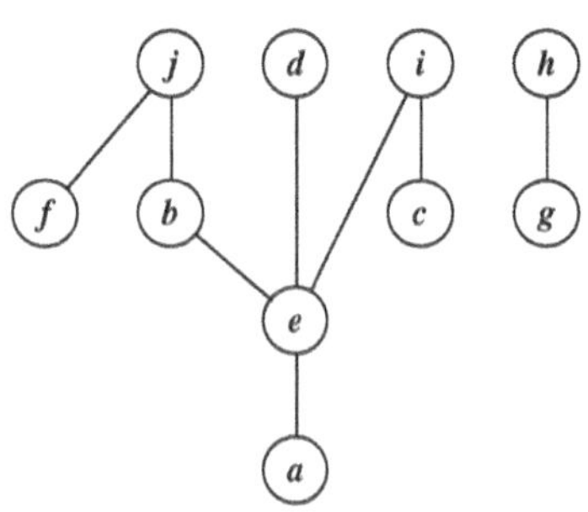

	q_1	q_2	q_3
a	1	2	3
b	3	2	5
c	2	5	2
d	3	3	4
e	1	2	4
f	4	2	2
g	6	1	1
h	6	1	3
i	2	6	5
j	4	2	6

Fig. 10.1 Hasse diagram of $(X, \text{IB}) = (X, \{q_1, q_2, q_3\})$ for demonstrating the calculation of d_{coin1}

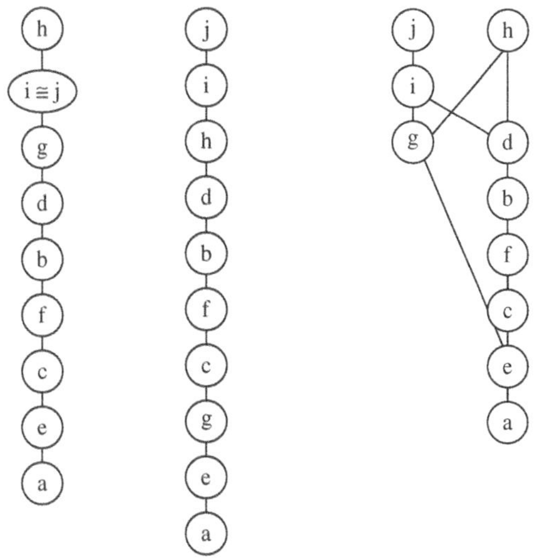

Fig. 10.2 (*LHS*) $(X, \{I_\Gamma\})$, (*middle*) $(X, \{I_{\text{poset}}\})$, (*RHS*) $(X, \{I_{\text{poset}}, I_\Gamma\})$

Both orders $(X, \{I_{\text{poset}}\})$ and $(X, \{I_\Gamma\})$ as well as $(X, \{I_{\text{poset}}, I_\Gamma\})$ are depicted in Fig. 10.2.

$U(X, \{I_{\text{poset}}, I_\Gamma\}) = 6$, hence $d_{\text{coin1}} = 1 - 0.1333 = 0.8666$, whereas $d_{\text{coin2}} = 1 - 0.27 = 0.73$. We see that both orders coincide pretty well. By looking at the Hasse diagram of $(X, \{I_{\text{poset}}, I_\Gamma\})$, we see that

- object g is incomparable to the objects d, b, f, c and
- object h is incomparable to the objects i, j.

What may be the reason for this? Looking back at Fig. 10.1, we see that the two objects g and h are forming own component in (X, IB). Therefore, g and h will contribute to be in $U(X, \{I_{\text{poset}}, I_\Gamma\})$ and be most prone to influences of the weight vector.

10.3 Spearman Correlation Analysis

10.3.1 Method

Spearman correlation applies if we have two linear or weak orders and we would like to know how far they are correlated. The correlation index tells us how much the two linear or weak orders coincide. So far as any single ranking position is considered, the Spearman correlation coefficient is pretty sensitive to rank inversion. We call ranks of the order 1 $R_1(i)$ and those of the order 2 $R_2(i)$, where $i = 1, \ldots, n$, with number of objects n.

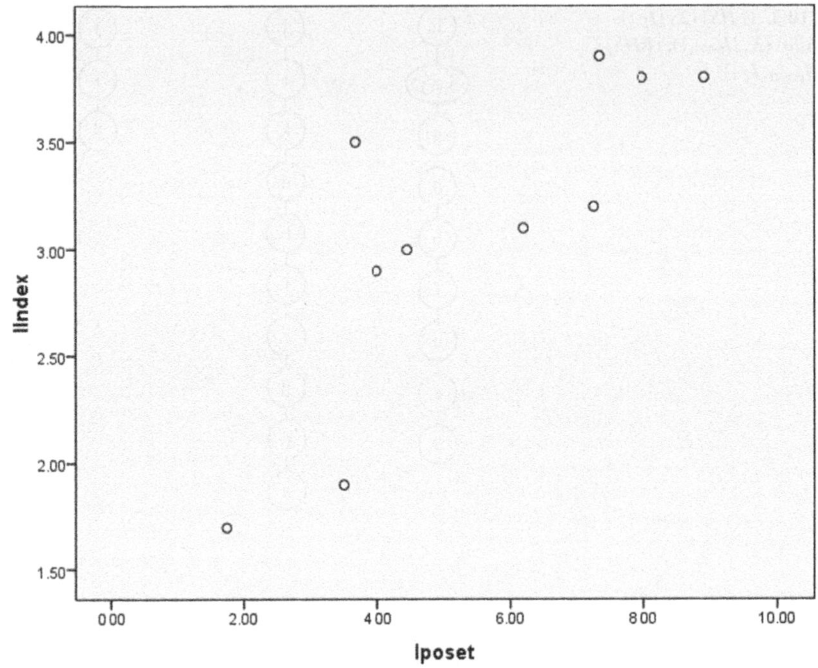

Fig. 10.3 Scatter plot of $I_\Gamma(= I_{\text{Index}})$ and I_{poset} of example in Section 10.2

Writing $d(i) := R_1(i) - R_2(i)$, the Spearman correlation is given by

$$r_s = 1 - \frac{6 \cdot \sum_{i=1}^{n} (d(i))^2}{n \cdot (n^2 - 1)} \tag{10.2}$$

$$r_s \in [-1, 1].$$

10.3.2 Illustrative Example

As order 1 we apply I_{poset}, and as order 2, I_Γ of the example in Section 10.2. The Spearman correlation coefficient is $r_s = 0.839$, indicating a good correlation, hence a good coincidence of both orders. In Fig. 10.3, the scatter plot of I_Γ (ordinate axis) vs I_{poset} (abscissa) is shown.

10.4 Concordance Analysis

10.4.1 Method

The concordance analysis is a robust and intuitive tool to compare one weak or linear order with another one. For example, using an index Γ, we may get five

Fig. 10.4 Principle of concordance analysis

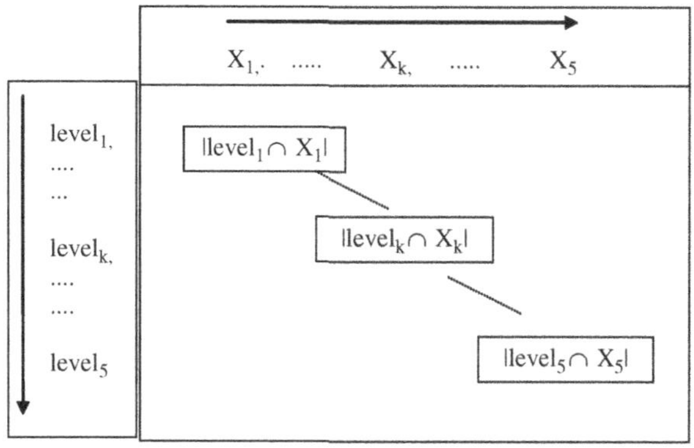

subsets $X_1, X_2, \ldots, X_5, X_i \subset X, X_i \cap X_j = \emptyset$, for $j \neq i$, which can be interpreted as "very bad," "bad," "medium," "good," "very good" and by the partial order, five levels (see Chapter 9) level_1 ("very bad"), level_2 ("bad"), ..., level_5 ("very good") are provided and we want to compare the level sets with the subsets. Patil (2005) introduces this intuitive technique to perform this comparison (Fig. 10.4). The arrows in Fig. 10.4 indicate the orientation (from very bad to very good) and we count the elements occurring in the main diagonal. In order to get a measure, we normalize this number by dividing by the number of objects.

The basic idea can be represented by a square $d \times d$ matrix cd (see Fig. 10.4) as follows: Let

$$P_{ki} = \{x \in X: \text{ height } i \text{ in } k\text{th order}\}, \text{ then } cd_{ij} = |P_{1i} \cap P_{2j}| \tag{10.3}$$

As motivated by Fig. 10.4, the two orders coincide more, as the entries in the diagonal of the concordance matrix are more. However, we accept some slight deviations as concordant: Therefore, the two diagonals neighboring the main diagonal are also taken into account, however with a lower weight κ (0.5 is recommended). Hence we arrive at

$$\text{con} = \left(\sum cd_{ii} + \kappa^* \sum cd_{|i-j|=1}\right) / n, n \text{ being } |\text{X}| \tag{10.4}$$

The expression $cd_{|i-j|=1}$ counts for the two diagonals neighboring the main diagonal and n is the number of objects. Patil (2005) finds by simulation studies a threshold value T.

$$T = 1/d, d \text{ being the number of subsets } X_i \text{ (levels)} \tag{10.5}$$

We speak of concordance between two rankings if

$$\text{con} > \text{T} \tag{10.6}$$

A fictitious example follows; real-life examples will be found in the case study chapters.

10.4.2 Illustrative Example

In Fig. 10.5, a Hasse diagram together with the data matrix is shown.

Assuming all weights equal, the index yields the weak order:

$$a < d < e < b \cong h < c < g \cong i < f$$

There are three levels (see Chapter 9):

$$\text{level}_1 = \{a\}, \text{level}_2 = \{c, e, i\}, \text{level}_3 = \{g, h, b, f, d\}$$

Correspondingly, we form three disjoint subsets:

$$X_1 = \{a, d, e\}, X_2 = \{b, h, c\}, X_3 = \{g, i, f\}$$

Corresponding to Fig. 10.4, we obtain Table 10.1.

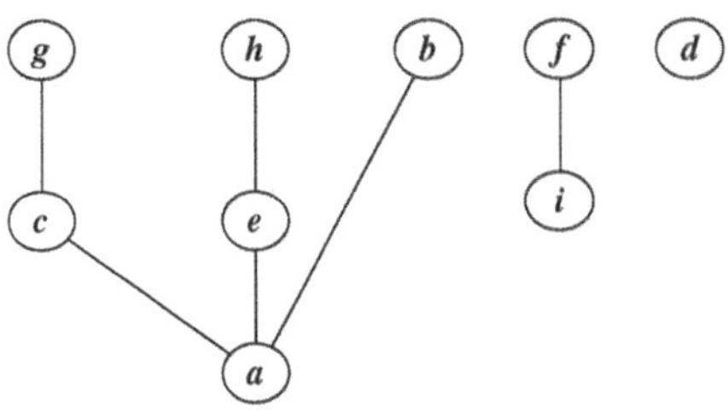

	q_1	q_2	q_3
a	1	2	3
b	3	2	5
c	4	6	3
d	1	7	0
e	2	3	4
f	0	8	9
g	6	6	3
h	2	3	5
i	0	7	8

Fig. 10.5 Illustrative Hasse diagram and the data matrix

Table 10.1 Intersections (top) and concordance matrix *cd* (bottom)

	$\{a, d, e\}$	$\{b, c, h\}$	$\{f, g, i\}$
$\{a\}$	$\{a\}$	Ø	Ø
$\{c, e, i\}$	$\{e\}$	$\{c\}$	$\{i\}$
$\{b, d, f, g, h\}$	$\{d\}$	$\{b, h\}$	$\{f, g\}$

	$\{a, d, e\}$	$\{b, c, h\}$	$\{f, g, i\}$
$\{a\}$	1	0	0
$\{c, e, i\}$	1	1	1
$\{b, d, f, g, h\}$	1	2	2

10.5 Intersection of Partial Orders

10.5.1 Motivation

Often two posets arise from different sets of indicators and it is of interest to relate the two posets. One way to do this is to combine both indicator sets and to get an extended information base $= \mathrm{IB}_1 \cup \mathrm{IB}_2$, then see what comparabilities remain in $(X,\ \mathrm{IB}_1 \cup \mathrm{IB}_2)$.

10.5.2 Method

In $(X,\ \mathrm{IB}_1 \cup \mathrm{IB}_2)$ only those comparabilities occur, which are present at the same time in (X, IB_1) and (X, IB_2). In other words

$$(X,\ \mathrm{IB}_1 \cup \mathrm{IB}_2) = (X, \mathrm{IB}_1) \cap (X, \mathrm{IB}_2) \tag{10.6b}$$

The two partial orders coincide more as larger the intersection in Eq. (10.6b) is.

The evaluation of the intersection operation in Eq. (10.6b) is best done if the representation of posets by ordered sets is applied (Section 2.5): If $x < y$ in (X, IB), then $(x, y) \in \mathbf{X} = (X, \mathrm{IB})$.

As in Chapter 7, V is the number of comparabilities. We call V_1 the number of comparabilities of (X, IB_1), V_2 of (X, IB_2), and V_{12} of $(X,\ \mathrm{IB}_1 \cup \mathrm{IB}_2)$.

Then obviously

$$V_{12} \leq \min(V_1, V_2) \tag{10.7}$$

If $(X, \mathrm{IB}_1) \subset (X, \mathrm{IB}_2)$, then $V_{12} = V_1$. Useful results by intersection can be expected if only one of the posets is included in the other one.

10.5.3 Illustrative Example

Consider the three Hasse diagrams in Fig. 10.6.

As in Chapter 2, we disregard the pairs which are in the diagonal of X^2:

$$(X, \mathrm{IB}_1) = \{(a,b), (a,d), (c,b), (c,d), (b,d)\}$$
$$(X, \mathrm{IB}_2) = \{(a,d), (c,b), (c,d), (b,d)\}$$
$$(X, \mathrm{IB}_3) = \{(c,b), (c,a), (c,d), (b,d), (b,a)\}$$

Inclusions:

$$(X, \mathrm{IB}_2) \subset (X, \mathrm{IB}_1) \text{ and } V_{12} = V_2 = 4$$

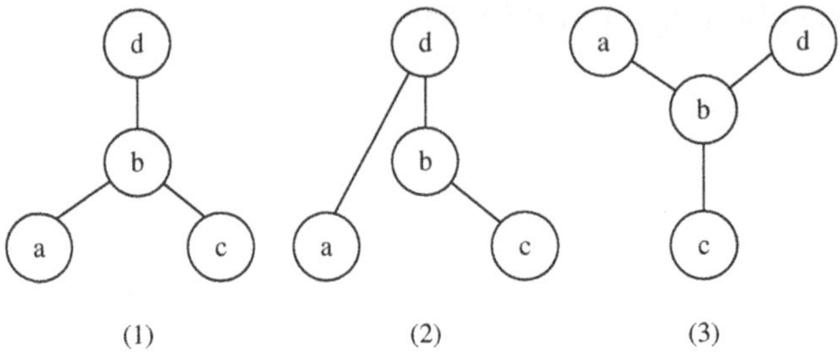

Fig. 10.6 Three visualizations: (*1*) (X, IB_1), (*2*) (X, IB_2), (*3*) (X, IB_3)

The ordered pair (b, a) is neither in (X, IB_1) nor in (X, IB_2). Furthermore, the ordered pair (a, d) which is in (X, IB_1) and (X, IB_2) is not in (X, IB_3). Therefore, no other $\subset$ relation can be found among the three posets.

Intersections:

$(X, \mathrm{IB}_1) \cap (X, \mathrm{IB}_2) = \{(a,d),(c,b),(c,d),(b,d)\} = (X, \mathrm{IB}_2), V_{12} = 4$ as it must be.

$(X, \mathrm{IB}_1) \cap (X, \mathrm{IB}_3) = \{(c,b),(c,d),(b,d)\}, V_{13} = 3$, a chain $c < b < d$ results, object a is isolated.

$(X, \mathrm{IB}_2) \cap (X, \mathrm{IB}_3) = \{(c,b),(c,d),(b,d)\}, \mathrm{V}_{23} = 3$, a chain $c < b < d$ results, object a is isolated.

10.6 Comparison of Two Partial Orders as a Multivariate Problem

10.6.1 Motivation

Here we want to count what is different between any two pairs (x, y) obtained from the one and the other partial order. We aim to visualize these counts in a histogram-like diagram.

10.6.2 Method

Let us take two elements $x, y \in X$, then the following constellations appear while comparing two empirical posets (Table 10.2).

From Table 10.2 we see that 4*4 different constellations are possible: (1*a*) with (2*a*), (1*a*) with (2*b*), etc.

Table 10.2 Possible constellations when two partial orders are compared, taken $x, y \in X$

Identifier	$x, y \in X$ in (X, IB_1)	Identifier	$x, y \in X$ in (X, IB_2)
1*a*	$x < y$	2*a*	$x < y$
1*b*	$x > y$	2*b*	$x > y$
1*c*	$x \parallel y$	2*c*	$x \parallel y$
1*d*	$x \cong y$	2*d*	$x \cong y$

We call any constellation out of the 16 situations a matching, m_i, $i = 1, \ldots 16$, and denote it by the corresponding symbols out of the list $\{<, >, \parallel, \cong\}$. (10.8)

For example, the constellation $(1a), (2c) : (<, \parallel)$.

As any pair $(x, y) \in X^2$ has exactly one of the 16 matchings, we can also write $m(x, y)$ in order to describe which concrete matching appears for pair x, y by comparing two partial orders. Only two matchings, namely (<, <) and (>, >), will contribute to the partial order $(X, \mathrm{IB}_1 \cap \mathrm{IB}_2)$. The information about 14 other matchings will be lost. Therefore, the theoretical idea is to count the frequencies of matchings as we browse through the object set:

$$F(\text{matching } i) = \text{count of } m_i, \text{ for all } (x, y) \in X^2 \tag{10.9}$$

The evaluation of Eq. (10.9) can best be explained as in Table 10.3.

Counts of some matchings like (<, <) and (>, >) as well as (>, <) and (<, >) separately are not meaningful if we have a comparison in mind. Therefore, instead of taking care of all 16 matchings, we group them in "behavior classes," $B_1, \ldots, B_5$, as follows (Fig. 10.7).

We describe now the degree of coincidence of two partial orders by performing the following steps (Eq. (10.9)):

1. Count the m_i by checking a matrix like that in Table 10.3.
2. Add up those m_i which belong to behavior class B_1.
3. Repeat step 2 for B_2, B_3, B_4, and B_5.
4. Denote the frequency of B_i by $F(B_i)$.
5. Normalize $F(B_i)$ by dividing by $n^*(n - 1)$ and call the resulting number $f(B_i)$.

Table 10.3 Counting matchings

Objects	Objects				
	1	...	k	...	n
1	$m(1, 1)$	...	$m(1, k)$	...	$m(1, n)$
...	....	...	...	...	...
k	$m(k, 1)$		–		$m(k, n)$
...	...	...	...	...	...
n	$m(n, 1)$	...	$m(n, k)$	...	$m(n, n)$

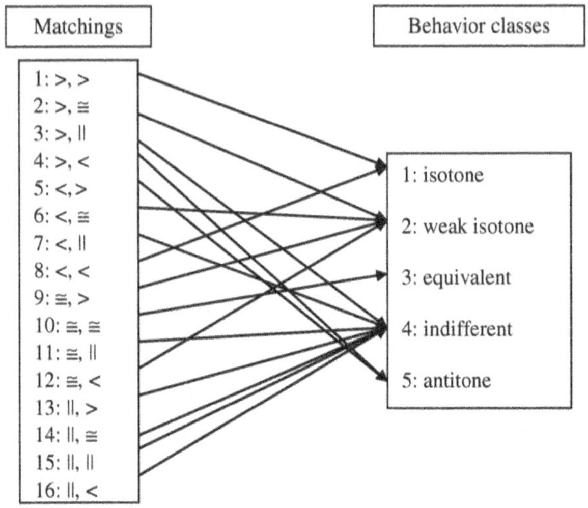

Fig. 10.7 Assignment of matchings m_i to behavior classes B_i

There are the following typical cases:

- $(X, \mathrm{IB}_1) \subset (X, \mathrm{IB}_2)$: $F(B_5) = 0, F(B_4) \neq 0, F(B_1) = 2^* V_1$ "good coincidence"
- $(X, \mathrm{IB}_2) \subset (X, \mathrm{IB}_1)$: $F(B_5) = 0, F(B_4) \neq 0, F(B_2) = 2^* V_2$ "good coincidence"
- $|(X, \mathrm{IB}_1) \cap (X, \mathrm{IB}_2)| = V_{12} << \min(V_1, V_2)$ (Eq. (10.7)): $F(B_5) \neq 0, F(B_4) \neq 0, F(B_1) = 2^* V_{12}$ "medium to poor coincidence"
- (X, IB_1) = dual of (X, IB_2) (see Chapter 4): $F(B_5) = 2^* V_1 = 2^* V_2, F(B_4) \neq 0$, $F(B_1) = 0$ "no coincidence, countercurrent behavior"

In order to describe the behavior of two partial orders in a compact way, we use the wording:

- isotone: matchings (<, <) and (>, >)
- antitone: matchings (>, <) and (>, <)
- weak isotone: the following matchings: (<, $\cong$), (>, $\cong$), ($\cong$, <), ($\cong$, >)
- indifferent: all matchings where || is part of the pair
- equivalent: matching ($\cong$, $\cong$)

It is convenient to present the comparison of two partial orders by a bar diagram of $f(B_i)$. This multivariate consideration of the comparison of partial orders is called "proximity analysis."

10.6.3 Illustrative Example

In Fig. 10.8 two Hasse diagrams (a) and (b) are shown which visually present two partial orders (X, IB_1) and $(X, \mathrm{IB2})$. What is the result of the proximity analysis?

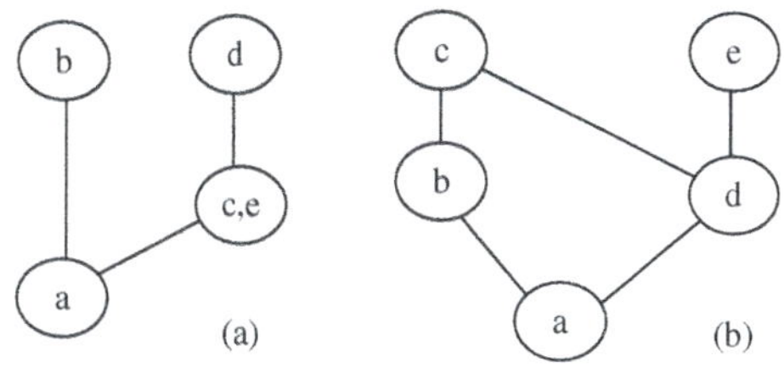

Fig. 10.8 Example for proximity analysis with two Hasse diagrams (a) and (b)

In Table 10.4 we fill out the cells by the matchings $m_1, \ldots, m_{16}$: In the cells first the result of the Hasse diagram (a) and then that of (b) are written. The matchings of the same type are counted and assigned to one of the five B_i classes, following the lines of Eq. (10.9).

The normalized frequencies $f(B_i)$ are presented as a bar diagram (Fig. 10.9).

Table 10.4 Comparison matrix among the five objects of the Hasse diagrams shown in Fig. 10.8 (only the upper triangle is shown)

	a	*b*	*c*	*d*	*e*
a	–	$<, <$	$<, <$	$<, <$	$<, <$
b		–	$\|, <$	$\|, \|$	$\|, \|$
c			–	$<, >$	$=, \|$
d				–	$>, <$
e					–

B_1, isotone: 4; B_2, weak isotone: 0; B_3, equivalent: 0; B_4, indifferent: 4; B_5, antitone: 2

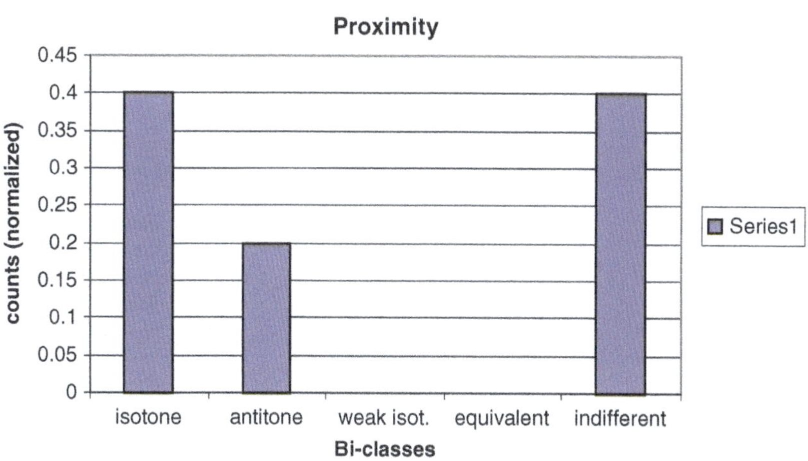

Fig. 10.9 Proximity analysis of the two Hasse diagrams of Fig. 10.8

How the normalized counts are combined to get a final scalar, expressing the proximity, depends on the application. For a real-life example, see Chapters 14 and 15.

10.7 Summary and Commentary

So, actually the tools at hand to compare orders (see Table 10.5) are the following:

1. Hasse diagram of two linear or weak orders, d_{coinc}
2. Spearman correlation analysis, r_s
3. Concordance analysis, con
4. Proximity analysis of two partial orders

There is another way of comparing linear or weak orders which we do not mention so far but for which here is a good place.

Imagine that the empirical composite index is formulated by a set of weights, which we abbreviate as g(emp). This set of weights bears all the experiences of stakeholders and decision makers. Another set of weights called g(poset) may be derived such that an index with weights g(poset) induces the same order as that derived by methods explained in Chapter 9, i.e., by LPOM, Bubley Dyer, CRF, and lattice theoretical methods. If such a set of weights g(poset) can be derived, we can compare it with g(emp).

Table 10.5 Advantages and disadvantages of comparison tools

	Advantages	Disadvantages
Hasse diagram of two linear or weak orders	Coincidences and non-coincidences can be visualized. Objects which are incomparable to many others can be easily identified	Sensitive to any single ranking inversion
Spearman correlation analysis	Easily applicable. Software is generally available Test statistic is provided	Sensitive to any single ranking inversion
Concordance analysis	Intuitive concept Test statistic A PyHasse module is available	Need of finding the same number of subsets for both rankings. The parameter κ may influence the result
Proximity analysis	Detailed information about the matchings arising from two partial orders. A PyHasse module is available	There is no single number telling us about the proximity of two partial orders

Now we are confronted with four cases:

(1) Such a set of g(poset) does not exist, which draws serious attention to the data matrix (indicator selection, measurement errors, and rounding procedures).
(2) By a suitable distance measure, both sets of weights are sufficiently close to each other. Then the partial order method justifies the set of weights g(emp).
(3) The distance is large. Then a re-examination of the data matrix and the weighting procedure to obtain the composite indicator is recommended.

As a software-supported approach is still not available, we let this kind of comparison be open for future work.

Reference

Patil, G.P. (2005). Cross-disciplinary class room notes. Center for Statistical Ecology and Environmental Statistics, Penn State University.

Chapter 11
Illustrative Case Studies

11.1 Overview

Here we demonstrate some of the tools outlined in Chapters 2, 3, 4, 5, 6, 7, 8, 9, and 10. The illustrative case studies are based on "real-life" data matrices. The sections are organized as follows (Table 11.1).

Table 11.1 Organization of Chapter 11

Tool	Sections	Case study	Related to
Hasse diagram	2.5	Pollution in Baden-Wuerttemberg	Environmental chemistry
Discretization	6.3		
p-algorithm	6.5		
POSAC	3.5	Internet sources about drinking water quality	Environmental health
Attribute-related sensitivity	4.2	Fish communities in wetlands	Biology
Ambiguity and antagonism	4.3, 4.4, 5.5.2	Ranking of high-production chemicals	Environmental chemistry
Attribute value-related sensitivity	6.6	Ecological value of communes	Ecology
Dominance among subsets	5.6	(a) Chemicals in a river (b) Human environment index	(a) Environmental chemistry (b) Environmental sciences
Separability	5.4, 5.6	Management in a river basin	Hydrology
Stepwise aggregation	7.4	Management in a river basin	Hydrology
Navigation	3.6, 5.3	Human environment index	Environmental Sciences
Fuzzy partial order	6.4	Biomanipulation in a lake	Limnology

R. Brüggemann, G.P. Patil, *Ranking and Prioritization for Multi-indicator Systems*, Environmental and Ecological Statistics 5, DOI 10.1007/978-1-4419-8477-7_11,

11.2 Illustrative Case Study: Pollution in Baden-Wuerttemberg (Environmental Chemistry)

11.2.1 Introduction

For monitoring the pollution status of the German state Baden-Wuerttemberg, the Environmental Protection Agency divided Baden-Wuerttemberg into 60 regions, which are the objects of our analysis (EPA Baden-Wuerttemberg, 1994; Bruggemann et al., 1997).

11.2.1.1 Hasse Diagram of (X, IB)

- X, the object set, consists of 59 regions, where data are available.
- IB, the information base, consists of four indicators, c_{Pb}, c_{Cd}, c_{Zn}, and c_S, the concentrations of Pb (lead), Cd (cadmium), Zn (zinc), and S (sulfur) in the herb layer in mg/kg dry mass. As shorthand notation, we write simply: IB = {Pb, Cd, Zn, S}.
- Orientation: The larger the concentration, the larger the loading of the region.

For convenience, the Hasse diagram based on the original data matrix, already shown in Chapter 3, is displayed once again in Fig. 11.1.

11.2.2 Further Tools of Partial Order Analysis

11.2.2.1 Minimum Rank Graph

In Fig. 11.2, the minimum rank graph is shown. We select two regions, namely regions 48 and 52, both of which are proper maximal elements (see Chapter 2).

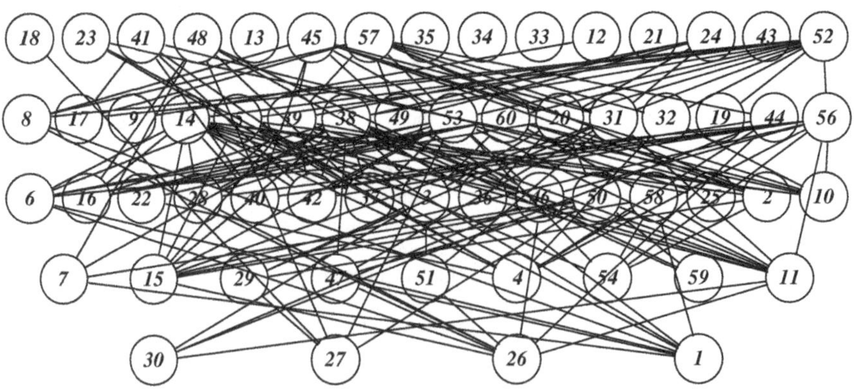

Fig. 11.1 Baden-Wuerttemberg. 59 regions. Herb layer, indicators Pb, Cd, Zn, and S (mg/kg dry weight)

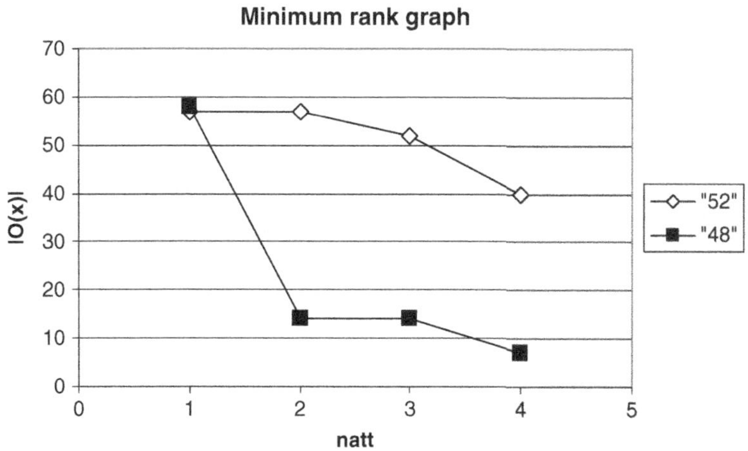

Fig. 11.2 Minimum rank graph of the two regions 48 and 52. Canonical sequence: Pb ≅ S > Cd > Zn

Both regions are maximal elements; however the minimum rank graph shows remarkable differences: Region 48 has more successors compared to region 52, because the concentration of Pb in region 48 is larger than that in region 52. Adding indicator S reduces |O(48)| drastically, because the concentration of sulfur is pretty low. Adding further indicators has only slight effects on |O(48)| and therefore on its minimum rank.

Region 52 has less successors compared to region 48 because of its lower concentration of Pb. Adding the indicator S and Cd reduces |O(52)| slightly, whereas adding indicator Zn to the data matrix has the strongest effect on region 52. The reason is that the concentration of Zn in region 52 is pretty low. Therefore, many regions are eliminated as elements of the down set of 52 after the last step.

11.2.2.2 Dominance Degrees

There is information available on the following characteristics:

1. Contribution forests
2. Degree of agricultural activity
3. Industrial density
4. Traffic density
5. Settlement density

The experts scored these five characteristics from 1 to 3, whereby value 3 indicates a bad status, i.e., a high pressure (in the sense of the DPSIR concept of the OECD; see Kristensen, 2004) on the ecosystem. We select regions having in

Table 11.2 Pressures

Pressure	Identifier	Regions
In three characteristics	H: high pressure	18, 52
In two characteristics	M: medium pressure	19, 22, 59, 1, 30, 47, 49, 56
In one characteristic	L: Low pressure	54, 4, 7, 16, 41, 45, 50, 55, 60, 3, 43, 44, 31, 39, 42

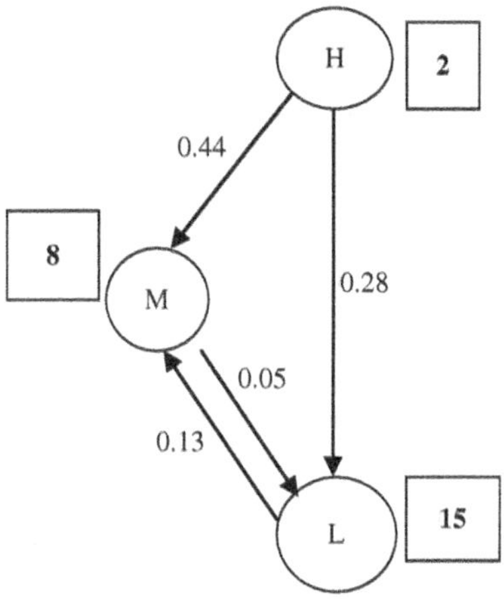

Fig. 11.3 Directed graph. Evaluation of the edges by the dominance degrees $\neq 0$

one, two, or three characteristics a score 3. Table 11.2 informs about the loadings of regions according to the pressure indicators.

The calculation of the dominance degrees of contextual defined subsets $X_i \subset X$ can be conveniently displayed by a directed graph and is shown in Fig. 11.3.

Figure 11.3 (number of regions belonging to different degrees of pressure is given in bold numbers; see Table 11.2) shows that Dom(H, M) = 0.44. Therefore, we may hypothesize that the degree of pressure governs the pollution level. However, if we compare regions of medium pressure to those of low pressure, the dominance analysis does not support this hypothesis. The reason may be that the pressure indicators provide a description on a regional scale, whereas the pollution may also be affected by long-range airborne transport processes.

11.2.2.3 Transformations of the Data Matrix

Discretization Scheme

The K values (see Chapter 6) were given by the scientists of the Environmental Protection Agency (Dr Kreimes: personal communication) as follows:

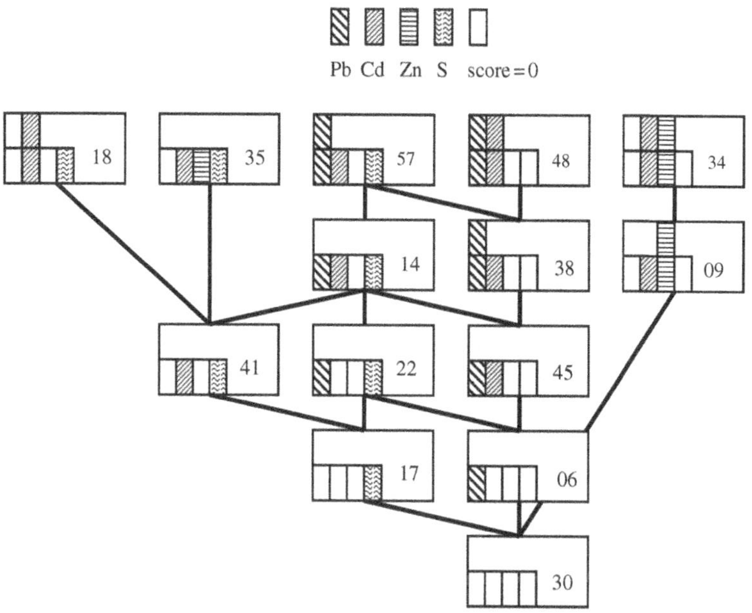

Fig. 11.4 Partial ordering of the regions of Baden-Wuerttemberg (see text)

$$K(\text{Pb}) = K(\text{Cd}) = K(\text{Zn}) = 3 \text{ with the scores } 0,\ 1,\ 2,\ K(\text{S}) = 2.$$

The minimum and maximum values are taken from the columns of the normalized data matrix (Table A.3).

11.2.2.4 Hasse Diagram

Figure 11.4 shows the resulting partial order. Instead of circles and identifiers as graphical elements, we draw small bar diagrams, which indicate the pollution profile.

11.2.2.5 Interpretation

In Fig. 11.4 the numbers to the right of the pollution profile are identifiers of the regions and the bars show their pollution status with respect to lead (Pb), cadmium (Cd), zinc (Zn), and sulfur (S) in the herb layer (mg/kg dry mass). For the equivalence classes, see Table A.4). The Hasse diagram makes evident that the following:

- Pollution increases in different manner when starting from the bottom (region 30) and moving upward along the lines.

- Any bifurcation tells us that the pollution pattern (like moving upward from region 17 to 41 on the one hand and 22 on the other hand) is qualitatively different: 41 is additionally loaded by cadmium, whereas 22 is loaded by lead.
- Any union of lines tells us that the pollution load is so large that qualitative differences in the lower part of the diagram are of no concern for all objects upward.
- In comparison to Fig. 11.1, we identify the separated subset {regions 34 and 09}. These regions cannot be compared with the most other regions, because they have high scores of the metal Zn, together with a medium score of the rather toxic but broadly technically used metal Cd. This pollution pattern will not be found for other regions. The graphical display by a Hasse diagram shows this peculiar property. The causal background for this high degree of separability may be the mining activities in former centuries in those regions (Kreimes, 1996).
- There is a triangular shape (see Chapter 5): Going upward on the Hasse diagram, one sees how the different profiles evolve, and how more and more incomparabilities appear and we can see why an object is and where it is located because we can see the data profile.
- There is a need to remedy the pollution status of many regions, but the strategy of remediation will be different, as each maximal element has another pollution profile.
- Finally, the component {12, 9} found in the Hasse diagram, Fig. 11.1 is not reproduced. Indeed the numerical differences leading to the two nontrivial components in Fig. 11.1 are very small.

11.2.2.6 p-Algorithm

We selected the cut values q_{i0} such that with respect to each attribute, 90% of the objects are sent into the swamp (see Chapter 6). In Fig. 11.5, the resulting Hasse diagram (equipped with the profiles of the maximal elements) is shown.

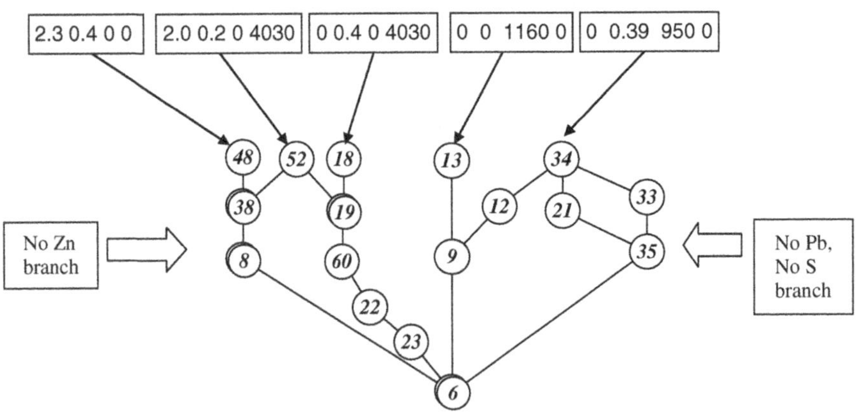

Fig. 11.5 The same Hasse diagram after applying the p-algorithm. Equivalence classes: {8, 45, 20}, {38, 57, 24}, {19, 43}, and the swamp SW (see text)

Following the lines of Chapter 5, we give some examples of navigation: Starting from the maximal elements of the left part, we see there is no Zn (in terms of the p-algorithm). Applying Eq. (5.9), we identify the objects in the left part of the diagram as being not polluted by Zn. Similarly the right part is that there is no Pb pollution.

11.3 Illustrative Case Study: Internet Sources About Drinking Water Quality (Environmental Health, IT)

11.3.1 Introduction

In a study performed by Voigt and Welzl (2002), the question was about the extent of informativeness of Internet sources about drinking water quality. Drinking water is extremely important. Its contamination by active pharmaceutical substances becomes a serious matter (see Freier et al., 2007). Hence it is of interest to know as to how we get information about the quality of drinking water. Voigt and Welzl (2002) investigated Internet sources of the 16 states of Germany. Five indicators were worked out:

1. Number of chemicals reported, NU
2. Kinds of chemicals, KC
3. Other properties like microbial studies, hardness of water, OP
4. Number of monitoring sites in cities, MS
5. Degree of explanations and the contexts, EX

Hence the information base is IB = {NU, KC, OP, MS, EX}.

11.3.2 Data Matrix and Partial Order

The indicator values are 0, 1, 2 and the orientation is that high value indicates a good information status. The object set $X = \{$BAW, BAY, BER, BRE, BRA, HAM, HES, MEC, NIE, NOR, RHE, SAA, SAN, SHO, THU$\}$. In Table 11.3, the data are summarized.

In short, Fig. 11.6 shows that a unique ranking of subsets of the 16 states is possible, although more than one indicator is needed to characterize them. For example, BRE < HES < BRA < SAN < BAW < BAY. We see furthermore that SHO and BAW have good positions as they are near the top of the Hasse diagram. However, they differ in their attribute values: SHO has value 2 in four of five indicators but 0 in indicator MS. BAW, however, has only good values in NU and KC, and medium values for the residual indicators, but no worst value. The Hasse diagram makes us aware of such data profiles.

Table 11.3 Sixteen states of Germany and the information status about drinking water

Id	State in Germany	NU	KC	OP	MS	EX
BAW	Baden-Württemberg	2	2	1	1	1
BAY	Bayern	2	2	2	1	2
BER	Berlin	1	2	1	2	1
BRA	Brandenburg	0	1	1	0	0
BRE	Bremen	0	0	0	0	0
HAM	Hamburg	0	0	1	0	1
HES	Hessen	0	0	1	0	0
MEC	Mecklenburg	0	0	0	0	0
NIE	Niedersachsen	0	0	1	0	0
NOR	Nordrhein-Westfalen	2	2	1	1	1
RHE	Rheinland-Pfalz	2	2	1	1	1
SAA	Saarland	0	0	0	0	0
SAC	Sachsen	1	1	1	1	1
SAN	Sachsen-Anhalt	1	2	1	0	1
SHO	Schleswig-Holstein	2	2	2	0	2
THU	Thueringen	0	0	1	1	0

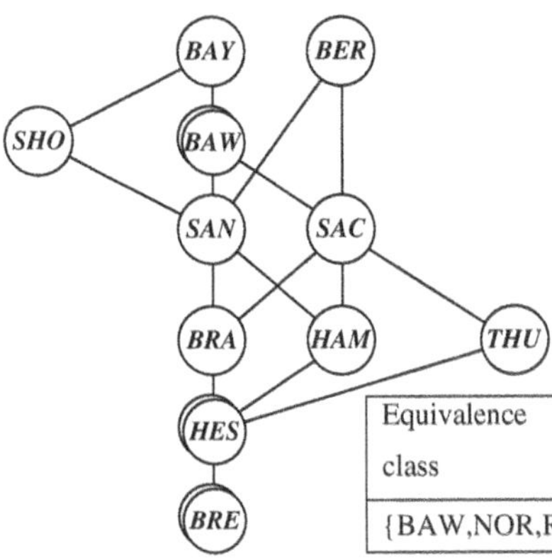

Equivalence class	Equivalence class	Equivalence class
{BAW,NOR,RHE}	{BRE,MEC,SAA}	{HES,NIE}

Fig. 11.6 Hasse diagram of (*X*, IB), together with a table of its equivalence classes

Several other chains of this length can be found. If we consider the representative elements of equivalence classes (see Chapter 2), then we find two linear extensions (Chapter 3) as follows:

le(1): (BRE, HES, THU, HAM, BRA, SAC, SAN, BER, BAW, SHO, BAY) and
le(2): (BRE , HES, BRA, HAM, SAN, SHO, THU, SAC, BAW, BAY, BER)

Do these two linear extensions reproduce ($X/\cong$, IB) implying dim ($X/\cong$, IB) = 2? With PyHasse software (Chapter 17) this can easily be checked and answered with "yes."

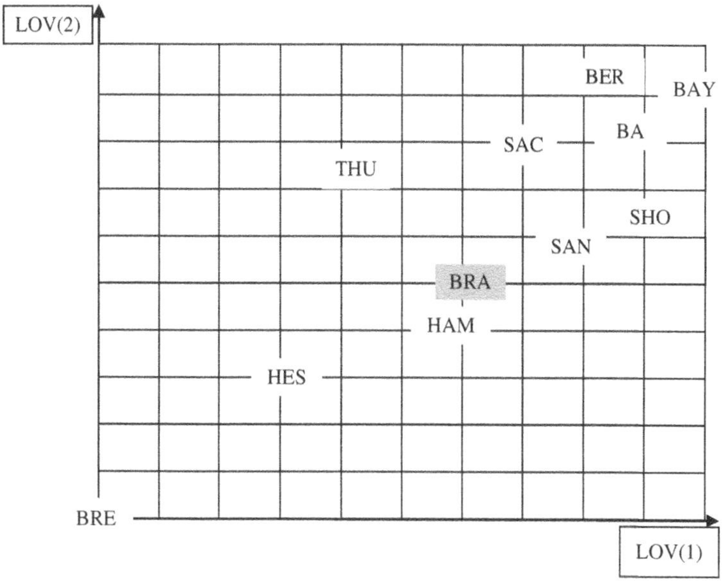

Fig. 11.7 A POSAC-like diagram, drawn after Voigt and Welzl (2002)

The two linear extensions allow a complete embedding of the objects in a two-dimensional coordinate system. The ranks of the two linear extensions can be taken as coordinate values. For example, THU would get (3, 7) and SAN (7, 5).

Now POSAC tries to find two coordinates preserving the comparabilities as much as possible (see Section 3.5). The procedure is based on an optimization algorithm, hence it may obtain the correct coordinate-wise representation only approximately. Indeed, the POSAC routine, as provided in the statistical software SYSTAT, finds a solution with 98% accuracy. The POSAC result is shown in Fig. 11.7.

Figure 11.7 shows the representatives. One can see that BRA is comparable to HAM, according to the POSAC diagram. However, in reality, it is incomparable.

This example shows that dimension theory (see Chapter 3, Section 3.5) has some useful applications here. Voigt and Welzl show that LOV(1) is mainly determined by KC, whereas for LOV(2), the indicators MS, OP, and KC contribute nearly to the same extent.

11.4 Illustrative Case Study: Fish Communities in Wetlands (Biology)

11.4.1 Introduction

Wetlands of Gosen are located southeast of Berlin, capital of Germany. There are 12 creeks whose maintenance is cost intensive. There are many considerations for being "important," for example, rare macrophytes and the riparian zone as ecotone.

Here, however, the fish communities are of main interest, because some of the fish species belong to the "red list species." That means there is a risk that closing a creek may cause the extinction of rare fish species. Scientists of the Leibniz-Institute of Freshwater Ecology and Inland Fisheries investigate these 12 creeks with respect to their fish communities (Bruggemann et al., 2002).

Hence:

- Object set $X = \{$gs, gv, gl, gm, ga, gz, A, F, G, K, M, T$\}$.
- IB consists of nine indicators measuring the abundance of nine fish species.
- Orientation of the attributes: A creek with more individuals of any of the nine fish species is considered as more important than a creek with less.

Thus a 12×9 matrix of abundance measurements was obtained and is to be evaluated.

11.4.2 Attribute-Related Sensitivity Study

Figure 11.8 shows the Hasse diagram of this data matrix. There are seven maximal elements. These seven creeks should be maintained because there are no other creeks that are better.[1]

There clearly arises one question: Which fish species influences that result most? Perhaps the Hasse diagram collapses to only some few maximal elements if the indicator of one fish species could be deleted from the data matrix. The attribute-related sensitivity study by means of the matrix W showed that the most important indicator is the number of individuals of a small fish, called "crucian carp."

Why is this little fish so important for the structure of the Hasse diagram? The reason is that the crucian carp is, on the one hand, very weak in competition for nutrients compared to the other eight fish species. On the other hand, the crucian

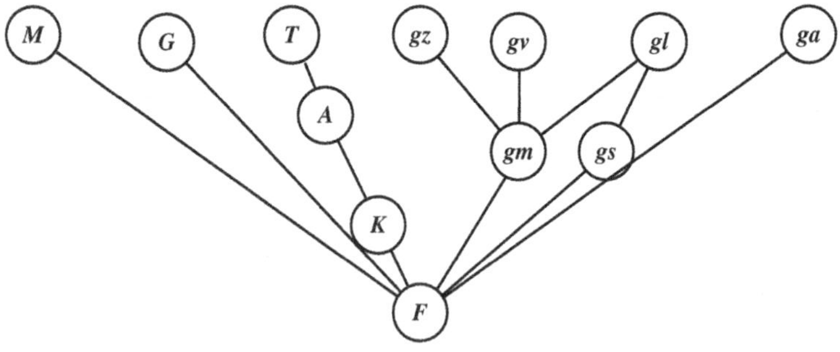

Fig. 11.8 Creeks of the wetlands of Gosen, ordered by the abundances of nine fish species

[1] Whether or not the remaining five creeks can be closed depends on the topology of the networks of creeks and is here of minor interest.

carp tolerates bad conditions, i.e., very shallow and warm, i.e. oxygen-deficient creeks. Other fish species avoid these creeks. Hence there is a trade-off: If the crucian carp is present, then the other fish species are not or almost not present, or when other fish species prefer a certain creek, then the crucian carp tends to stay in other ones. Therefore, this small fish induces many incomparabilities. Deleting the column "abundance of crucian carp" from the data matrix will replace many of these incomparabilities. Hence, the abundance of the crucian carp is the most important indicator for the Hasse diagram.

11.5 Illustrative Case Study: Ranking of High Production Volume Chemicals (HPVCs) (Environmental Chemistry)

11.5.1 Introduction

The evaluation of marketed chemicals is confronted with around 1,00,000 already used chemicals. Yearly around 1,000 chemicals are appearing newly on the market. The current number of existing substances marketed in volumes above 1 ton is estimated to be 30,000. With REACH (registration, evaluation and authorization of chemicals) a new impact was given to rank chemicals (see, for instance, Ahlers et al., 2008; Führ and Bizer, 2007): Before sophisticated but rather expensive and time-consuming risk assessment studies (for instance, by application of the simulation model EUSES; see, e.g., Attias et al., 2005) are performed, one wants to rank with easily available indicators in order to find out the most important chemicals to save time and costs.

11.5.2 Partial Order

As an example, 12 high production volume chemicals (HPVC) were selected (Lerche et al., 2002). Let us repeat the main questions and steps in a ranking study:

What is the aim of ranking? Environmental hazard

How can we describe the environmental hazard?

By attributes like the production volume (prod.vol), toxicity (tox.), accumulation tendency (acc), and probable lifetime of a chemical (degrad.).

What orientation should be selected?

- *Production volume*: We let it as it is; large values indicate an hazard
- *Toxicity*: We have to revert the data (for example, by multiplication with −1)
- *Accumulation*: We let it as it is; large values indicate an hazard
- *Degradation*: In the literature, one finds biodegradation in percentage per day. That means the larger the number, the higher the degree of degradation, and the lower the lifetime of a chemical in our environment, the lesser their adverse impact on the environment. Therefore, we have to revert the data.

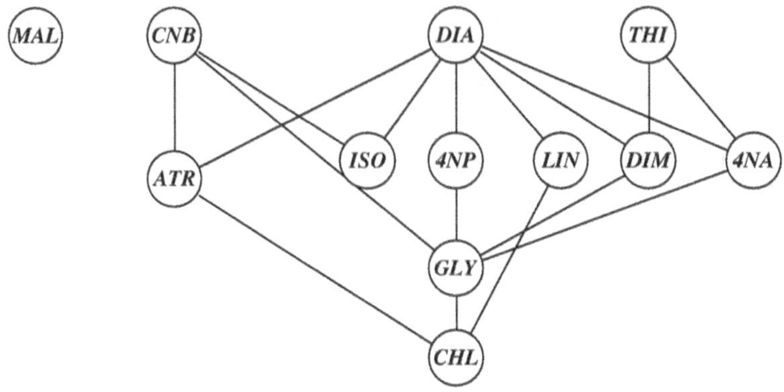

Fig. 11.9 Hasse diagram of high production volume chemicals (HPVCs) under accumulation, toxicity, and lifetime

What are the objects?

Twelve chemicals with a rather high production volume, for which abbreviations like MAL, CHL, GLY, and ISO are used to identify them in the Hasse diagram.

The following example should illustrate the role and the use of CAM, the cumulative ambiguity maximum. Therefore, we simulate the effect of adding an indicator. We omit for the moment the information production volume and see how the Hasse diagram looks like and which value we get for CAM (Fig. 11.9).

11.5.3 Cumulative Ambiguity Maximum (CAM)

Software WHASSE renders the value 0.621 for $CAM_{object\ set}$.

Following the lines of Chapter 4, an impact on the Hasse diagram is to be expected if an indicator is either deleted from or added to the data matrix. Therefore, it might be good to look for further indicators to characterize the objects. Indeed we have one indicator left in our background, the production volume.

Figure 11.10 shows the Hasse diagram, which is obtained by inserting the corresponding data column "production volume" in the data matrix.

Now, $CAM_{object\ set} = 0.76$.

CAM increased from 0.621 to 0.76. Hence the impact on a Hasse diagram by adding new indicators is decreased. Inspection of Fig. 11.10 shows three components (compare Chapter 2). Therefore, the high number of incomparabilities is plausible. More attributes would further reduce the number of comparabilities and introduce more ambiguity into the ranking study. Thus – if there are no urgent contextual requirements for the introduction of further indicators – we do not need to find more of them.

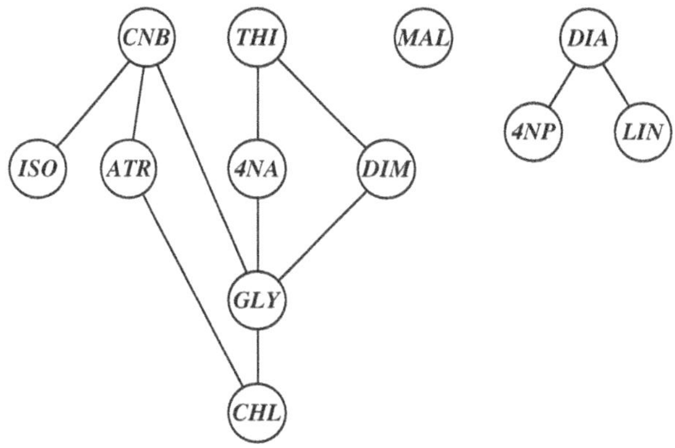

Fig. 11.10 Hasse diagram of HPVCs under production volume, accumulation, toxicity, and lifetime

11.5.4 Antagonism

Inspecting the Hasse diagram in Fig. 11.10, we may wonder as to how the separation $X_1 = \{\text{DIA, LIN, 4NP}\}$ from $X_{res} = X - X_1$ can be explained. Using methods explained in Chapter 5

$$\text{Sep}(X_1, X_{res}, \{\text{PV, log KOW}\}) = 0.815$$

Therefore, we can display the order relations by an approximate scatter plot (Fig. 11.11).

In Fig. 11.11, the objects of X_{res} which are not minimal, maximal, or isolated elements are located within the grey field. As the separation is not complete, some comparabilities among elements of X_1 and X_{res} are still present. Some of these relations are indicated by ●——● lines.

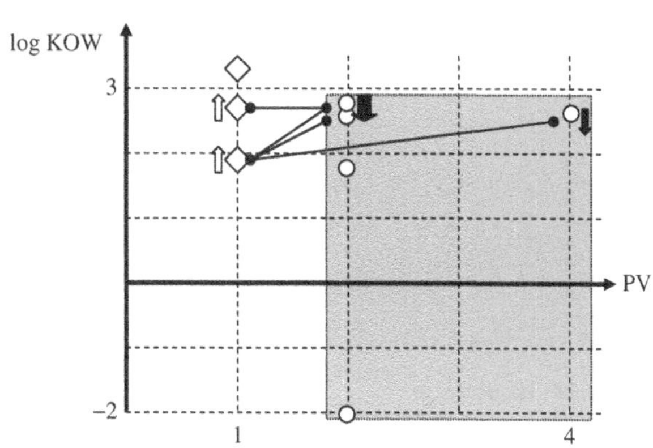

Fig. 11.11 The objects of X_1 are denoted as *diamonds*, whereas the *circles* are the elements of MIN, MAX, and ISO of (X_{res}, IB) (see text)

The indicator BD (lifetimes of chemicals) completes the separation. The block arrows indicate how adding BD breaks the comparabilities such that

$$\text{AIB} = \{\text{PV, log KOW, BD}\} \text{ and } \text{Sep}(X_1, X_{\text{res}}, \text{AIB}) = 1.$$

11.6 Illustrative Case Study: Ecological Value of Communes (Ecology)

11.6.1 Introduction

For a study, 15 out of 108 communes in Italy (Val Baganza near Parma) were arbitrarily selected and denoted as a, $b, \ldots, o$.

In Val Baganza, the most frequent CORINE Biotope habitats are

- lowland hay meadows
- Medio-European rich soil thickets
- subalpine thermophile siliceous grasslands
- northern Apennine Mesobromion grasslands.

The task is to estimate the ecological value of the 15 communes. However, there is no measure to quantify the ecological value. Hence we need proxies by which the unknown ecological value may be quantified (Fig. 11.12, hierarchy of proxies).

Rossi et al. (2008) defined the following indicators as proxies for ecological value (see Rossi, 2001 for background material):

size_ha: All the other things being equal, the biodiversity tends to increase with the habitat size and is therefore indicating an ecological value.

vert_rich: All the other things being equal, the value of a habitat seems to be positively correlated with the number of vertebrates, whose ranges cover the habitat.

h_rarity: Value of a Corine Biotope habitat within the size of the area studied.

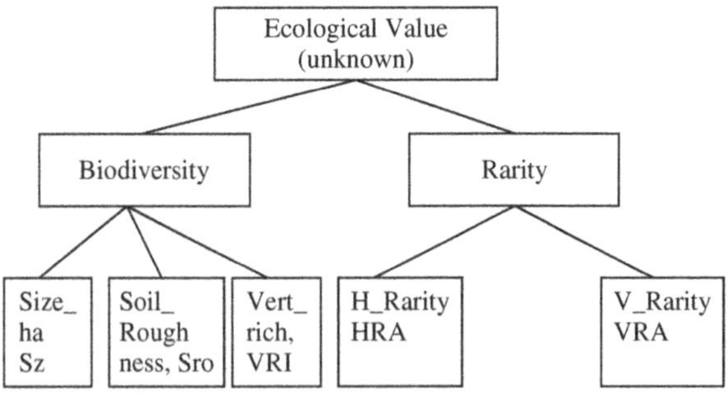

Fig. 11.12 Hierarchy of criteria to describe ecological value. Abbreviations, such as Sz and Sro, are used

v_rarity: Involvement of the Corine Biotope habitats in those areas which host rare vertebrates.

soil_rough: Value of a habitat with reference to its soil roughness. The irregular topography of each Corine Biotope habitat has been computed as a coefficient of variation (CV):

$$\text{CV} = [\text{std. dev. (altitude)}/(\text{mean(altitude)})]^{*}100 \tag{11.1}$$

11.6.2 Partial Order

The data matrix consists of 15 rows and 5 indicators, $|X| = 15$, $|\text{IB}| = 5$. In Fig. 11.13, the Hasse diagram of (X, IB) is shown.

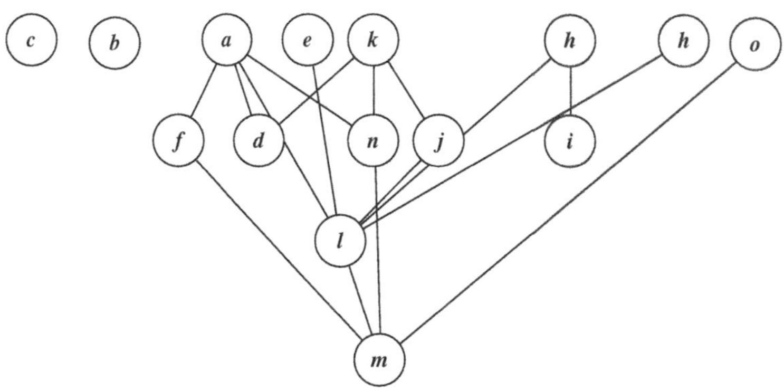

Fig. 11.13 Hasse diagram of 15 Italian communes, IB = {VRI, HRA, VRA, Sro, Sz}

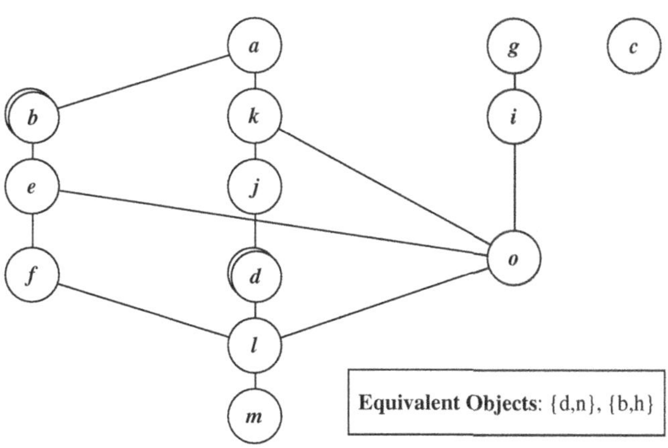

Fig. 11.14 Hasse diagram of 15 arbitrarily selected communes (out of 108) and five indicators {VRI, HRA, VRA, Sro, SZ}, each one with the scores 0,1,2

Following the principle of "ordinal modeling," we also perform a discretization with the discretization scheme $K = 3$, with minimum and maximum values taken from the data matrix (see Chapter 6) and Table A.6. The resulting Hasse diagram is shown in Fig. 11.14.

We see that the Hasse diagram (Fig. 11.14) has many comparabilities, hence the selection of the five indicators seems to describe a common concept, which we interpret as "ecological value" of these communes.

We see furthermore that there is one commune, *c*, which is isolated, hence this commune may be more intensively analyzed, applying, for example, the tool of antagonism (Chapter 5). As we already applied antagonism in several application chapters, and as the isolation of commune *c* may just arise from the arbitrariness of the selection of the communes, we exclude this analysis.

11.6.3 Attempts to Improve the Position in the Partial Order (Attribute Value Sensitivity)

Now assume that the communes would like to try to improve their ecological status. Let us select those communes which are presently located at the fifth level (one level below the top one).

The representative communes are *h*, *k*, *i*.

Indicators which already have the score 2 are not changed, because they are in the best state. In Table 11.4, applying $\Delta=1$, the actual and the simulated tuples of indicators are shown together with the effects on successors and predecessors.

Figure 11.15 visualizes the results for the commune *h* following the data in Table 11.4.

Figure 11.15 shows the change for commune *h* in terms of its successors and its predecessors if the indicator value is increased by $\Delta=1$.

Table 11.4 Simulated data and their effects on characteristics of the partial order

Object	Standard VRI, HRA, VRA, Sro, Sz	Simulated tuple	Change of successors[1]	Change of predecessors
h	21210	**2**2210	5	−1
		212**2**0	2	−1
		2121**1**	2	0
k	22110	22**2**10	5	−1
		221**2**0	0	−1
		2211**1**	1	−1
i	21011	2**2**011	2	−1
		21**1**11	0	0
		210**2**1	0	0
		2102**2**	0	0

The simulated value is in bold literals
[1]Equivalent elements are counted as successors

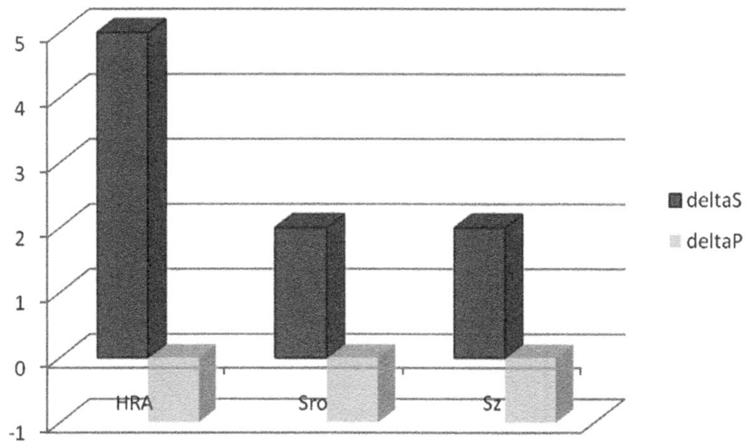

Fig. 11.15 Attribute value sensitivity (avs) (Chapter 4) of the commune *h*

From Table 11.4 one can deduce that for commune *h*, the most important effect is to change for the attribute HRA from score 1 to 2. In this case it gets five more successors. Hence, in any index ranking, these five additional successors must be below commune *h*. Somewhat worse but still efficient is the change of the other two attributes, Sro and Sz. Commune *k*: Most efficient is the change in attribute VRA, where *k* wins five additional successors. One additional successor is obtained if Sz is enhanced from 0 to 1.

Commune *i*: Here, only attribute HRA improves the situation. Commune *i* gets two more successors and becomes a maximal element.

11.7 Illustrative Case Study: Chemicals in a River (Environmental Chemistry)

11.7.1 Introduction

The background may be that an accident happens which releases a mixture of substances. Here we select chemicals whose systematic name is "alkanes." In Fig. 11.16, some simplified chemical formulas are shown.

Fig. 11.16 Chemical formulas of three alkanes. *From left to right*: propane, 2-methylbutane, and 2,2-dimethylpropane

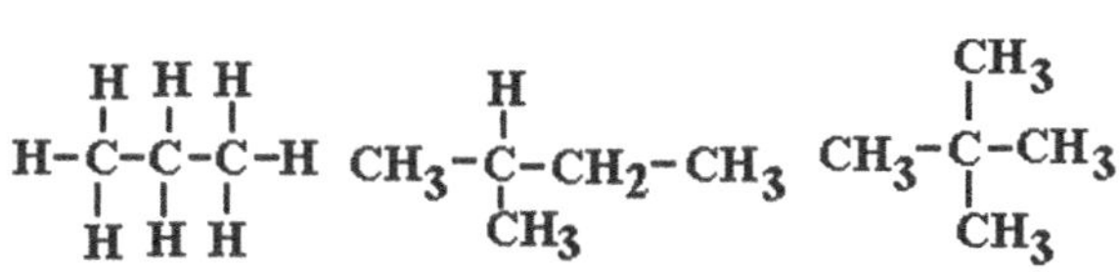

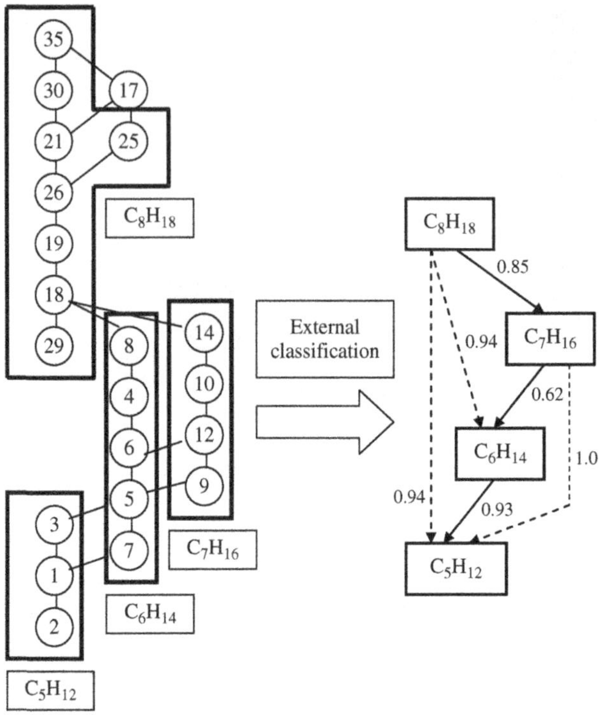

Fig. 11.17 (*LHS*) Hasse diagram of the quotient set of alkanes. (*RHS*) The resulting dominance graph (see text)

Restrepo et al. (2007) analyzed the chemical class of alkanes. In Fig. 11.17 (LHS), the Hasse diagram of (X, IB) is shown. (The numbers within the circles indicate different molecules. The rectangles indicate the compounds having the same sum formula C_nH_m.)

In the partial order (X, IB), X is the object set consisting of alkanes with carbon number between 5 and 8, and IB is the set of indicators describing the sedimentation, downstream transport, and volatilization of the chemicals. The indicator values are calculated by means of EXWAT, assuming some environmental data of a river (Matthies et al., 1989; Bruggemann and Drescher-Kaden, 2003; Bruggemann et al., 2006). Orientation: The larger the values of the indicators, the higher the hazard the chemicals exert.

11.7.2 Dominance

We pose the question: Is the fate of chemicals in the river governed by molecular weight, or branching of a chemical structure, or the maximal length of the carbon chain? To answer this question, classify the chemicals into subsets of compounds according to their sum formula. Thus molecules with different chemical structure belong to the same class, because they have the same number of carbon and hydrogen atoms. Thus the chemical structural information allows us to assign an additional structure to the Hasse diagram, namely that of chemical classes (rectangles in the diagram). Now among these chemical classes, the dominance values for any pair can be calculated applying the software.

PyHasse: The result is shown in Fig. 11.17 (RHS). The directed edges are evaluated by $\max(\mathrm{Dom}(X_1, X_2), \mathrm{Dom}(X_2, X_1))$. Broken lines correspond to transitivity relations. We find the dominance sequence $C_8H_{18} > C_7H_{16} > C_6H_{14} > C_5H_{12}$.

In detail:

- The directed edges indicate the prevailing fraction of order relations. For members of the chemical class C_6H_{14}, x, and members of C_5H_{12}, y in 93.3% of all cases $x \geq y$.
- We interpret the diagram as follows: Independent of the branching or other structural peculiarities of the molecules, the environmental loading is mainly determined by the molecular weight.
- The larger the weight, the more hazardous the chemical with respect to its fate descriptors in rivers. The dominance analysis established a canonical sequence of classes of molecules corresponding to their molecular weight.

11.8 Illustrative Case Study: Management in a River Basin

11.8.1 Background Information

Let us consider an example from water management in the river Elbe basin which is located in middle/east Europe (Behrendt et al., 2002).

The water management in the watershed of river Elbe is faced with

- regional consequences (as one of the sustainability principles)
- different loadings (pressure indicators, see OECD: http://de.wikipedia.org/wiki/DPSIR, see also Kristensen (2004): http://enviro.lclark.edu:8002/servlet/SBRead?ResourceServlet?rid=1145949501662_742777852_522)
- attempts to apply different measures, aiming toward a reduction of pressures on the river Elbe and its tributaries.

Forecasting the impacts of different scenarios of water management strategies on the Elbe river basin cannot realistically be simulated by field experiments. Therefore, a mathematical simulation model is necessary. The model MONERIS (Behrendt et al., 2002) is a regional water quality model, which takes into account different inputs within a watershed and estimates retardation factors and degrees of elimination by reactions or volatilization. Eight indicators, concerning different speciations and pathways of nitrogen into surface waters, were calculated in order to characterize the scenarios. Following the DPSIR concept of the OECD, the eight indicators are classified as pressure indicators. Their orientation is as follows: High pressures are expressed by high values of the indicators and indicate a bad status of the surface waters in the river Elbe basin.

11.8.2 The Hasse Diagram

Following Behrendt (personal communication), 14 scenarios of water management strategies are selected (see Table 11.5).

For any scenario, the eight indicators are estimated by means of MONERIS. Additionally the measured eight indicators for the years 1985, 1995, and 1999 were included into the final data matrix as reference years. The structure of the 17 × 8 data matrix as basis for the partial order analysis is shown in Fig. 11.18.

Table 11.5 Fourteen water management scenarios

Scenario	Type	Explanation (Behrendt, Opitz)
1	Rural	10% reduction of tile drained area
2	Rural	20% reduction of tile drained area
3	Rural	25% of arable land will be cultivated without plough
4	Rural	50% of arable land will be cultivated without plough
5	Rural	75% of arable land will be cultivated without plough
6	Marketing	Detergents with P will be replaced by P-free detergents in Czech Republic
7	Technical/urban	All particulate sewage from population not connected to sewers is transported to wastewater treatment plants (wwtp's)
8	Technical/urban	99% of population with sewer connection are connected to wwtp's
9	Technical/urban	50% storage for combined sewers (50% storage corresponds to 11.6 m^3 storage volume per hectare paved urban area)
10	Technical/urban	100% storage for combined sewers (100% storage corresponds to 23.2 m^3 storage volume per hectare paved urban area)
11	Wwtp	All wwtp's are in agreement with the EU wastewater guideline
12	Wwtp	All wwtp's with more than 1,00,000 inhabitants implement an additional microfiltration. P-effluent concentration lower than 0.050 mg/l P
13	Retention	In addition to the surface waters, all wetland areas (according to Corine 346 km^2) are used for retention
14	Retention	0.5% of agricultural area (according to Corine 450 km^2) is transferred to retention areas

Fig. 11.18 Structure of the 17 × 8 data matrix

	$I_1, I_2, I_3, \ldots\ldots I_8$
scenario 1 ... ... scenario 14	Estimation by MONERIS
year 1985 year 1995 year 1999	Measured values

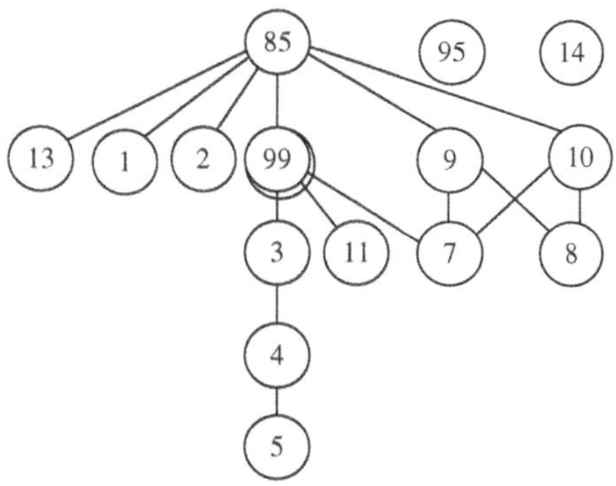

Fig. 11.19 Scenarios 1–14 and the years 1985, 1995, and 1999 ("85," "95," and "99"). Equivalence class: {99, 6, 12}

Thus the analysis of (X, IB) is based on (i) object set X of 17 scenarios; (ii) information base IB of eight indicators; and (iii) orientation: The larger the value, the higher the pressure. Figure 11.19 shows the Hasse diagram.

Figure 11.19 shows the following:

- There is a simultaneous decrease of pressure values for the chain 85 > 99 > 3 > 4 > 5.
- There are isolated elements, namely the year 1995 and the scenario 14.
- The scenarios, intended to improve the water quality in the future, are not necessarily better than reference years.
- Many scenarios are incomparable to the recent year, 1999, of measurements.
- Rural scenarios {1, 2, 3, 4, 5} and technical scenarios {7, 8, 9, 10} are separated subsets (Chapter 5).

11.8.2.1 Use of Superindicators

By an antagonism study, the following result was obtained: $X_1 = \{1, 2, 3, 4, 5\}$, the rural scenarios, $X_2 = \{7, 8, 9, 10\}$, the technical scenarios, $\mathrm{AIB}(X_1, X_2) = \{I_3, I_4, I_7\}$. If the set X_1 is reduced to X_1' to have only the rural scenarios 3, 4, 5, with 25, 50, or 75% of arable land cultivated without plough, then

$\mathrm{Sep}(X_1', X_2, \{I_4, I_7\}) = 1$. The two indicators I_4 and I_7 describe the nitrogen release into surface waters by erosion (I_4) and from wastewater treatment plants (I_7). As these two indicators are responsible for the separation of X_1' and X_2, a combination of both to a superindicator (see Chapter 7) may allow us to compare scenarios of X_1' with those of X_2. The normalized indicators of nitrogen input due to erosion, I_4, and due to point sources, I_7, were combined as follows:

case 1: $0.2^*I_4 + 0.8^*I_7$, case 2: $0.4^*I_4 + 0.6^*I_7$,
case 3: $0.6^*I_4 + 0.4^*I_7$, case 4: $0.8^*I_4 + 0.2^*I_7$

Therefore, four new data matrices were obtained, where the remaining six indicators $\{I_1, I_2, I_3, I_5, I_6, I_8\}$ are not changed but the four superindicators included from four weight combinations. From Fig. 11.20, we see that the relative configuration of scenarios 8, 9, and 10 remains unchanged, while the weights used for the superindicator are varied. Scenario 9 is in all cases worse than the rural scenarios of X_1'. Scenario 7 is comparable with all three rural scenarios and gets its best position relative to the scenarios 3, 4, 5 in case 1, where the indicator I_7 (nitrogen release due to wastewater treatment) has a large weight. Obviously then the good values of I_7 can compensate bad values of I_4. We suspect that the technical needs to improve wastewater treatment plants are easier to fulfill than the needs for improving the

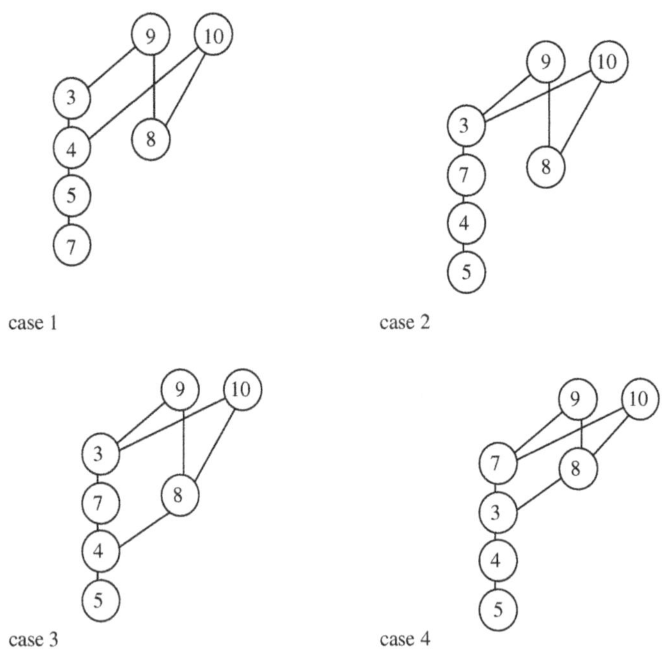

Fig. 11.20 Hasse diagrams of the scenarios {3, 4, 5, 7, 8, 9, 10} corresponding to the four cases (see above)

input due to erosion, which is a process depending on factors, some of which cannot be influenced by technology.

We see that a stepwise aggregation to superindicators (the very idea of METEOR, Chapter 7) can be helpful. The partial order is enriched without averaging over all indicators.

11.9 Illustrative Case Study: The Human Environment Interface Index (HEI) (Environmental Sciences)

11.9.1 Overview and Data Matrix

The human environment interface (HEI) index (Singh, 2008; Patil and Taillie, 2004) is a composite index based on three leading indicators, namely the following:

Land indicator (*L*): The land indicator *L* considers the change in the percentage of the forested land to the total land area with respect to the reference (base) year's characteristic.

Air indicator (*A*): The amount of carbon dioxide emissions per capita of a country for a year denotes the level of the air indicator for that year.

Water indicator (*W*): This indicator is the arithmetic mean of the percentage of population with sustainable access to an improved water source and improved sanitation.

The indicators capture the human progress toward the environmental management. Being expressed in different units, these indicators are first transformed into dimensionless indices. Then an aggregation with equal weights yields the HEI. Lower value reveals less of a country progress toward environmental protection goal. Hence, HEI reflects the managerial efforts a country makes to maintain and improve the greenness of land, blueness of sky, and cleanness of drinking water (Patil, 2000). The ranking-based information is expected to stimulate the countries for the improvement of the existing environment.

All in all the number of countries is 151 for which the HEI can be computed, hence the object set *X* consists of 151 countries and the information base (IB) encompasses three indicators. The case study aims at comparing HEI with the outcomes of partial order.

The complete data matrix, the countries, and the abbreviations used, as well as the HEI, are shown in the appendix (Table A.5).

11.9.2 Ordinal Approaches

The analysis is based on the raw data matrix. The Hasse diagram of (*X*, IB) is shown in Fig. 11.21:

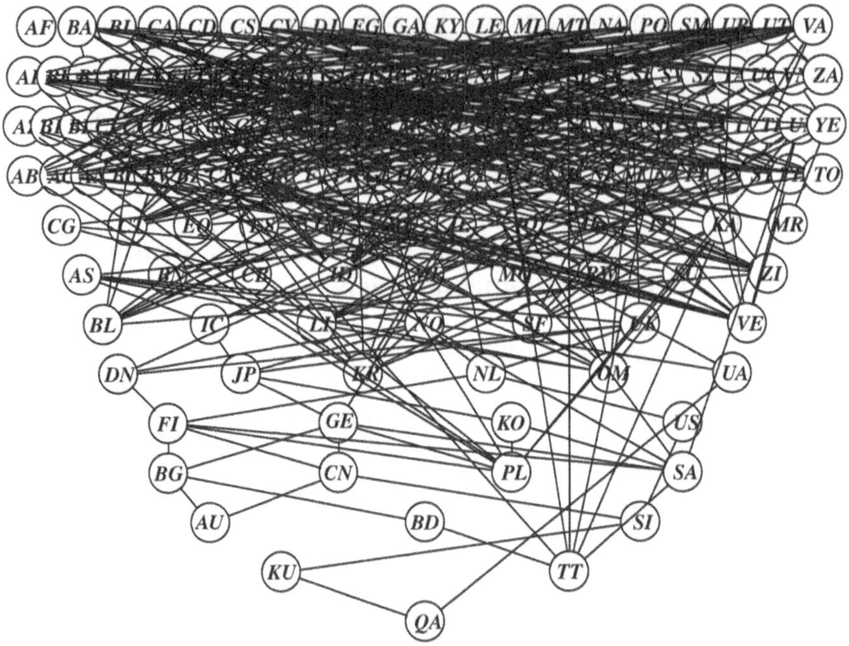

Fig. 11.21 Hasse diagram for 151 countries, based on the indicators *L*, *A*, *W*

- The object set *X* consists of 151 countries.
- The information base IB is $\{L, A, W\}$ and indicators are normalized.
- The orientation: The larger the indicator value, the better the status of the country.

11.9.2.1 Shape

First of all, its shape is striking: The Hasse diagram seems to have a triangular shape (see Chapter 5). With greater values in the indicators, the number of incomparabilities among the countries seems to increase. As we are aware that the shape also depends on the convention of how to draw a Hasse diagram, we apply the analysis tool $U(L(i))$ and the result is shown in Fig. 11.22.

This diagram shows that there is no trend in the number of incomparabilities if we compare the different levels. Indeed there are more minimal than maximal elements.

11.9.2.2 Navigation

The tools are up sets and down sets. For example, when we want to know the position of Germany with respect to other countries, we can look for up sets and down sets (Fig. 11.23).

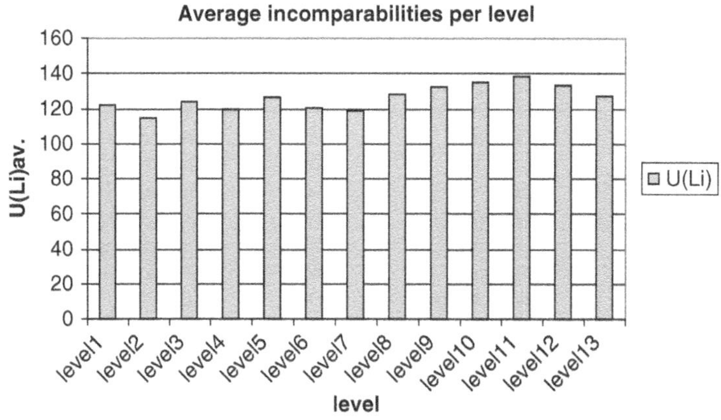

Fig. 11.22 Average incomparabilities per level

Fig. 11.23 (*LHS*): *F*(GE) (up set of GE); (*RHS*): *O*(GE) (down set of GE) (software PyHasse)

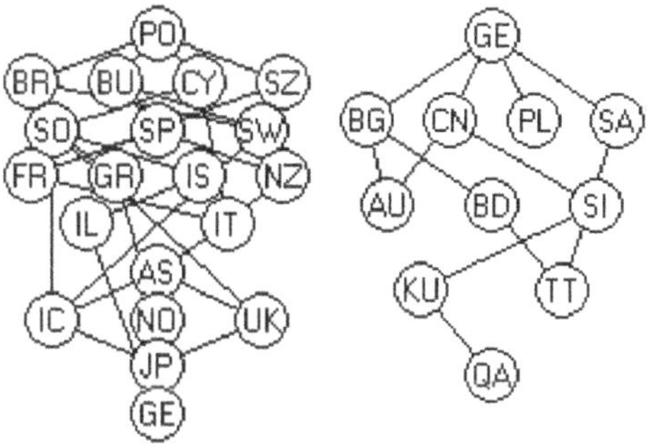

There are 19 other countries in which all three indicators are better (F(GE)), and there are 10 countries in which all three indicators are worse (O(GE)) than those in Germany. There are no connections to 121 other countries (U(GE) = 121), therefore the profile of Germany based on *L*, *A*, and *W* must be rather peculiar.

11.9.3 Dominance Degree of Contextual Subsets

Consider, for example, the European nations (Table 11.6). We pose the following question: Is the highly industrialized middle Europe dominated by the lower industrialized and hence less polluted south Europe? We address this question by applying the dominance-separability approach as explained in Chapter 5.

We calculate the dominance degree and separabilities. In Table 11.7, the dominance degrees (Dom(*i*,*j*) and Dom(*j*,*i*)) and the separabilities Sep(*i*,*j*) can be found (i, j = SE, ME, ..., NE).

Table 11.6 Countries of Europe, classified to belong to north Europe (NE), west Europe (WE), middle Europe (ME), south Europe (SE), and East Europe (OE)

Country	Subset	Country	Subset	Country	Subset
Albania	SE	Iceland	WE	Germany	ME
Austria	ME	Ireland	WE	Greece	SE
Belgium	WE	Italy	SE	Hungary	OE
Bulgaria	OE	Netherlands	WE	Switzerland	ME
Denmark	NE	Norway	NE	United Kingdom	WE
Finland	NE	Portugal	SE	Slovakia	SE
France	WE	Rep. of Moldova	OE	Spain	SE
Sweden	NE	Ukraine	OE		

Table 11.7 First figure Dom(*i*, *j*) (row *i* dominates column *j*), Dom(*j*, *i*) (column *j* dominates row *i*), and the symmetric separability

	SE	ME	OE	WE	NE
SE	–	0.5, 0.05, 0.44	0.125, 0.08, 0.79	0.61, 0.02, 0.36	0.67, 0, 0.33
ME	–	–	0.08, 0,17, 0.75	0.55, 0.28, 0.17	0.58, 0.17, 0.25
OE	–	–	–	0.21, 0, 0.79	0.25, 0, 0.75
WE	–	–	–	–	0.33, 0.25, 0.42

If $\text{Dom}(x, y) \geq \varepsilon$, with filter ε being 0.5, we draw a directed edge from x to y and obtain the following directed graph (i.e., an extremely small network), see Fig. 11.24.

As can be seen from Fig. 11.24, there is an isolated element, OE. For the other subsets, two maximal chains (dominance sequences, compare Chapter 5) can be found: SE > ME > NE and SE > ME > WE.

In any case, south Europe (SE) has a top position among the countries of Europe.

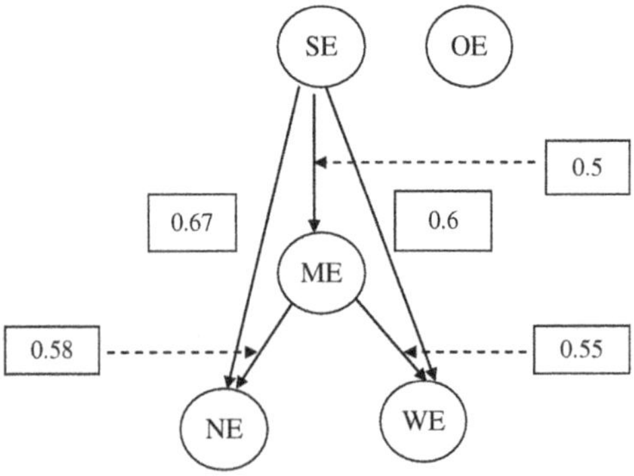

Fig. 11.24 Based on the indices *L*, *A*, and *W*, a dominance diagram is constructed (filter $\varepsilon = 0.5$). For details, see Tables A.19 and A.20

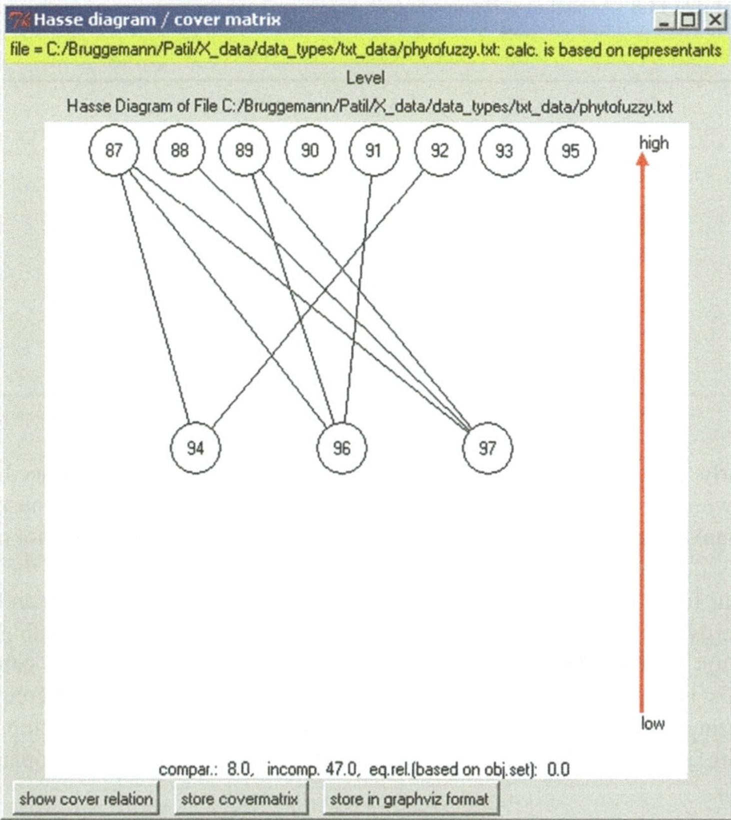

Fig. 11.25 Hasse diagram, based on the data of Table 11.8 (software PyHasse)

11.10 Illustrative Case Study: Analysis of Lake Restoration and Biomanipulation: Example Phytoplankton Community Structure (Biology)

11.10.1 Introduction

The status of a lake (Feldberger Haussee, Germany) needs to be improved (Krienitz et al., 1996). There is a high phytoplankton population and one wants to reduce it by inserting predator fish into the lake. The motivation for this biomanipulation lies in food web theory, but does it work in practice? To answer this question, we applied partial order on the data matrix, where the years 1987 (start of biomanipulation) until 1997 are the objects. The concentrations of five phytoplankton species were selected as indicators. The response of phytoplankton to the changed conditions reflects the success of the biomanipulation measures.

Table 11.8 Annual mean value of phytoplankton group concentrations (mg/l)

Year	Cl	Ba	Cr	Di	Cy	Sum
87	5.5	2.3	5.3	0.8	4.0	17.9
88	3.4	0.6	1.3	1.8	7.0	14.1
89	3.6	1.6	1.3	0.2	6.0	13.7
90	3.2	0.2	0.3	0.1	15.0	18.8
91	3.5	1.8	1.7	0.1	13.0	20.1
92	2.7	0.4	3.9	0.1	21.0	28.1
93	6.7	1.4	1.3	0	8.0	17.4
94	2.6	0.3	2.8	0	2.0	7.7
95	0.8	1.4	3.5	1.7	7.5	14.9
96	1.7	1.5	1.2	0	2.0	6.4
97	1.8	0.2	0.6	0.2	0.1	2.9

Clearly, it is of interest as to how the phytoplanktonic biomass is reduced. First of all, we can see by means of an indicative function (sum of the biomass over phytoplankton species, see Table 11.8) that the phytoplanktonic mass did not monotonically decrease. Second, the reduction may not impact all species in the same way: Our focus, however is not on the phytoplankton species distribution and their intricate dynamics but on how we can rank the years due to the responding phytoplankton biomass. By means of Hasse diagrams, we can do both: We can rank the years but also make evident that the phytoplanktons respond differently to the grazing stress due to the enhanced zooplanktonic population. Incomparable years are just the order theoretical expression for that different phytoplankton behavior.

11.10.2 Methods and Materials

In this study, we have compiled the annual mean values of the main phytoplankton groups: Chlorophyceae (Cl), Bacillariophyceae (Ba), Cryptophyceae (Cr), Dinophyceae (Di) and Cyanophyceae (Cy); the abbreviations of these phytoplankton groups are indicated in parenthesis. For details of phytoplankton successions in Feldberger Haussee, see Krienitz et al. (1996).

11.10.2.1 Data in the Poset Approach

The years of biomanipulation are considered as our objects and will be comparatively evaluated. Hence the object set is $X = \{87, 88, 89, 90, 91, 92, 93, 94, 95, 96, 97\}$.

The concentrations of five main phytoplankton groups (mg/l) are selected as the indicators, by which the years of biomanipulation are characterized: Therefore, the information base is $\text{IB} = \{\text{Cl, Ba, Cr, Di, Cy}\}$. The phytoplankton data set as well as the indicative sum of their biomass is shown in Table 11.8.

Related on the sum (Table 11.8 last column) the ranking of the years would be

$$92 > 91 > 90 > 87 > 93 > 95 > 88 > 89 > 94 > 96 > 97$$

The order of years indicates that the expectation of the longer the biomanipulation, the smaller the phytoplanktonic biomass is not correct. Was biomanipulation successful?

11.10.2.2 Partial Order

Based on the data set of Table 11.8, the Hasse diagram encompassing all years is shown in Fig. 11.25.

We see two levels and three isolated objects (90, 93, 95). The year 1987, when the biomanipulation started, is in the same level as six subsequent years. Only three years, 94, 96, and 97, show the desired dependency. What happens? Once again: Was the biomanipulation successful? However, we must take care of the ordinal character of Hasse diagrams. So we follow the idea of ordinal modeling (see Chapter 6): We could perform a discretization of data or a fuzzy analysis. Here we will apply the concept of fuzzy partial order.

11.10.3 Results of Fuzzy Partial Order

In fuzzy partial order (Chapter 6), the degree of what should be considered as "noise" is mapped onto the tolerance level α. Correspondingly, we can find a series of Hasse diagrams, beginning with a very high degree of tolerance and ending with the lowest degree of tolerance, where any measurement detail is ordinal interpreted.

There are 31 α cuts with the lowest at 0.406 and the highest at 1:

- With the α less than 0.406, we consider all data differences as irrelevant. Hence, all years are put into one equivalence class. We do not see any differentiation and hence we cannot decide whether the biomanipulation was successful.
- If we select $\alpha = 0.45$, then all differentiations are still neglected, except the greatest one: The years 87, 88, ..., 96 form one equivalence class. Year 97 is a singleton. The Hasse diagram based on this tolerance level (see Fig. 11.26) tells us that within this crude ordinal modeling, indeed there was an improvement from the starting year 1987 compared with the final year 1997!
- If we selected $\alpha = 0.55$, then a chain of three elements is obtained $97 < 94 < 87$ (Fig. 11.26).
- Further increasing α values leads to a nonlinear structure of the partial order which indicates that nature does not react linearly, but due to different phytoplankton types differently on the grazing pressure. Still a chain of years corresponding to the expectation $97 < 96 < 94 < 88 < 87$ can be identified.

If α is selected higher or equal to 0.9, then we see a breakdown of the order. We can no more conclude that the biomanipulation works as expected over the years.

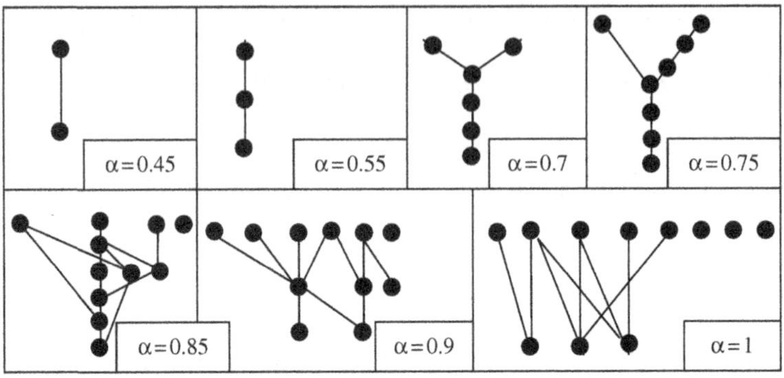

Fig. 11.26 Evolution of (not labeled) Hasse diagrams (PyHasse, see Chapter 17)

There are many possible reactions which even lead to incomparability between the last two years, i.e., between 96 and 97. Even worse, isolated objects occur. Hence we may say that now the final two Hasse diagrams are a result of the biological complexity, which masks the general trend of the years of biomanipulation.

In Fig. 11.26, the Hasse diagram corresponding to $\alpha = 1$ is what we already have seen: It is just the Hasse diagram of the original data, i.e., if any measurement detail is brought into evidence by the partial order concept. Taking the results shown in Fig. 11.26, together with the tendency to render 97 as a minimal element, there is a clear evidence that the biomanipulation should be considered successful.

References

Ahlers, J., Stock, F. and Werschkun, B. (2008). Integrated testing and intelligent assessment – New challenges under REACH. ESPR-Environ. Sci. Pollut. Res., 15, 565–572.

Alkanes. http://www.docbrown.info/page06/DFalkanes.htm.

Attias, L., Boccardi, P., Boeije, G., Brooke, D., de Bruijn, J. and Comber, M., et al. (2005). European Union system for the evaluation of substances: The second version. Chemosphere, 59, 473–485.

Behrendt, H., Kornmilch, M., Opitz, D., Schmoll, O. and Scholz, G. (2002). Estimation of the nutrient inputs into river systems – Experiences from German rivers. Reg. Environ. Change, 3, 107–117.

Bruggemann, R. and Drescher-Kaden, U. (2003). Einfuehrung in die modellgestuetzte Bewertung von Umweltchemikalien – Datenabschaetzung, ausbreitung, verhalten, wirkung und Bewertung. Berlin: Springer.

Bruggemann, R., Fredrich, F., Wolter, C., Pudenz, S. and Steinberg, C. (2002). Partielle ordnungen: Ein hilfsmittel zur beschreibung von artengemeinschaften. In A. Gnauck (Ed.), Theorie und modellierung von oekosystemen, Workshop Koelpinsee 2000 (pp. 173–200). Aachen: Shaker-Verlag.

Bruggemann, R., Pudenz, S. and Kreimes, K. (1997). Oekologische Bewertung der Regionen Baden-Wuerttembergs mit neueren mathematischen Techniken. In Landesanstalt fuer Umweltschutz Baden-Wuerttemberg (Ed.), 5. Statuskolloquium Projekt "angewandte Oekologie" 18. und 19. Maerz 1997 Schloss Ettlingen (pp. 335–343). Karlsruhe: Landesanstalt fuer Umweltschutz Baden-Wuerttemberg.

Bruggemann, R., Restrepo, G. and Voigt, K. (2006). Structure – fate relationships of organic chemicals derived from the software packages E4CHEM and WHASSE. J. Chem. Inf. Model., 46, 894–902.

DPSIR. http://de.wikipedia.org/wiki/DPSIR.

Freier, K.P., Bruggemann, R. and Nützmann, G. (2007). Pharmazeutisch aktive Substanzen in kleinen Flieβgewaessern – Modellierung unter Beruecksichtigung des Einflusses von Grundwasser. UWSF – Z.Umweltchem.[TM]kotox., 19(3), 189–196.

Führ, M. and Bizer, K. (2007). REACh as a paradigm shift in chemical policy – responsive regulation and behavioural models. J. Cleaner Prod., 15, 327–334.

Kreimes, K. (1996). Oekologisches Wirkungskataster Baden-Wuerttemberg – Bewertung und zusammenfassende Darstellung von Untersuchungsergebnissen. In U. Arndt, A. Fomin, and S. Lorenz (Eds.), Bio-indikation; neuere Entwicklungen – Nomenklatur – Synoekologische Aspekte; Beitraege und Diskussion 1. Hohenheimer Workshop zur Bioindikation am Kraftwerk Altbach-Deizisau, 1995 (pp. 160–169). Ostfildern: Guenter Heimbach.

Krienitz, L., Kasprzak, P. and Koschel, R. (1996). Long term study on the influence of eutrophication, restoration and biomanipulation on the structure and development of phytoplankton communities in Feldberger Haussee (Baltic Lake District, Germany). Hydrobiologia, 330, 89–110.

Kristensen, P. (2004). The DPSIR framework. http://enviro.lclark.edu:8002/servlet/SBReadResourceServlet?rid=1145949501662_742777852_522.

Landesanstalt fuer Umweltschutz Baden-Wuerttemberg (Ed.). (1994). Signale aus der Natur, 10 Jahre Oekologisches Wirkungskataster Baden-Wuerttemberg. Ettlingen: Kraft Druck GmbH.

Lerche, D., Bruggemann, R., Sorensen, P.B., Carlsen, L. and Nielsen, O.J. (2002). A comparison of partial order technique with three methods of multicriteria analysis for ranking of chemical substances. J. Chem. Inf. Comput. Sci., 42, 1086–1098.

Matthies, M., Bruggemann, R., Muenzer, B., Schernewski, G. and Trapp, S. (1989). Exposure and ecotoxicity estimation for environmental chemicals (E4CHEM): Application of fate models for surface waters and soils. Ecol. Model., 47, 115–130.

Patil, G.P. (2000). UNEP workshop on human environment interface index. Washington, DC.

Patil, G.P. and Taillie, C. (2004). Multiple indicators, partially ordered sets, and linear extensions: Multi-criterion ranking and prioritization. Environ. Ecol. Stat., 11, 199–228.

Restrepo, G., Bruggemann, R. and Voigt, K. (2007). Partially ordered sets in the analysis of alkanes fate in rivers. Croatica Chem. Acta, 80(2), 261–270.

Rossi, O. (Ed.) (2001). Cartografia multiscalare della natura – testo delle relazioni. IX Congresso Nazionale Della Societa Italiana Di Ecologia, Lecce Settembre 1999, University of Parma, Parma, Italy.

Rossi, F., Pecci, A., Amadio, V., Rossi, O. and Soliani, L. (2008). Coupling indicators of ecological value and ecological sensitivity with indicators of demographic pressure in the demarcation of new areas to be protected: The case of the Oltrepo Pavese and the Ligurian–Emilian Apennine area (Italy). Landsc. Urban Plann., 86, 12–26.

Singh, A. (2008). UNEP workshop on human environment interface index. Nairobi, Kenya.

Voigt, K. and Welzl, G. (2002). Drinking water analysis systems in German cities: An evaluation approach combining Hasse diagram technique with multivariate statistical methods. In K. Voigt and G. Welzl (Eds.), Order theoretical tools in environmental sciences – Order theory (Hasse diagram technique) meets multivariate statistics (pp. 113–127). Aachen: Shaker-Verlag.

Chapter 12
Case Study: Child Development (Sociology)

12.1 Overview

Starting point is the data matrix made of six indicators describing different aspects of child development and 21 nations, mainly of Europe. A ranking of the 21 nations is based on a composite indicator. Using several methods, we try to assess the construction of the composite indicator of UNICEF. Both the concordance analysis (Chapter 10) and the canonical order (Chapter 9) support the construction of the UNICEF. The comparison with the canonical order is naturally more detailed and we find some rank inversions. With the help of the local partial order model (Chapter 9), we explain these. Without partial order, there is no reason to define separated subsets. The partial order constructed from the six indicators and the 21 nations shows several separated subsets (see Chapter 5). Most striking is the separation between {It, Pt} and the residual set of nations. Which indicators explain this separation and with which values? The partial order identifies the indicators "family" and "education" as the responsible ones. When an aggregation to a composite indicator is performed, the single indicators lose their individuality as they are just summands contributing to the value of the composite indicator. Similarly, one can construct new orders (called the m^r orders, see Chapter 7) which also do not take into account the individuality of the indicators. The resulting partial orders contain pretty long chains of nations which allow unambiguous ranking of many nations without crunching the indicators into one composite indicator. There is a natural question about as to how much the composite indicator-based ranking can be improved by changing the value of an indicator. We do not perform a complete analysis but illustrate the methodological steps with Ireland and Denmark. We show that Ireland can improve its ranking position best if it has better indicator values in "education."

R. Brüggemann, G.P. Patil, *Ranking and Prioritization for Multi-indicator Systems*, Environmental and Ecological Statistics 5, DOI 10.1007/978-1-4419-8477-7_12,

12.2 Basic Information, Data Matrix, and Results of UNICEF Study

This study is based on a report of UNICEF (Innocenti Research Centre, Report Card 7, 2007). A comprehensive assessment of well-being of "children and young people in 21 nations of the industrial world is given" (cited from the report).

The study provided 40 different indicators which are aggregated through several interim steps into six main indicators (Table 12.1).

From the data matrix (see Table A.7), UNICEF defines an index with equal weights for all six indicators, i.e.

$$\Gamma(x) = \Sigma(1/6)^* R_i(x), \text{ weight vector} = (1/6, 1/6, \ldots, 1/6) \tag{12.1}$$

where $R_i(x)$ is the rank by the ith indicator of nation x.

For example, Belgium (Be) has the following data (Table 12.2)

$$\Gamma(\text{Be}) = (1^*7 + 1^*16 + 1^*1 + 1^*5 + 1^*19 + 1^*16)/6 = 10.7$$

From Γ, the following ranking, O_Γ, is deduced (from the worst to the best):

(UK, US, Hu, Au, Pt, Fr, Cz, Pl, Gr, Ca, De, Be, Ire, It, No, Su, Es, Fi, Dk, Sw, Ne)

Table 12.1 Six indicators and their background information

Indicator	Abbreviation	Background information
Material well-being	wb	Relative income poverty, households without jobs, reported deprivation
Health and Safety	hs	Health at birth, immunization, mortality
Educational well-being	ed	Aspirations, achievements, participation
Family and peer relationships	fa	Family structure, family relations, peer relations
Behaviors and risks	br	Risk behavior, experience of violence, health behavior
Subjective well-being	sub	Health, personal well-being, school well-being

Table 12.2 Section out of Table A.7

		wb	hs	ed	fa	br	sub
		Material well-being	Health and safety	Educational well-being	Family and peer relationships	Behaviors and risks	Subjective well-being
Belgium	Be	7	16	1	5	19	16

The top third subset is Ne, Sw, Dk, Fi, Es, Su, No.
The middle third subset is It, Ire, Be, De, Ca, Gr, Pl.
The bottom third subset is Cz, Fr, Pt, Au, Hu, US, UK.

12.3 Motivating the Use of Partial Order

This is a detailed UNICEF study, where the peculiarities of any single nation are commented, and there is a broad discussion on how the six indicators were obtained.

Now any politician of a nation may see that his nation is "good" with respect to some indicator, even if his nation receives a bad overall position in the ranking. Thus Italy is good in the indicator "family," "fa." Naturally the question arises: Is not "family," "fa," more important than the others, say "ed," education, and give "fa" a higher weight? UNICEF, however, used the same weight for each indicator. Hence, the summation (Eq. (12.1)) implies that good points may compensate bad points and vice versa. If, however, such compensation is allowed, then questioning the uniform weight of any indicator in the index is indeed justified. Thus Italy would get a better overall position if the weight for "fa" would get a higher value. Such procedure would however make politicians of other nations unhappy. Poland, for example, is good in education and would therefore like to see this indicator given a higher weight.

There is another issue: The need for defining a composite indicator (like that in Eq. (12.1)) is understandable. However, as the UNICEF report indicates, there is in some of the six indicators a high degree of conceptual overlapping. For example, the indicator "he," health, is one of the six indicators. However, the indicator health is also partly present in the indicator "sub," "subjective well-being." This kind of conceptual overlap means that health is more pronounced in the ranking, because it appears two times, once explicitly in "health" and once implicitly in "sub." Hence, it may be a good idea to keep the six indicators separated, but simultaneously analyzed rather than composited.

12.4 Partial Order Analysis

12.4.1 Aims of Partial Order Analysis

1. Can we find chains of nations, where the status of one country is comparably fixed with respect to some others? There may be a real need to improve child well-being in one or more of the six attributes for such countries which worry about their poor position.
2. Are there countries whose positions will severely depend on how the six indicators are combined? They may initialize an update of the study to show how different weight vectors can influence their positions.

12.4.2 Hasse Diagram of 21 Nations Based on Six Indicators

In Fig. 12.1, the Hasse diagram is shown based on the entries of Table A.7. We rearranged the table so that the "good" nations are on the top of the Hasse diagram. The information base, IB, is {wb, hs, ed, fa, br, sub}. In order to include USA, the missing value in the indicator "sub" was given the mean value taken from the 20 nations.

12.4.2.1 Structural Characterization

There are six components, four of which are trivial, i.e., are isolated elements (see Chapter 2). One nontrivial component consists of the majority of nations $X_1 = \{\text{Ne, Sw, No}, \ldots,\}$ and the other one consists of Italy and Portugal $X_2 = \{\text{It, Pt}\}$. The set ISO (see Chapter 2) contains the isolated nations Be, Ca, Pl, and Au. How different components are related with the data matrix is studied below. UK, Ne, and Dk are articulation points (Chapter 5). Removing, for example, UK from the data matrix would make Su an isolated element. Removal of Ne from the data matrix would generate two new components. Su is an example of a "loosely" connected object. Isolated and loosely connected ones need our attention because of their peculiar data profiles. The tool to find out the peculiarity is the search for antagonistic indicators.

12.4.2.2 Level

The Hasse diagram provides three levels. Generally speaking, this low number of levels means that there are many incomparabilities. Large $U(x)$ sets (see Chapter 3) in turn indicate that many nations have some indicator values which make them better and some other indicator values which make them worse than others. Here are the three levels (see Chapter 5):

$\text{level}_3 = \{\text{Ne, Su, No, Sw, Fi, Dk, It, Be, Ca, Pl, Au}\}$,
$\text{level}_2 = \{\text{Ire, Hu, Es, De, Cz, Fr, Pt}\}$, and
$\text{level}_1 = \{\text{Gr, UK, US}\}$.

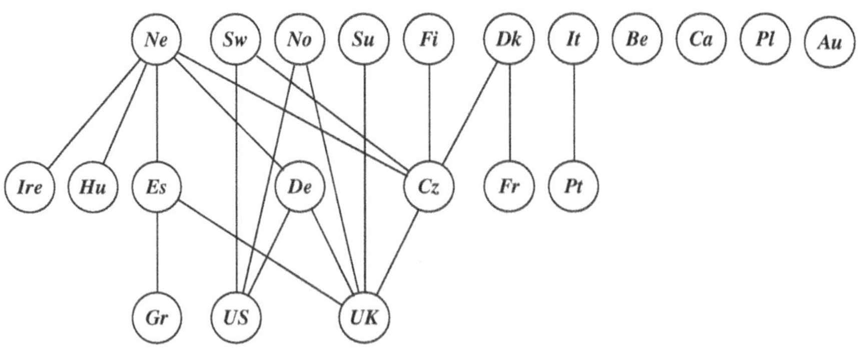

Fig. 12.1 Hasse diagram of 21 nations, IB = {wb, hs, fa, ed, br, sub}

There is the set of isolated elements ISO = {Be, Ca, Pl, Au} and a nontrivial component Pt $\leq$ It.

12.4.2.3 Concordance Analysis

In Chapter 2, we have learned that the drawing of a Hasse diagram is not unique. Therefore, we must examine two scenarios using concordance analysis (see Chapter 10):

Scenario H: The objects are given the highest level possible.
Scenario L: The objects are given the lowest level possible.

In Table 12.3, the number of objects related to scenario H is in bold, while that of scenario L is in italic letters. The concordance indices, con, referring only to the main diagonal (because of only three subsets) are as follows:

Scenario H: con = 10/21 = 0.48 > T = 0.333 (d is the dimension of concordance matrix = 3)
Scenario L: con = 12/21 = 0.57 > T = 0.333 (d is the dimension of concordance matrix = 3)

Thus the level provided by partial order theory corresponds pretty well to the classification by means of Γ.

Table 12.3 Concordance analysis for scenarios *H* and L

	Subsets in UNICEF		
Subsets in partial order	Ne, Sw, Dk, Fi, Es, Su, No	It, Ire, Be, De, Ca, Gr, Pl	Cz, Fr, Pt, Au, Hu, US, UK
Ne, Sw, No, Su, Fi, Dk, It, Be, Ca, Pl, Au	**6**	**4**	**1**
Ne, Sw, Dk, Fi	*4*	*0*	*0*
Ire, Hu, Es, De, Cz, Fr, Pt	**1**	**2**	**4**
Es, De, Cz, Su, No, It	*3*	*2*	*1*
Gr, US, UK	**0**	**1**	**2**
Ire, Hu, Gr, US, UK, Fr, Pt, Be, Ca, Pl, Au	*0*	*5*	*6*

12.4.2.4 Chains

The maximal chain length equals 3. There are eight chains of maximal length 3 and eight chains of maximal length 2. The identification of chains is an important tool to find the invariant mutual order among the nations. Let us take one three-element chain like UK < De < Ne. As discussed in Chapter 7, the relative ranking of the elements of a chain will be invariant relative to the weight vector. Thus Germany, De, is in all indicators worse than the Netherlands. Clearly, for Germany, it is not possible to suggest any weight vector to get a better ranking result than Netherlands. Germany must improve the situation for children, leading to better values for the indicators. In Section 12.9.2, we will have more discussion on this.

12.4.2.5 Antichains

There are more and longer antichains than chains, indicating that incomparability is the dominant factor. Isolated elements or weakly connected elements like Su or Fr, or the chain Pt < It, will have large U(x) sets and large ranking intervals. Following Chapter 3, large ranking intervals imply high influence of weights on the final ranking positions (see Eq. (3.19)).

12.5 Indicator Set

12.5.1 Attribute-Related Sensitivity

In Fig. 12.2, the values $W(X, \text{IB}, \text{IB} - \{q_i\})$, $i = 1, \ldots, 6$ (for details, see Chapter 4), are shown.

Figure 12.2 shows that the most important indicator is fa, "family and peer relationships," and the least one is br, "behavior and risks." If indicator fa is deleted from the data matrix, then the Hasse diagram (Fig. 12.3) is obtained.

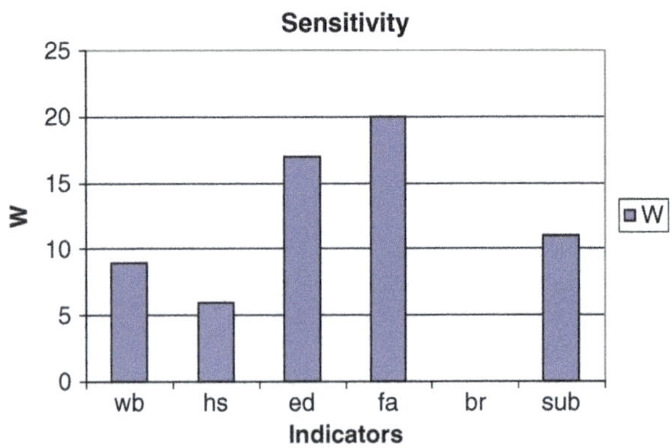

Fig. 12.2 Attribute-related sensitivity of the six indicators to the Hasse diagram

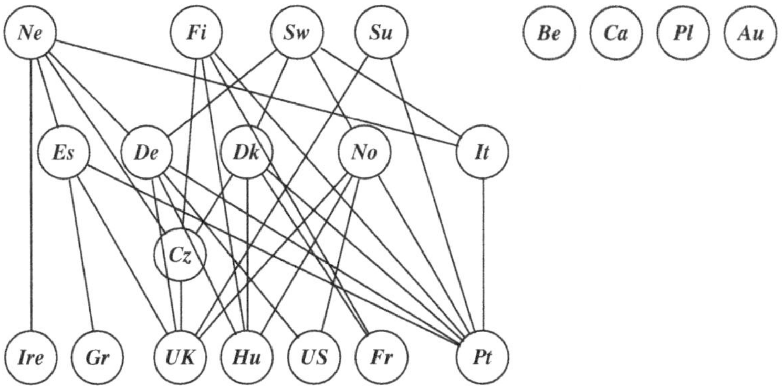

Fig. 12.3 Effect of deleting indicator fa from the data matrix

We note the following:

- The longest chain contains UK $\leq$ Cz $\leq$ Dk $\leq$ Sw, hence four levels can be identified.
- The four isolated elements Be, Ca, Pl, and Au remain.
- The component Pt $\leq$ It is now connected and Italy "moves down" because its strong indicator "fa" is deleted from the data matrix and its weaker indicators prevail.
- Su, Switzerland, is still "loosely" connected (Chapter 5), and all other proper maximal elements (Ne, Fi, and Sw) are covering four or more nations.

Some other nations "move down" too, which were originally in $level_3$ or $level_2$ (Fig. 12.1). For example, in Fig. 12.3, we find Dk $\leq$ Sw. Hence, with respect to all five indicators wb, hs, ed, br, and sub, Dk has worse values than Sw. Now look at Fig. 12.1: Here Dk is incomparable to Sw and is an element of the first level. Only in the indicator "family," Denmark is definitely better than Sw. Therefore, adding the indicator fa to the data matrix makes Denmark incomparable to Sw.

12.5.2 Ambiguity, Cumulative Ambiguity, and Minimum Rank Graphs

According to Chapter 4, we calculate CAM to be 0.881. As CAM can only vary between 0 and 1, this means adding new indicators to the data matrix will not change the Hasse diagram much: New indicators may break some of the comparabilities making the Hasse diagram (Fig. 12.1) still more flat. We conclude that on the one hand, the given six indicators provide a sufficient diverse picture and on the other hand, deleting some indicators from the data matrix may change the Hasse diagram (as can be seen when Fig. 12.1 is compared with Fig. 12.3). We see that adding indicators ed and sub to the column of "fa" leads to CAM = 0.75, which is 85% of the final value of 0.88. The partial order due to {fa, ed, sub} contains 85% of the incomparable pairs of the partial order found in Fig. 12.1. The remaining indicators he and br may be seen as fine-tuning the partial order, because their contribution to the final CAM value is rather small.

12.5.2.1 Cumulative Ambiguity Graph

In Fig. 12.4, the cumulative ambiguity graph (Chapter 4) is shown.

12.5.2.2 Minimum Rank Graph

As explained in Chapter 4, we start with the most important indicator fa and add successively the less important ones.

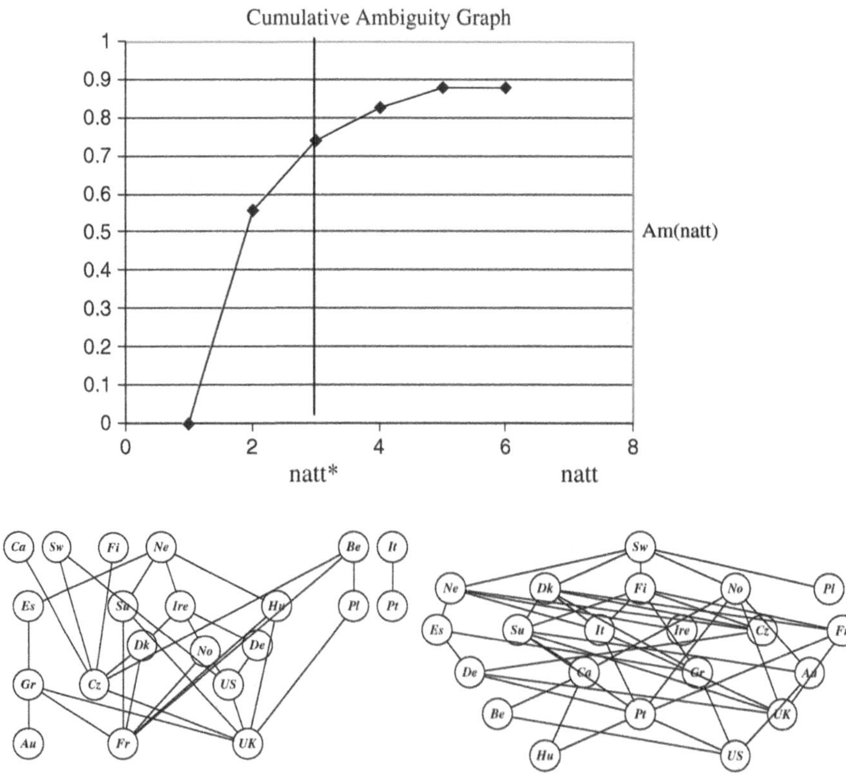

Fig. 12.4 Am(natt) and the decomposition of IB at natt* = 3 (see Chapter 4). *(Bottom) LHS*, $IB^{(1)}$ = {fa, ed, sub}; *RHS*, $IB^{(2)}$ = {wb, hs, br}

The indicator fa ranks the nations from worst to best as follows:

fa: UK < US < Cz < Ca < Fi < Au < Sw < Pl < De < Fr < Gr < No < Dk < Es < Ire < Hu < Be < Su < Ne < Pt < It

The result of adding the next indicator, ed, reduces the length of the maximal chain.

Italy

Instead of 20 successors in the chain, induced by "fa," Italy has now only one successor, namely Pt. Adding indicator ed reduces the minimum rank and increases the number of possible positions depending on the actual selection of weights.

Belgium

Due to the indicator fa alone, Belgium has 16 successors. Adding the indicator ed, the number of successors of Be remains the same. The minimum rank graph summarizes the effect of successively adding the indicators to the data matrix. Figure 12.5 provides the minimum rank graph for Belgium and Italy.

12.5.3 Antagonism

Let us select two subsets $X_1 = \{\text{It, Pt}\}$ and $X_2 = X - X_1 - \text{ISO}$.

Through software WHASSE, we find the set of antagonistic indicators AIB = {ed, fa}. The indicators ed and fa completely separate the two subsets It, Pt on the one hand and Ne, Sw, Su, …, US on the other hand (see Fig. 12.6), $\text{Sep}(X_1, X_2, \text{AIB}) = 1$).

Once again the indicator "family," fa, plays a distinctive role: Together with ed, it separates X_2 {Italy, Portugal} from X_1, i.e., from 15 other nations.

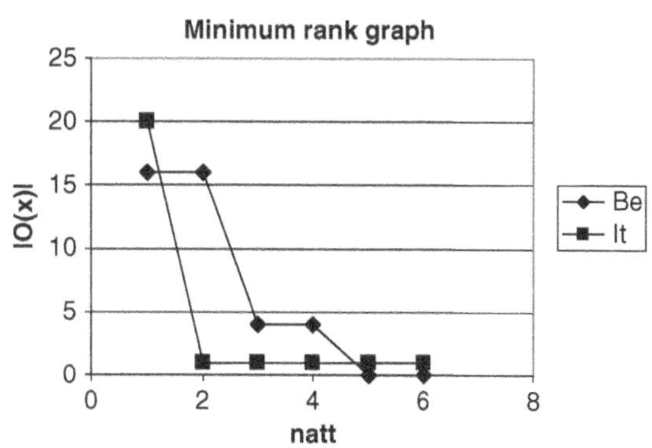

Fig. 12.5 Minimum rank graph of Be and It

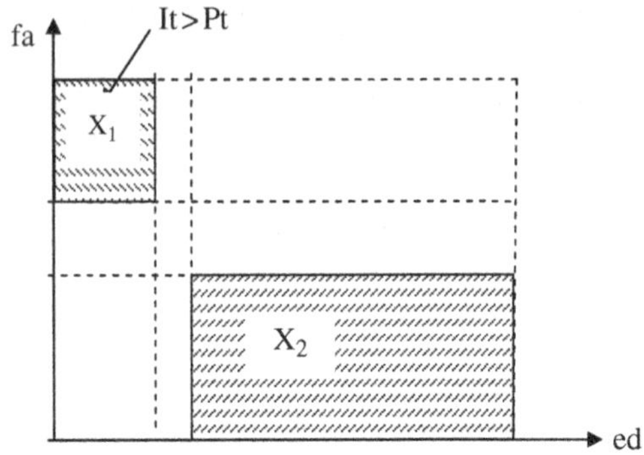

Fig. 12.6 Relation of Italy, It, and Portugal, Pt, to the other non-isolated nations X_2 (not scaled)

12.6 Partial Orders Based on Rank Orders of Attributes

The idea is to try to find orders which are not based on an averaging over all indicator values but retain the information about their disparity. The Hasse diagram due to the m^3 order (Chapter 7) is shown in Fig. 12.7).

In contrast to Fig. 12.1, we now get pretty long chains. For example

$$\text{US} < \text{UK} < \text{Cz} < \text{Ire} < \text{Es} < \text{Sw} < \text{Ne or US} < \text{UK} < \text{Hu} < \text{Ca} < \text{Es} < \text{Sw} < \text{Ne}.$$

Thus a comparison of nations on the basis of their worst, median, and best ranks is much simpler. We can even identify a greatest (Netherlands) and a least element (USA) (see Chapter 2). We may discard the median (being used as a fine trigger)

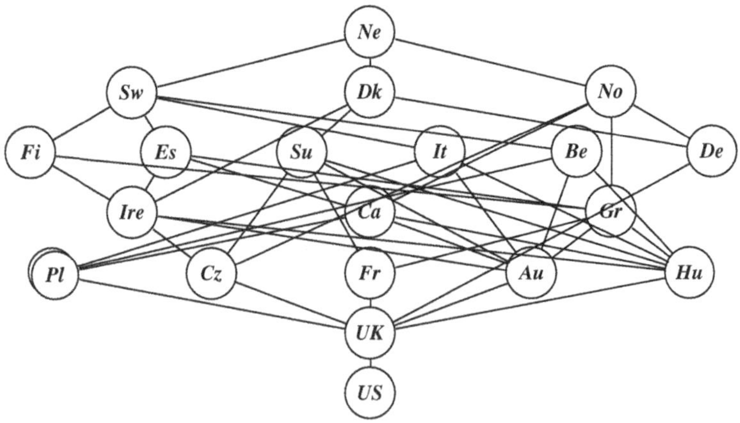

Fig. 12.7 Hasse diagram of m^3 order. Pl ≅ Pt

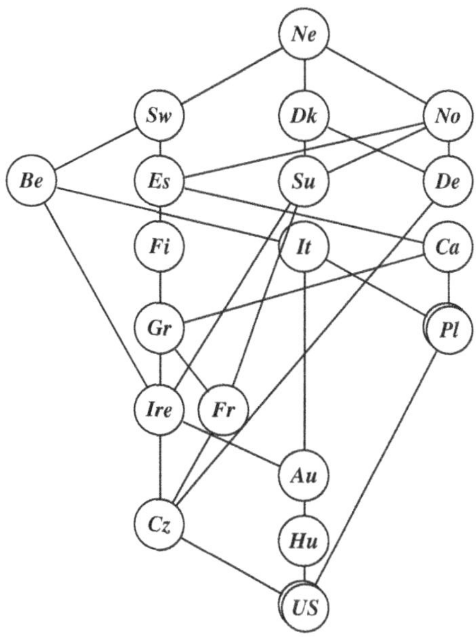

Fig. 12.8 Hasse diagram of the m^2 order (equivalent: {US, UK} and {Pl, Pt})

and examine the Hasse diagram, based on the m^2 order alone. Instead of the individual indicators we now compare nations on the basis of their worst and their best indicator values simultaneously (Fig. 12.8).

What do we see in Fig. 12.8?

1. Gr $<_{m^2}$ Fi: The worst indicator value of Gr is less than the worst indicator value of Fi. The best indicator value of Gr is less than the best indicator value of Fi.
2. Ne is at the top of the m^2 order. From this we know, independent of how large actually the interval [min(q(Ne)), max(q(Ne))] is, that all other min values as well as all other max values are less than or equal to those of Netherlands.
3. Es $||_{m^2}$ Su: The disparity due to m^2 in indicator values of these two nations is different.

Furthermore, we explained in Chapter 7 the role of incomparabilities in m^2 order. There we learned that incomparability in m^2 implies an inclusion order of the [min(q), max(q)] intervals. Hence an antichain like Be, Es, Su, De is a chain in the $\subseteq$ order according to increasing intervals [min(x), max(x)] (Fig. 12.9).

Germany, De, has the smallest interval. Therefore, Germany has a pretty sharp distribution of the six indicator values. Any variation of the weight vector for index calculation would lead to only a small variation in Γ. No political influence on the weight vector will help Germany to get a better position than Su or Es or Be. Belgium has the greatest interval within this subset of countries. This fact means

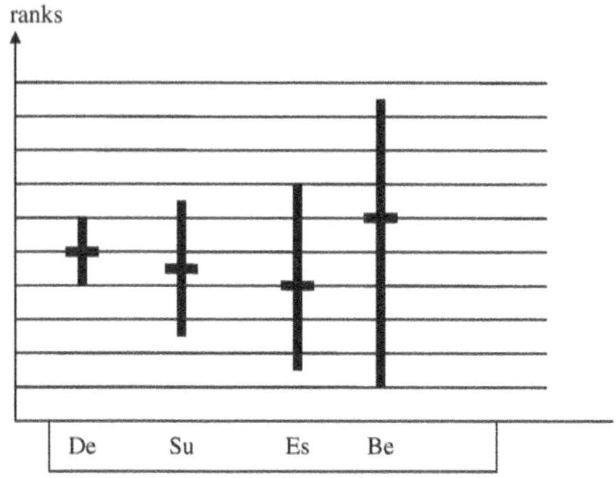

Fig. 12.9 Analysis of one of the antichains of diagram Fig. 12.8. The medians were taken from the data matrix

that Belgium has many choices in the selection of weight vectors to improve its ranking position.

12.7 Linear Orders

12.7.1 Where Are We?

The partial order analysis began with the data matrix, as can be found in Table A.7.

The Hasse diagram was rather flat because of many incomparabilities. Nevertheless, a sensitivity analysis could be performed and we showed how to find out why there are separated subsets (for example, {It, Pt} vs other nations). A decision about a mutual ranking among nations is difficult to make because of the shortness of chains. We know that Gr < Es < Ne without crunching the six indicators into a composite indicator. However, there is no answer for a mutual ranking between, say, Es and Cz. A step forward in decision making is to analyze the m^2 or m^3 orders where much of individual information about the indicators is lost but the information about disparities among their values retained. With this, many longer chains can be obtained, and we found that, for example, Es > Cz without worrying about weights. We continue this line of argumentation and derive weak orders among the nations based on purely order theoretical information as can be found in the Hasse diagram of Fig. 12.1.

12.7.2 Averaged Height Estimated by the Local Partial Order Model

The essential parameters of this model are $U(\mathrm{x})$, the set of successors, $S(x)$, and the set of predecessors, $P(x)$ (see Chapters 3 and 9). In Table 12.4, the characteristics of the LPOM model are summarized.

Table 12.4 Characteristics of the 21 nations w.r.t. LPOM taken from Fig. 12.1

Nation	*U*	*S*	*P*	Nation	*U*	*S*	*P*
Ne	12	8	0	Es	17	2	1
Su	19	1	0	De	17	2	1
No	18	2	0	Cz	15	1	4
Sw	17	3	0	Ire	19	0	1
Fi	18	2	0	Hu	19	0	1
Dk	17	3	0	Gr	18	0	2
It	19	1	0	UK	11	0	9
Be	20	0	0	US	16	0	4
Ca	20	0	0	Fr	19	0	1
Pl	20	0	0	Pt	19	0	1
Au	20	0	0				

The LPOM model finds the following weak order:

(UK < US < Cz < Gr < Fr ≅ Pt ≅ Ire ≅ Hu < Au ≅ Pl ≅ Ca ≅ Be < De ≅ Es < It ≅ Su < Fi ≅ No < Dk ≅ Sw < Ne)

The top seven are Ne, Sw, Dk, No, Fi, Su, and It. Compared with the top seven of the UNICEF, Italy is included, whereas Spain is located in the middle group. In its simplest form, LPOM generates many ties. Therefore, we also apply a canonical order which, however, will result in some ties too because of the inherent symmetry of the Hasse diagram (Fig. 12.1).

12.7.3 Canonical Order

Following the lattice theoretical method explained in Chapter 9, the ranking is as follows:

O_{poset}: (UK < US < Gr < Cz < Pt < Fr < Ire ≅ Hu < Ca ≅ Au ≅
≅ Pl ≅ Be < De < Su < Es < No < Fi < It < Sw < Dk < Ne)

In comparison to the order obtained by the composite indicator of UNICEF, there are some rank inversions such as Hu vs Gr, Au vs Cz, or It vs Su.

We apply the method explained in Section 10.2 to see quantitatively the degree of coincidence between the two orders (canonical order and UNICEF ranking). The partial order analysis shows that 27 incomparable pairs appear between O_Γ and O_{poset}, therefore $d_{\text{coinc}} = 1-(27/210) = 0.87$. The Spearman correlation index (see Section 10.3) is 0.88. Both numbers indicate that the general trend is rather well coincident for both approaches.

12.7.4 Analysis of Rank Inversions: An Example

Why is in the canonical order Su < It, whereas in the UNICEF ranking Su > It? By application of LPOM, where Su ≅ It, we can outline the reason.

In Fig. 12.10, the rank-ordered rows, qo, of the data matrix of Su and It (see Chapter 7) are shown.

Averaging due to the UNICEF method leads clearly to Su > It. The high value of Italy in the indicator fa cannot compensate all the low values in the other indicators. Why we arrive at Su < It in the canonical order? In Fig. 12.11, a scheme according to the LPOM approach is shown.

In the Hasse diagram (Fig. 12.1) approximately Su and It have the same order theoretical configuration. Both have only one successor and no predecessor. However, Italy has 19 nations which can take all of the three positions in the $S-x-P$ chain (see Chapter 9), whereas Switzerland, Su, has only 6. Italy tends to get a higher position in the weak order of canonical order because there are more nations to realize lower positions than for Switzerland.

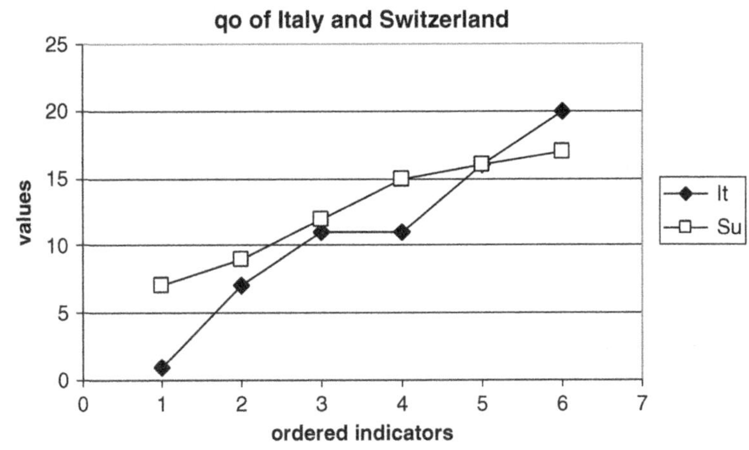

Fig. 12.10 Rank-ordered attribute values qo(It) and qo(Su), see Chapter 7

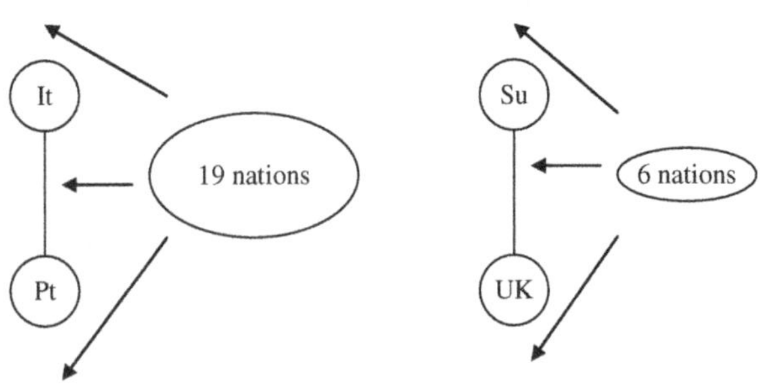

Fig. 12.11 Scheme to explain Su < It in canonical ranking (see text)

12.8 Sensitivity of the Single Nations to Indicators

So far we have discussed partial orders, having complete set X in mind. Now we take the point of view of a stakeholder who would like to learn more about his country $x \in X$.

One question is: What is the sensitivity of a single nation x to the indicators? For an answer, we have to select the singleton $\{x\}$ for X' in Eqs. (4.2) and (4.4). The results are shown in Table A.8. We see, for example, that wb is important for Ne, fa for Sw, and De, ed for Su, and It and sub for Dk ($W(\{\text{Ne}\}, \text{IB}, \text{IB-}\{\text{wb}\}) = 5$, W({Sw}, IB, IB-{fa}) = 7, etc.). Figure 12.12 illustrates the influence of wb on Ne by displaying the down sets.

Deleting indicators from the data matrix is certainly not possible when a ranking of nations is ahead. However, a high sensitivity of a nation to an indicator R_i may motivate to improve the value of $R_i(x)$. The question is, the improvement of which indicator R_i is most helpful. Here we perform an attribute value sensitivity study (see Section 6.6) which may be more straightforward.

12.9 Attribute Value Sensitivity

12.9.1 Preliminaries

What happens if a certain indicator value is changed by a unit, Δ, in particular 1? For which indicator out of the six will this have the best effect in terms of partial order?

If there is a change in partial order, what consequences can be drawn for linear orders?

The six indicators of this study are ranks. Therefore, to keep the computational effort tractable, a simulation study needs to be performed in the following.

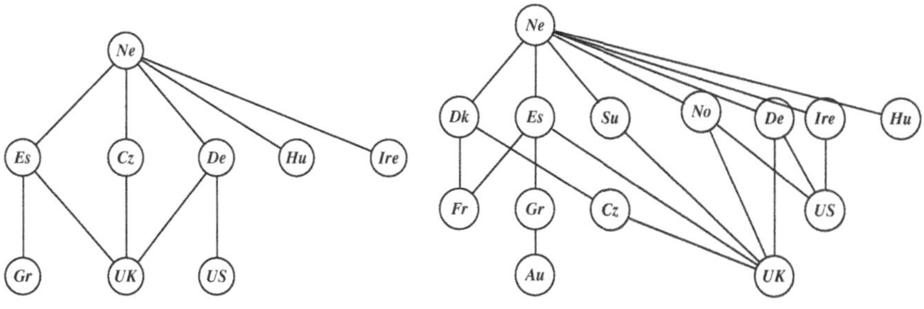

O(Ne, IB) O(Ne, IB-{wb})

Fig. 12.12 Down sets of Ne according to different information bases

Let x be the nation of interest and $R_i(x)$ the rank of the ith indicator and y that nation for which $R_i(y) = R_i(x) + 1$. Simulating now a change for nation x in R_i, by Δ, we consider the following:

(1) x: change of ranks according to $R_i(x) \rightarrow R_i(x) + \Delta$
(2) y: change of ranks according to $R_i(y) = R_i(x) + \Delta \rightarrow R_i(x) = R_i(y) - \Delta$.

Now, with the example of Ireland, we study Δ=1 for all single indicators one after another (Section 12.9.2), and with the example of Denmark, we study the influence of changing Δ on certain indicators (Section 12.9.3).

12.9.2 Ireland

The question is: Which kind of improvement of one of the six indicators might be the most efficient one (Table 12.5)?

12.9.2.1 Changes in Hasse Diagram

Table 12.5 shows that changing the indicator values of ed or br by $\Delta = 1$ affects the position of Ireland in the Hasse diagram: By changing the ranks for ed or br, Ireland becomes an isolated element.

12.9.2.2 Changes in Linear Orders O_Γ and O_{poset}

O_Γ: While $|U|$ is increasing, Ireland becomes an isolated element. Indeed the ranking interval of 20 and following the lines of Section 3.7, Ireland has the chance to get the top position in O_Γ through an appropriate weight vector. The lowest possible rank in O_Γ is 1 and the highest possible rank is 21.

O_{poset}: As several other nations are isolated elements, Ireland becomes equivalent to many others in the final weak order. As there is no weight vector which can be varied, Ireland's ranking position as an isolated element is slightly better!

Table 12.5 Simulation of the ranks of Ireland. The term "standard" refers to the Hasse diagram, Fig. 12.1

Indicator	$\|P\|$	$\|S\|$	$\|U\|$	What happens
Standard	1	0	19	(See Fig. 12.1)
wb	1	0	19	–
hs	1	0	19	–
ed	0	0	20	Ire is an isolated element in the Hasse diagram
fa	1	0	19	–
br	0	0	20	Ire is an isolated element in the Hasse diagram
sub	1	0	19	–

12.9.2.3 Consequences for Management

As the indicator br may be the outcome of the situation of the child, which is also partially described by other indicators, the recommended activity should concentrate on the indicator ed. In fact, the indicator educational well-being has three more basic perspectives (see Table 12.1):

- achievement at age 15 with:
    1. average achievement in reading literacy
    2. average achievement in mathematical literacy
    3. average achievement in science literacy
- *aspiration*: percentage aged 15–19 remaining in education and
- *participation*: the transition to employment with
    1. percentage aged 15–19 not in education, training, or employment
    2. percentage of 15-year olds expecting to find low-skilled work

Therefore the activities to give Ireland better positions should be concentrated on educational well-being with all its aspects.

12.9.3 Denmark

We select three indicators:

(1) sub, the indicator where Denmark has its worst score
(2) ed, an indicator where Denmark gets a middle position and
(3) wb, an indicator where Denmark has the maximal score.

In the first two cases, we examine what happens if Δ is increased step by step.

In the third case, we reduce the indicator wb step by step. Once again we apply the two-step procedure as explained in Section 12.9.1.

The results are listed in Table A.9.

In Fig. 12.13, the threshold values of $|\Delta_u|$ and $|\Delta_d|$ (see Fig. 6.11) are shown.

Figure 12.13 shows, for example, that one has to invest more than five points into the indicator ed until a change in terms of partial order characteristics appears (in contrast to sub, where already two points are sufficient).

The study shows that

- improving sub by one point does not change the Hasse diagram; however, by a change of two points, Denmark gets four successors and consequently $|U|$ decreases.
- improving ed by five points does not change the characteristics of Denmark. When Denmark gets in ed, the rank 20 $|S(\text{Dk})|$ increases by one unit.

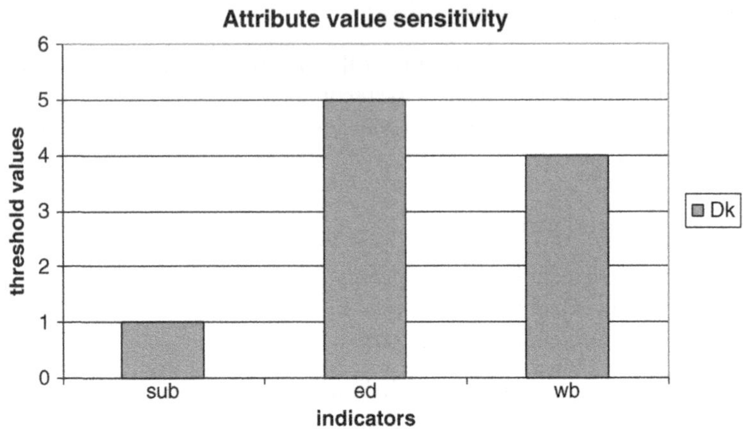

Fig. 12.13 Threshold values of $|\Delta_u|$ and $|\Delta_d|$ of Dk

- a change for the worse in indicator wb, material well-being, by four points does not change the Hasse diagram. If, however, the rank of wb is changed to the value 13, Denmark loses one successor and $|U|$ increases by one.

12.10 Summary and Commentary

This chapter dwells on two main lines of arguments:

1. How far can we verify the results of a study based on weight vectors by alternative methods?
2. Do we find additional insights by partial order?

We show that the results of UNICEF based on a weight vector are pretty coincident. The coincidence of levels, provided by partial order theory with three subsets derived from the UNICEF ranking, can be questioned because of the rather rough classification into three states. However, the linear orders derived from more sophisticated partial order techniques do not differ much from those based on an index. The partial order confirms the UNICEF results although they are based on an equal weighting of the indicators. If weights are considered as uncertain, then the application of Eq. (3.19) allows to check which nation would have a chance to get better ranking positions just by proposing other weighting schemes. Germany, for example, has little possibilities to improve its ranking position. The m^2 order shows this fact unambiguously.

Does an index hide important results? This second question can be answered with yes. When the partial order is considered, then its network of cover relations is of concern. This network of lines has much to do with "where is an object and why is it, where it is." Therefore, the importance of indicators for the Hasse diagram is to be considered and the indicator "family" is the most important one, whereas the indicator "behavior and risk" is least important.

Reference

UNICEF (2007). Child poverty in perspective: An overview of child well-being in rich countries. Innocenti report Card 7. Florence: UNICEF Innocenti Research Centre.

Chapter 13
Case Study: Stream Channel Stability Infrastructure at Bridge Crossings (Engineering Sciences)

13.1 Overview

Forty-nine bridge crossings were described by 13 indicators. As in Chapter 12, a composite indicator was suggested. The partial order analysis applied several tools in order to demonstrate its versatility. So, for example, formal concept analysis (Chapter 8) was applied resulting in a network of implications. These implications may be considered as hypotheses and should motivate further investigations concerning the problem of bridge stability in stream or channel crossings.

Four main questions were posed. Partial order analysis should be able to give an answer to them:

(1) Comparison of the composite indicator of Johnson (2005) with the result of partial order analysis. Is the composite indicator justified?
(2) Can the thresholds to classify stream/channel bridge crossings be verified?
(3) Which indicators are important?
(4) Can we reduce the costs of investigations by recommending a set of less expensive indicators?

By partial order analysis, the questions got the following answers:

(1) The composite indicator is confirmed by the partial order based on 13 indicators as well as on four superindicators.
(2) The thresholds can be verified.
(3) The "channel alignment" is the most important indicator.
(4) A reduced set of four indicators seems to be the most appropriate one. Two indicators belong to the level of expertise 1 and the other two belong to levels 2 and 3, respectively.

R. Brüggemann, G.P. Patil, *Ranking and Prioritization for Multi-indicator Systems*, Environmental and Ecological Statistics 5, DOI 10.1007/978-1-4419-8477-7_13,

13.2 The Data Matrix and Basic Results

The data set about 49 bridge crossing sites was provided by a study performed for the Federal Highway Administration (FHWA). The aim of the FHWA study was to develop a set of indicators for stream stability at bridge crossings. The stability of a stream channel near a bridge crossing has many implications for the risk posed to the bridge structure itself. The indicators used are described by Johnson (2005) and Newlin and Bhat (2007). "There is an important need to determine the causes of the failure of bridges over waterways, and the determination of the indicators most influential in stream stability is vital" (Newlin and Patil, 2010). There are 13 indicators that "describe watershed-scale factors, floodplain function, bank stability, and channel features." The indicators are scored with values between 1 and 12, where 1 is the best and 12 the worst. In Table 13.1, the indicators are listed and explained and in Table A.10, the data matrix can be inspected.

After a score is assigned for each of the 13 indicators, a total score $\Gamma(x)$ is obtained by a summation of the individual scores. This assumes that each of the indicators has equal weighting and that they independently describe channel stability. The total score is then given a classification of "Excellent," "Good," "Fair," or "Poor" based on threshold values that vary for different stream channel types (Johnson, 2005).

Furthermore, the 13 indicators can be categorized by level of expertise and necessary time for evaluation. For different indicators, varying levels of stream channel behavior knowledge is required. Three levels of expertise are assigned in the following manner:

(1) "observation and a moderate level of expertise are required,"
(2) "observation and a high level of expertise are required," and
(3) "measurement and a high level of expertise are required."

The indicators can also be grouped based on the particular feature of the stream–bridge intersection that it characterizes. The 13 indicators describe watershed/regional scale, local channel conditions, bank stability, and bridge alignment. The assignment to superindicators is shown in Table 13.2.

We refer to this aggregated set as "four-superindicator system." So the case study "bridges" can be analyzed with respect to different aspects, see Fig. 13.1.

The index (Johnson, 2005) used is

$$\Gamma(x) = \sum g_i{}^* \mathrm{I}_i(x),\ x \text{ bridge site},\ i = 1, \ldots, 13,\ g_i = 1/13 \text{ for all } i \tag{13.1}$$

For our purpose we inverted the indicator score values such that the bridge sites in the best condition get a large value in the corresponding indicator. Therefore, large values of $\Gamma(x)$ indicate sites in a good state. We refer to $\Gamma(x)$, according to Eq. (13.1), as score(total).

Table 13.1 Indicators of stream channel stability at bridge crossings

Indicator	Description	No.	Level of expertise	Feature category
Watershed and floodplain activity (FA)	Surrounding land use; forested, grazing, urbanization, logging, etc.	I_1	1	Watershed or regional
Flow habit (FH)	Perennial, intermittent, ephemeral streams, flooding behavior, stream order	I_2	2	Watershed or regional
Channel pattern (CP)	Straight, engineered, meandering, braided	I_3	2	Watershed or regional
Entrenchment or channel confinement (CC)	Connectivity of floodplain with channel, evidence of infrastructure undercutting	I_4	2	Watershed or regional
Bed material (BM)	Sediment size, packed or loose, fraction of sand	I_5	3	Local channel
Bar development (BD)	Narrow or wide, vegetated or newly deposited, grain size of deposited sediment	I_6	3	Local channel
Obstructions (Ob)	Bedrock outcrops, amour layer, LWD, grade control structures, revetment, vanes	I_7	1	Local channel
Bank soil texture (ST)	Clay, silt, loam, sand; cohesive or noncohesive	I_8	3	Bank stability
Average bank slope angle (BSA)	Bank slope for unconsolidated and consolidated materials	I_9	1	Bank stability
Bank protection (BP)	Vegetative (riparian zone width), engineered revetment	I_{10}	1	Bank stability
Bank cutting (BC)	Percentage of raw banks, undercutting	I_{11}	1	Bank stability
Mass wasting or bank failure (BF)	Scalloping of banks, slumping, tension cracks	I_{12}	2	Bank stability
Bridge–channel alignment (CA)	Upstream distance to bridge from meander impact point, bridge alignment with channel flow direction	I_{13}	2	Alignment

An abbreviation of the 13 indicators is also given in parentheses in the first column

The three best sites according to Γ are 48 (9.85), 52 (9.69), and 57 (9.62). The value of Γ is in parentheses. The three worst bridge sites are 15 (3), 17(3.23), and 44 (3.85).

Table 13.2 Superindicators

Superindicator	Superindicator is obtained as
Stream–bridge intersection on a regional scale	$I_1 + I_2 + I_3 + I_4$
Local channel characteristics	$I_5 + I_6 + I_7$
Bank stability	$I_8 + I_9 + I_{10} + I_{11} + I_{12}$
Alignment of the bridge with the stream channel that it crosses	I_{13}

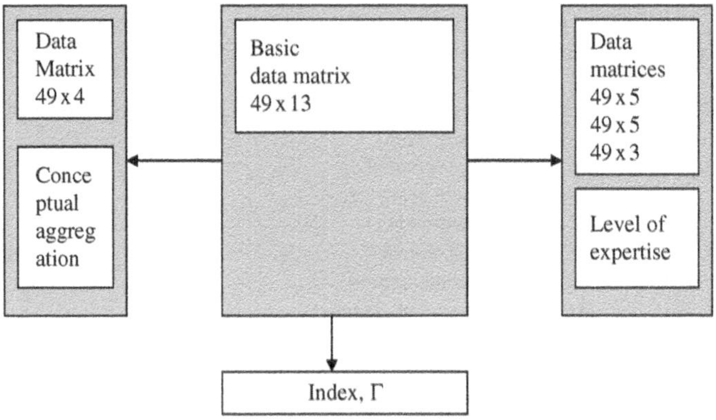

Fig. 13.1 Different aspects for studying the bridges. (*Left*) Superindicators, (*middle*) basic indicators $I_1, \ldots, I_{13}$, (*right*) three data matrices according to the three levels of expertise

13.3 Questions We Are Aiming to Answer

13.3.1 Questions

1. Johnson (2005) uses $\Gamma(x)$, the total score, to rank the stream channel stability near a bridge crossing. How does it compare with the ranking based on 13- or on the 4-superindicator system? Are there other ways of ranking and do they agree with each other?
2. The stream channel stability is assigned to one of the four conditions; "Excellent," "Good," "Fair," or "Poor" based on threshold values of the total score. Is this a good classification? Can it be supported by other methods?
3. In general, not all of the indicators are equally important. We are interested to know which indicators are more influential overall, which are more influential for specific stream types, and whether it is appropriate to reduce the number of indicators. Furthermore, we would like to know how indicators influence the position of single sites, and whether there are interrelationships among the indicators.

4. The 13 indicators can be further classified into three groups based on the level of expertise. Can we reduce the cost of implementing a stream stability assessment method by collecting only the less expensive indicators?

13.4 Toward Answers I

13.4.1 Thirteen Basic Indicators

The Hasse diagram (Fig. 13.2) is oriented so that excellent bridge sites are found in the top level, whereas poor bridge sites are found in the bottom level. According to the principles of how to draw Hasse diagrams (see Chapter 2), not all minimal elements appear at the bottom of the diagram. There are in fact 16 minimal elements (identified by site number):

$$\text{MIN} = \{2, 3, 6, 7, 15, 17, 18, 22, 23, 28, 32, 34, 36, 43, 44, 56\}$$

Among these 16 objects, three stream sites, 15, 17, and 36, are represented in the bottom level because they are the end members of chains of length 3 and belong therefore to the worst sites. Isolated elements can be considered as elements which are at the same time maximal and minimal elements. We identify that six out of the sixteen minimal elements are isolated objects:

$$\text{ISO} = \{2, 3, 6, 28, 32, 56\}$$

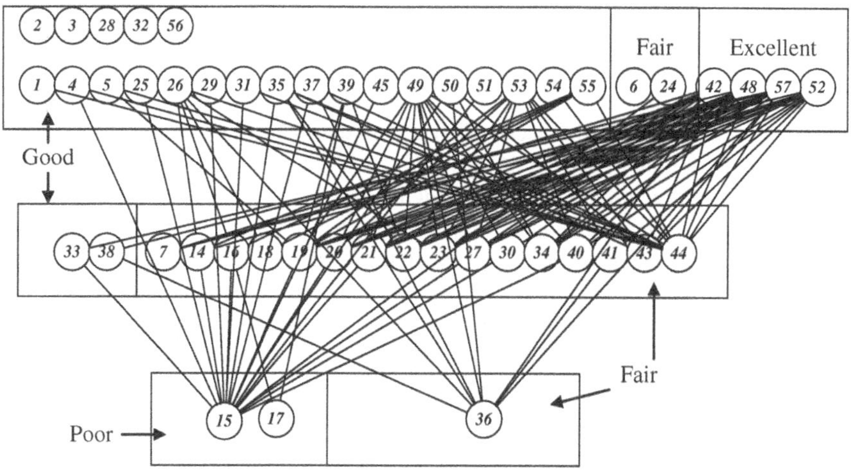

Fig. 13.2 Hasse diagram for 49 sites with 13 indicators (see text)

Table 13.3 Summary of the results by partial orders and of the engineering scientists (13 indicators)

	Level due to partial order		
Score (total)	Level 3	Level 2	Level 1
Excellent	4/4		
Good	22/24	2/24	
Fair	2/19	16/19	1/19
Poor			2/2

The elements of ISO should appear – following the drawing rules of PyHasse – in the top level. However, we arranged them in that way that they fit into the rectangle of "good" bridges. Any of the isolated elements, bridge site 2, bridge site 3,. . ., bridge site 56, cannot be compared to any other element (see Chapter 3). Considering their data profile, they are crisscrossing that of any other bridge site.

In Fig. 13.2, the rectangles encompass bridges of the same classification level after Johnson (2005). The higher the level, the better the bridge site condition.

We see that all "excellent" and most of "good" bridge sites are in level 3. Most of the "fair" bridges are in level 2 (counted from bottom to top) and all "poor" bridge sites are in level 1. Furthermore, by the partial order approach, we can identify chains and levels which we can compare with the results based on score (total). Bridges which are ranked differently due to the index or due to the partial order are of high interest: They indicate when averaging the indicators mask important details. In Table 13.3, the first value is the number of sites on a given level, and the value after the "/" is the total number of sites due to the classification of the engineering scientists.

13.4.2 Superindicator System Having Four Indicators

Figure 13.3 is the Hasse diagram for the four-superindicator system. It consists of seven levels and no isolated objects. There are nine maximal objects in the top level. Six objects are minimal, MIN $= \{6, 7, 15, 17, 36, 44\}$.

The partial aggregation (Chapter 7) which reduces the number of indicators from 13 indicators to four superindicators has resulted in an increase in comparability between study sites with 133 comparisons in the 13-indicator data set and 460 comparisons in the four-superindicator system, demonstrating the enrichment and the simplification of the partial order. The aggregation of indicators, either to one score, the score (total), or to the four-superindicator system, is order preserving. Therefore, it is clear that neither Fig. 13.2 nor Fig. 13.3 will show comparabilities that are not consistent with the order induced by the score (total). Nevertheless it should be kept in mind that the appearance of many incomparabilities indicates the strong compensating effect in obtaining the total score Γ. See, for instance, bridge sites 17 and 57. For both, the total score and the assignment to levels in partial order theory

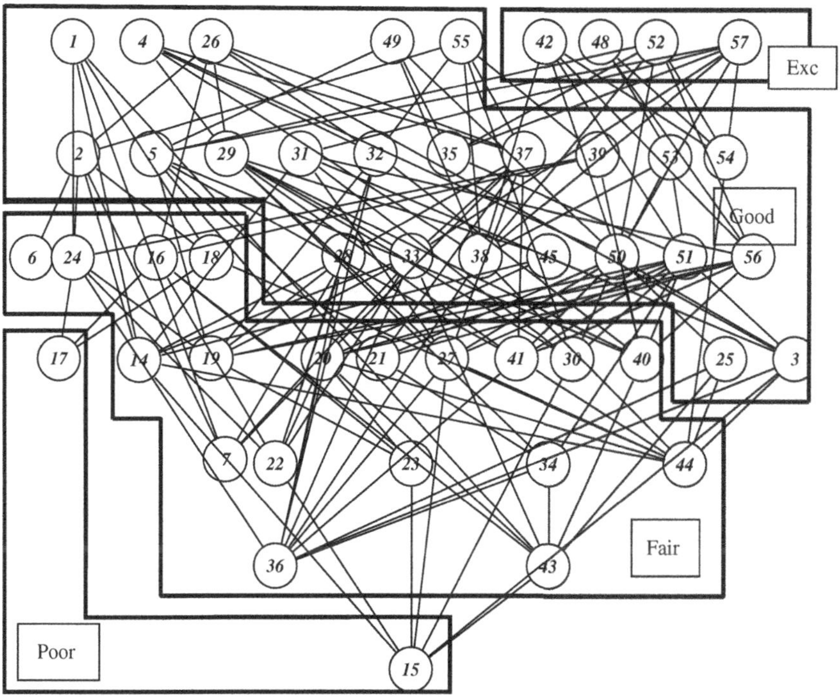

Fig. 13.3 Hasse diagram for 49 sites with the four-superindicator system

evaluate 17 worse than 57. Nevertheless, we find (applying up sets (see Chapter 2)) that 17||57. There must be at least one superindicator by which the "poor" bridge is better than the "excellent" bridge 57. Indeed, we find that $17 >_{I13} 57$.

In Fig. 13.3, the polygons from the left bottom to the right top represent the stream condition assigned to the sites based on the total score of summing all 13 indicators. The subset {42, 48, 52, 57} is evaluated as "Excellent" (Exc.)

As in Section 13.4.1, we compare the partial order approach (Hasse diagram in Fig. 13.3) with the classification derived from total score (Table 13.4). As in Table 13.3, the first number is the number of bridge sites in a certain level of the Hasse diagram, whereas the number after / is the number of bridges according to the classification by the engineers.

13.4.3 Summary

The Hasse diagram technique can best visualize the order relations among objects. As one of the most important outputs, Hasse levels can be produced to represent the relative position of an object against others. The object set is partitioned into

Table 13.4 Summary of the results by partial orders and of the engineering scientists (four-superindicator system)

	Level 7	Level 6	Level 5	Level 4	Level 3	Level 2	Level 1
Excellent	4/4						
Good	4/24	10/24	8/24	2/24			
Fair	1/19		3/19	8/19	5/19	2/19	
Poor					1/2		1/2

equivalence classes (the "levels") according to decreasing distance to the maximal elements (see Chapter 9). Those Hasse levels can be compared with the four intervals corresponding to "Excellent," "Good," "Fair," or "Poor" to see whether there is a need to adjust the threshold values defining "Excellent," "Good," etc. Both the partial order approach by 13 indicators and that by four superindicators justify the thresholds.

Question 1 can be answered with "yes." Question 2, which is a more technical one, can be answered with "yes" too. There is no need to adjust the threshold values.

13.5 Toward Answers II: Indicator Set

13.5.1 Overview

In this section, we attempt to answer question 3. We will first answer the question for the 13 indicators. Here we also take into account that the importance of the indicators for different contextual bridge sites sets can be different. The importance of the four superindicators will next be determined. In the section on stability and minimum rank graphs, we show how the consecutive cumulation of indicators changes the partial order and the minimum rank of certain objects. Finally, we demonstrate how by formal concept analysis an implication network of indicators can be established. This may help pose new hypotheses for engineering scientists.

13.5.2 Attribute-Related Sensitivity Analysis

PyHasse provides tools to perform a sensitivity analysis. Following Eq. (4.6) the channel alignment, I_{13}, is considered as the most important indicator. The next most important indicator is I_8, bank soil texture, which causes a change of 32 comparabilities from the Hasse diagram of all indicators. All results are shown in Table A.11 and the summary in Table 13.6.

The sensitivity analysis has also been applied to the four-superindicator system (Table A.12, summary in Table 13.6). The superindicator "channel alignment" again comes out to be the most important indicator, followed by local channel characteristics, watershed and regional characteristics, and bank characteristics.

13.5.2.1 Sensitivity Dependent on Different Stream Types (Dune Riffle, Riffle Pool, . . .)

In order to identify the most important indicators for specific stream types, the full data matrix has been divided according to the following stream subsets: dune ripple, riffle pool, plane bed, and modified (Montgomery and Buffington, 1997; US Army Corps of Engineers, 1994). In Table 13.5 the four possible subsets of stream types are explained.

The results of the attribute-related sensitivity are summarized in Table 13.6 for three influential indicators. The indicator for channel alignment appears as the most important indicator for all data sets summarized in Table 13.6.

The importance of indicators appears to be related to the correlation between indicators. Indicators that are the least correlated with other indicators appear to be more important according to the partial order analysis. For example, the most important indicator, channel alignment I_{13}, is poorly correlated with any of the other indicators, the maximal correlation value being 0.277 (correlation I_{13} with I_{11}).

In Fig. 13.4 the two sensitivities (13-indicator system vs. 4-superindicator system) are compared: Rather large sensitivities in the 13-indicator system will not

Table 13.5 Stream types, after Montgomery and Buffington (1997)

Stream type	Explanation	Site Nos
Dune ripple	Sand bed, low to moderate slope, response-type stream with bedforms	1, 2, 3, 6, 7, 31, 32, 39, 40, 41
Riffle pool	Gravel bed, low to moderate slope, response-type stream with bedforms	4, 5, 14, 15, 16, 17, 18, 19, 20, 21, 22, 23, 24, 30, 33, 35, 36, 37, 38, 39, 40, 42, 43, 44, 53
Plane bed	Gravel/cobble bed, moderate to steep slope, response-type stream without bedforms	25, 26, 27, 28, 29, 42, 45, 48, 49, 50, 51, 52, 53, 54, 55, 56, 57
Modified	The natural configuration has been severely modified by human intervention	5, 6, 14, 15, 16, 17, 21, 39, 44, 45, 54, 55, 57

Table 13.6 Summary of the attribute sensitivity analysis. 1 being the most important (see Chapter 4), 2 the next, and 3 the least important indicator

Data set	Importance 1	Importance 2	Importance 3
All sites	Channel alignment	Bank soil texture	Obstructions
Dune ripple	Channel alignment	Bank soil texture	Obstructions, bar development
Riffle pool	Channel alignment	Bank soil texture	Obstructions
Plane bed	Channel alignment	Obstructions	Bank protection
Modified	Channel alignment	Bank soil texture	bed material, obstructions

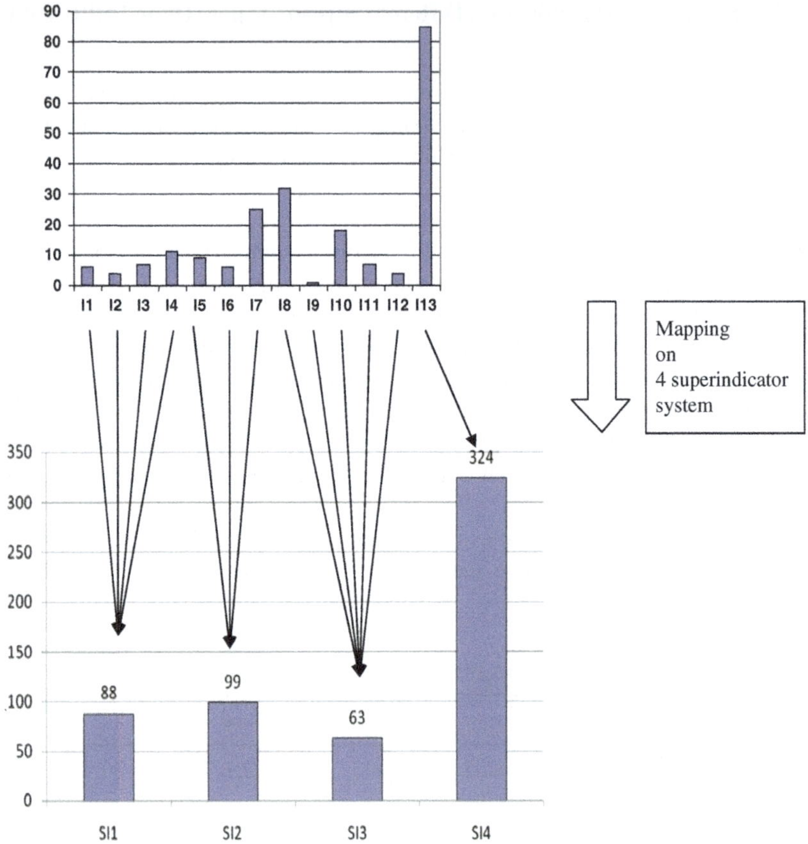

Fig. 13.4 Sensitivities in the 13-indicator and the 4-superindicator systems

necessarily imply large sensitivities in the four-superindicator system. For example, I_8 and I_{10} have sensitivity values 32 and 18, respectively (see Table A.11). Nevertheless, the index I_2 (of the four-superindicator system), quantifying "local channel" aspects, has the lowest sensitivity. The aggregation may compensate two indicators with low correlation (0.234).

13.5.3 *Ambiguity, Cumulative Ambiguity, and Minimum Rank Graph*

CAM for the 13-indicator system equals 0.887. This value, rather near 1, indicates that the indicator set is sufficiently complete. In Fig. 13.5, the cumulative ambiguity graph is shown.

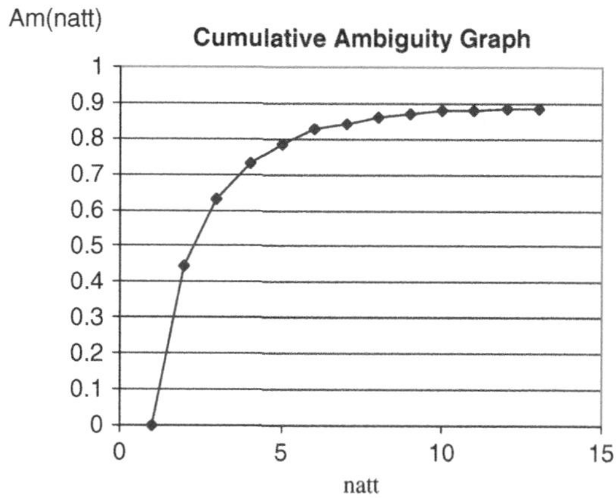

Fig. 13.5 Cumulative ambiguity graph for bridges based on 13 indicators ($I_{13} > I_8 > I_7 > I_{10} > I_4 > I_5 > I_{11} > I_3 > I_6 > I_1 > I_{12} > I_2 > I_9$. Ties: $I_2 \sim I_{12}, I_1 \sim I_6, I_3 \sim I_{11}$)

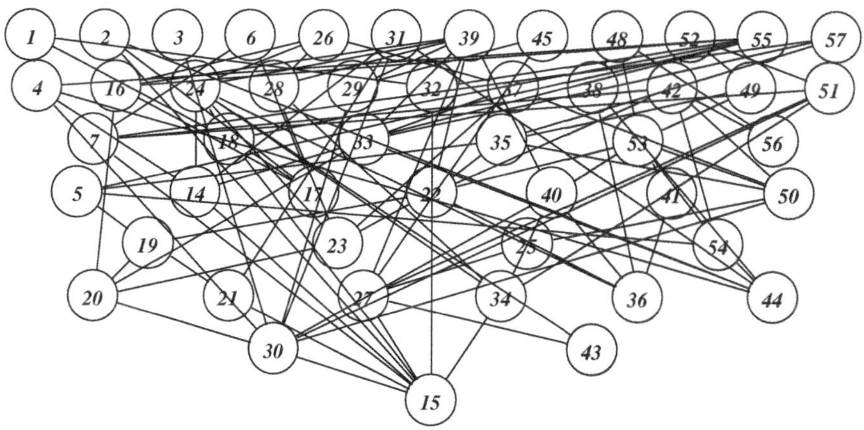

Fig. 13.6 Hasse diagram based on the set of indicators that generate 82% of the maximum value of CAM

Figure 13.6 shows that at natt* $= 4$, a selection of the indicators I_{13}, I_8, I_7, I_{10}, which provide 82% of the maximum value reached Am(natt*) $= 0.73$. Thus following the decomposition $\text{IB} = \text{IB}^{(1)} + \text{IB}^{(2)}$ at natt = natt*, the poset $(X, \text{IB}^{(1)})$ is an approximation to (X, IB) in the sense that more indicators would only induce minor changes.

13.5.3.1 Concordance Analysis

In Table 13.7 the concordance analysis is shown (see Chapter 10). The eight levels of the Hasse diagram (Fig. 13.6) are pairwise aggregated so that four consecutive evaluation scores by the Hasse diagram are obtained. As before, the indicator by Johnson was used to evaluate the bridge sites as poor, fair, good, and excellent.

Table 13.7 Concordance analysis

	Hasse poor	Hasse fair	Hasse good	Hasse excellent
Poor	1		1 (bridge site 17)	
Fair	3	8	6	3
Good		2	6	16
Excellent				3

If only the main diagonal is considered, then concordance index = 18/49 = 0.37. If, as was proposed in Section 10.4, the two parallel diagonals are counted and weighted by 0.5, then we obtain concordance index = (18 + 0.5*30)/49 = 0.67. Following the lines of Chapter 10, the concordance can be considered as significant.

The striking exception is bridge site No. 17, which is evaluated by partial order as good but got an evaluation as poor by the total score. Note, however, that bridge site No. 17 has $|U(17)| = 44$, i.e., it is highly incomparable and has a large ranking interval.

The main message of this section is that we may use a reduced set of indicators I_{13}, I_8, I_7, and I_{10}. This set contains two indicators of expertise level 1, one of level 2, and one of level 3. We consider the inclusion of an indicator of level 3 as a disadvantage. As a supplement to answering question 4, we can offer another suggestion to reduce the number of indicators, keeping the costs reduced.

13.5.3.2 Minimum Rank Graph

In Fig. 13.7, the minimum rank graph (see Chapter 4) is shown for four objects: sites 4, 24, and 48 are maximal elements , whereas site 33 is located in the middle level of the Hasse diagram (Fig. 13.2).

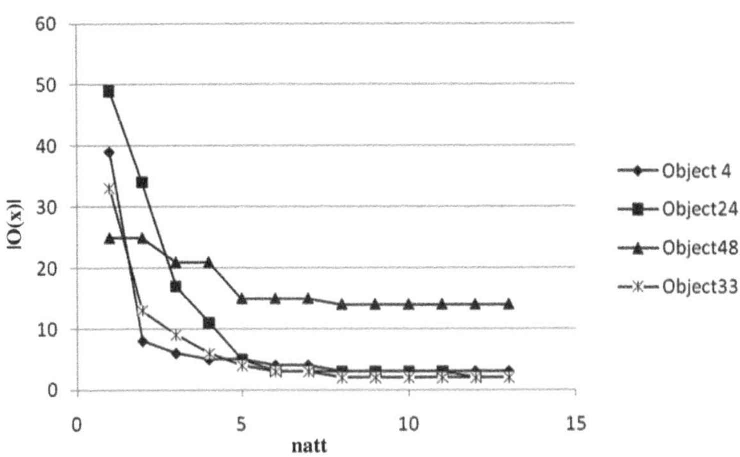

Fig. 13.7 Minimum rank graph of four sites: 4, 48, 33, and 24

Fig. 13.8 Partial order model

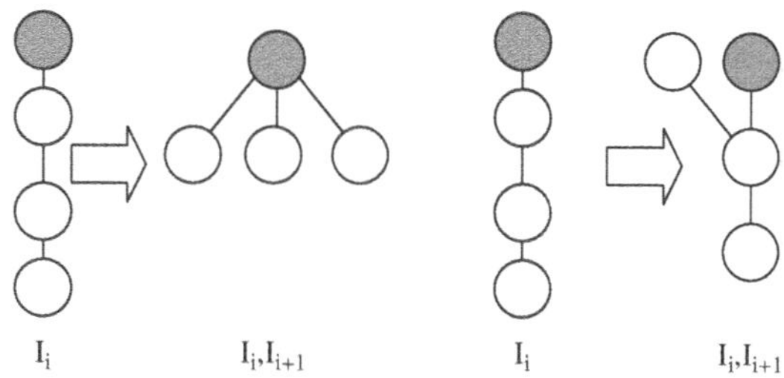

Site 48: The indicators I_8, I_7, and especially I_{10} have only a slight influence, although these indicators with sensitivity values of 25 and 18 are still important with respect to the total set of objects. A partial order model for such behavior is provided in Fig. 13.8 (LHS).

Figure 13.8 (LHS) shows a partial order model for invariance of a minimum rank graph while adding an indicator, the shaded object being actually considered. The number of successors is the same, while the structure of the partial order is changing. Adding indicators reduces the number of successors and increases the number of incomparable pairs (Fig. 13.8, RHS).

Site 4: According to score (total), site 4 is a good site. Site 4 is ranked pretty high if only the indicator I_{13}, alignment, is applied. However, with increasing set of indicators, the minimum rank graph of site 4 rapidly decreases to low values, making its position in any numerical aggregation model very uncertain. Because all successors in the case of I_{13} alone are now incomparable with site 4, the ranking interval becomes large (Eq. (3.19)).

Site 33: Starting with a rather high position due to indicator I_{13} (alignment), the next four indicators reduce the number of successors. Hence, any successor of site 33 in the case of I_{13} becomes incomparable with site 33 when more indicators are added to the data matrix.

Site 24: The site is evaluated with respect to indicator I_{13} as one of the best. Inserting indicators reduces the number of successors first rapidly, later only slowly. After inserting the fifth indicator, site 24 remains in a position with less than five successors.

A partial order model is shown in Fig. 13.8 (RHS). We see this as confirmation of 24 as a weak site, although the indicators for channel alignment and I_8, bank soil texture, assure site 24 a good position.

13.5.4 Implication Network

Discussing indicator sets should not be restricted to the analysis of the importance of indicators for a Hasse diagram and therefore for the possible location of objects, but should also find out the interrelationships among the indicators. Here we do this for those bridges which are in poor alignment with the channel: We select that set of bridge sites having low values in the indicator I_{13} ("Poor alignment bridges"). We

Table 13.8 Poor alignment bridge sites classified, median values

I_1	I_2	I_3	I_4	I_5	I_6	I_7	I_8	I_9	I_{10}	I_{11}	I_{12}	I_{13}
5	8	8	7	4	7	8	8	3	4	5	5	3

introduce binary attributes depending on whether the indicator value I_i is $\leq \text{median}_i$ or $> \text{median}_i$ $(i = 1, 2, \ldots, 13)$. The median values are shown in Table 13.8.

13.5.4.1 Line Diagram

When interrelationships of indicators is of interest, then formal concept analysis (Chapter 8) is the appropriate tool. The line diagram of the formal concept analysis is shown in Fig. 13.9 and the context table in Table A.13.

We are mainly interested in the implications. Therefore, we give here only two examples of how to read the lattice:

(1) Bridge site 15 has the properties CA and FA, whereas bridge site 36 has the properties BSA, BP, and BM.
(2) Which bridge sites are common for the properties CA and ST? Due to the infimum which is above sites 34 and 43, we find additionally sites 25 and 27.

13.5.4.2 Implications

It is not meaningful to discuss all 75 associations which can be obtained from the formal concept analysis. Instead we concentrate (a) on associations with EoA = 100, i.e., on implications and (b) on those whose list of realized premises contains only one property. Table 13.9 (Id is the identification number and N_{realiz} is the number of objects for which the premise of the implication is true) shows that selection.

The implications should now read as follows:

Rule 13: A good flow habit FH implies a good value for the bank slope angle BSA.
Rule 15: A good value for channel pattern, CP, implies good values for channel confinement (CC) as well as for bank slope angel (BSA).

13.5.4.3 Directed Graph of Implications

These rules refer only to the poor alignment bridge sites and to the median classification among them and enlighten the interrelationships of the indicators which might be of interest for engineers. We can visualize the interrelationships by a directed graph (Fig. 13.10).

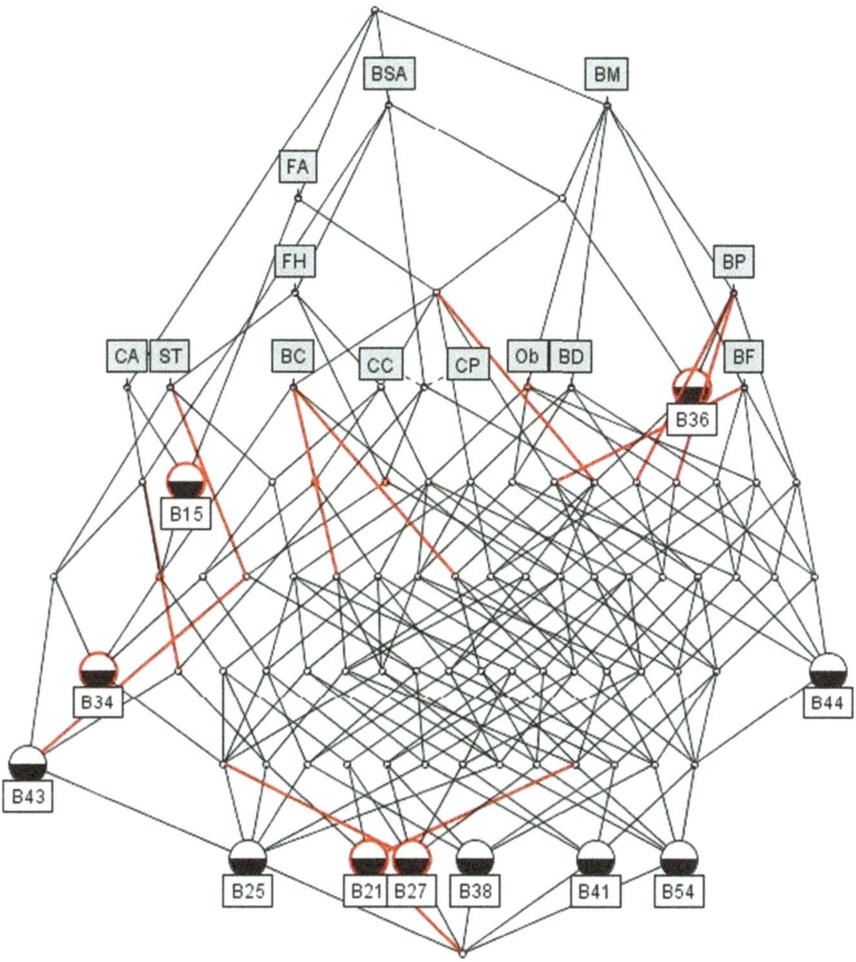

Fig. 13.9 Line diagram of the formal concept lattice of the "poor alignment bridge sites." Note, we selected a layout modus saving space

Table 13.9 Examples of implications for bridges in bad condition with respect to I_{13}

Id	N_{realiz}	Implication	Id	N_{realiz}	Implication
13	7	FH => BSA	23	6	ST => FH, BSA
15	6	CP => CC, BSA	24	7	BP => BM
16	6	CC => CP, BSA	25	6	BC => FA, BM, BSA
21	6	BD => BM	26	6	BF => BM
22	6	Ob => BM			

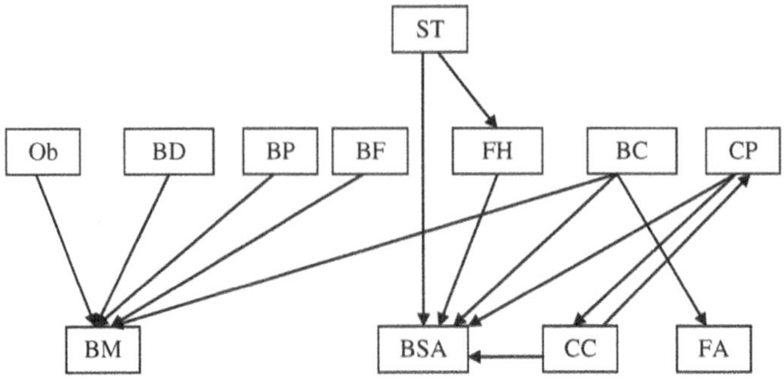

Fig. 13.10 Implication network among the 12 indicators for poor alignment bridge sites and a median classification

13.5.4.4 How Should We Use These Implications?

First of all, the rules are here very restricted, as we selected poor alignment bridge sites and – beyond this – classified the indicators by the median. Granted these (severe) restrictions, the implications are nothing else than what was given by the (binary) data matrix! The tool of formal concept analysis is precisely to find out such relations from the table. The implications should be considered as a working hypothesis. For example, bed material (BM) gets values above the median, if either Ob (obstruction), or BD (bar development), or BP (bank protection), etc. (see Fig. 13.9) got indicator values which are larger than the median within the poor alignment bridge sites subset. One may hypothesize that the indicators Ob, BD, BP, BF, and BC correlate with BM, – at least for poor alignment bridge sites!

13.6 Canonical Orders

13.6.1 Where Are We?

The sections of this chapter were so far concerned with comparative knowledge discovery: We looked at the position of objects in various Hasse diagrams, identified levels, and made use of stability and minimum rank graphs to see how the indicators are working. In doing this we followed the very principle of partial order analysis not to intermingle the indicators but to see what they can tell us, keeping them separated. Central point is the system of order relations among the bridge sites. The fourth question, however, cannot be answered easily because of the many incomparable pairs. In Chapter 9, we make use of the linear extensions (Chapter 3) whose multitude expresses the appearance of many incomparable pairs and from which linear or weak orders can be obtained. The answer to the fourth question as well as to the first one will be provided in the next section.

13.6.2 Application of Linear Extensions

Since assigning equal weight to each indicator is rather arbitrary, we are discussing an alternative: An alternative is provided in Chapters 3 and 9. We will apply the canonical order due to the Bubley Dyer (BD) and the LPOM algorithms for all 49 and additionally the lattice theoretical method for 15 bridge sites. We are interested to compare the averaged ranks obtained from them with the values of the total score Γ. Table 13.10 shows the results for 49 sites of different indicator constellations (all indicators, only indicators of level 1, etc.). We apply the Spearman correlation analysis to compare the 10 linear or weak orders with that due to the index Γ.

Note that among the five sets of indicators, the scenario (4) yields slightly better results in comparison to that of level 1 or level 2 indicators. In Fig. 13.11 a scatter plot of BD vs. Γ (L.H.S.) and of LPOM vs. Γ (R.H.S.) is shown (all indicators).

To include the lattice theoretical method, we selected 15 bridge sites pretty arbitrarily and calculated the linear order of these bridge sites by means of lattice theoretical methods (Section 9.6). In Table 13.11, the indicator constellations together with their Pearson correlation with Γ are shown (15 bridge sites).

In all the three methods, the correlation between O_Γ and O_{poset}, based on indicators of level 1, are the best. The correlation between O_Γ and O_{poset} based on three

Table 13.10 Spearman correlation indices of Γ vs. the heights (see Chapter 3) due to the 10 partial order variants, based on all 49 bridge sites

Scenario	Bubley Dyer	LPOM
(1) 13 basic indicators	0.92	0.92
(2) Level 1 indicators	0.86	0.87
(3) Level 2 indicators	0.85	0.87
(4) Level 1 and level 2 indicators together	0.9	0.9
(5) Superindicators	0.91	0.9

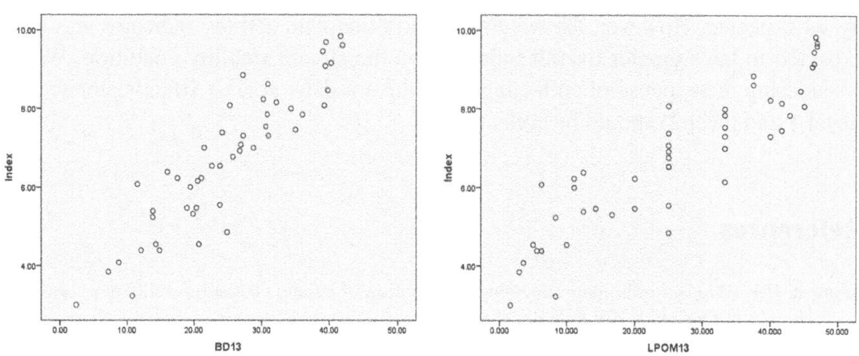

Fig. 13.11 Comparison of the rank of sites based on score (total) and based on canonical orders

Table 13.11 Spearman correlation of the linear or weak orders of three partial order methods with the total score of Johnson for the six indicator constellations

Indicator configuration	Lattice theoretical-derived averaged ranks and its order	Bubley Dyer-derived averaged ranks and its order	Averaged ranks derived by the local partial order model and its order
Level 1	0.93	0.92	0.89
Level 2	0.81	0.81	0.80
Level 1 + level 2	0.76	0.70	0.80
Level 3	0.84	0.85	0.85
Four superindicators	0.79	0.80	0.83
$\{I_{13}, I_8, I_7\}$[a]	0.62	0.66	0.70

[a]Three most important indicators as outcome of the sensitivity study

indicators $\{I_{13}, I_8, I_7\}$ is worst. Generally the linear or weak orders due to partial order are in pretty good agreement with O_Γ. The main message of this section is that – based on the canonical order (see Chapter 9) – costs and time could be saved, by using only those indicators which belong to the expertise level 1.

13.7 Summary and Commentary

For the stream channel bridge crossing case study, assigning stream condition based on score (total) is satisfactory. Also, grouping all 13 indicators into four indices does not have a large effect on the order relations of the stream sites. The sites show reasonable agreement with the Hasse diagram and the canonical ranks for both data matrices. Based on the score (total), the threshold values that assign the stream sites into four categories are supported by the levels of partial order theory. Channel alignment is one of the most influential indicators for overall stream stability, as expected. However, the watershed and floodplain activity indicator was also expected to have greater overall influence on the stream stability condition. When considering the expense of collecting the indicator data, at least 10 indicator scores (level 1 and level 2) should be collected.

References

Johnson, P.A. (2005). Preliminary assessment and rating of stream channel stability near bridges. J. Hydraulic Eng., 131(10), 845–852.

Montgomery, D.R. and Buffington, J.M. (1997). Channel-reach morphology in mountain drainage basins. Geol. Soc. Am. Bull., 109(5), 596–611.

Newlin, J.T. and Bhat, K.S. (2007). Identification and prioritization of stream channel maintenance needs at bridge crossings. Proceedings of the International Bridge Conference, IBC 07–18, Pittsburgh, PA.

Newlin, J.T. and Patil, G.P. (2010). Application of partial order to bridge engineering, stream channel assessment, and infra structure management. Environ. Ecol. Stat., 17, 437–454.

US Army Corp of Engineers (1994). Engineering and design-channel stability assessment for flood control projects. EM 1110-2-1418, Washington, DC.

Chapter 14
Case Study: Watershed Analysis (Hydrology)

14.1 Overview

Twenty-one watersheds were characterized and ranked on the basis of two multiple indicator systems, level 1 (least expensive) and level 2 (expensive). Furthermore, level 3 indicators are defined which need investigations in the field and are pretty expensive and only six watersheds are characterized.

Composite indicators are defined on the basis of level 1 indicators, called LSI, and level 2 indicators, called SWR. LSI and SWR are thought of as two different means to rank the watersheds with respect to the environmental health. The indicators on the three levels are considered as proxies to describe the abstract and not measurable concept of "environmental health."

One task in the poset analysis is the verification or the falsification of the two composite indicators.

Whereas LSI is fairly justified by the partial order analysis, the SWR needs more attention, as its weighting scheme differs from that derived from a partial order analysis, applying the POSAC method (Chapter 3). Furthermore, it is observed that the partial order based on level 1 indicators differs remarkably from that based on level 2 indicators. Finally, it is striking that a proximity analysis (see Chapter 10) favors level 1 indicators as proxies of level 3, albeit for this study only six watersheds were available.

By the sensitivity study, it turns out that the indicator "impervious surface in watersheds" was most important under the level 1 indicators, whereas "invasive cover class" was most important under level 2 indicators.

As in the analysis of child development (Chapter 12), separated subsets are found, which are an outcome of a partial order analysis of the indicators of level 1. The indicator IMP (impervious surface in watersheds), CORFOR (percentage of total forest that is core forest in watershed) as well as FOR (percentage of forest in watersheds) explain this separation.

Special attention was given to the level 3 (environmental chemistry and biology) indicators: An examination of NO_3 vs biological parameters renders strongly differing sensitivity to the weights (of NO_3 vs biological parameters): The watershed

R. Brüggemann, G.P. Patil, *Ranking and Prioritization for Multi-indicator Systems*, Environmental and Ecological Statistics 5, DOI 10.1007/978-1-4419-8477-7_14,

"Saint Mary's A" (SM) is almost insensitive, whereas the ranking of "back river" (BR) varies strongly with the weights.

14.2 Background and Data Matrix

The data set of 21 watersheds obtained from the Atlantic Slope Consortium (ASC) will be analyzed with the goal of determining an accurate ranking of the health of the watersheds. See Brooks et al. (2007). As in Chapter 13 (bridge study), the data set has different levels of indicators, grouped into level 1 to level 3, increasing in the quality and accuracy of the data as well as in the amount of cost and effort needed to obtain the data:

Level 1: Landscape assessment using satellite data is the easiest to access and the least expensive (data matrix, see Table A.14).

Level 2: Rapid field assessment is obtained from on-site sampling. Certain level of expertise is involved in the field assessment (data matrix, see Table A.15). Generally, level 2 data is relatively inexpensive compared to the level 3 data.

Level 3: Intensive field assessment needs to be purchased from the US Environmental Protection Agency (EPA). It is the most expensive and best quality of data among the three levels. Due to the money and effort in the procedure of obtaining this data, it is available for only six watersheds (data matrix, see Table A.16).

The orientation of all these indicators is as follows: The higher the indicator value, the better the watershed.

We provide an overview of the three-level indicator system in Table 14.1 and the names of the watersheds in Table 14.2.

The investigators combined the five level 1 indicators and the seven level 2 indicators to indices: The composite level 1 index is called the landscape index (LSI):

$$\mathrm{LSI} = [\mathrm{FOR} + (\mathrm{IMP} + \mathrm{LDI})/2 + (\mathrm{MPAT} + \mathrm{CORFOR})/2]/3 \tag{14.1}$$

The composite level 2 index is called stream–wetland–riparian (SWR) index:

$$\mathrm{SWR} = (1/4)^{*}(\mathrm{FW} + \mathrm{SHA} + \mathrm{IR} + \mathrm{SS}) \tag{14.2}$$

$$\mathrm{FW} = (1/4)^{*}(\mathrm{BUW} + \mathrm{BA} + \mathrm{INV} + \mathrm{FPWL}) \tag{14.3}$$

The values of both indices can be found in the appendix (Table A.17).

Table 14.1 Meaning of the indicators of the three levels

Level 1		Level 2		Level 3	
Indicator	Definition	Indicator	Definition	Indicator	Definition
FOR	Percentage of forest in watershed	BUF	Buffer score	BIBI	Benthic IBI (index of biological integrity)
LDI	Landscape density index in watershed	IR	Incision ratio	FIBI	Fish IBI
IMP	Percentage of impervious surface in watershed	BA	Basal area of trees	NO_3	Concentration of nitrate[a]
MPAT	Mean forest patch size in watershed	INV	Invasive cover class		
CORFOR	Percentage of total forest that is core forest in watershed	SHA	Stream habitat assessment score		
		SS	Number of stream stressors		
		FPWL	Number of floodplain–wetland stressors		

[a]The orientation of NO_3 has to be reversed because a large value indicates a bad state of the watershed

Table 14.2 Watershed names and their identifier

Watershed	Identifier	Watershed	Identifier
Back River	BR	Conodoguinet A	CA
Cattail Creek	CC	Grindle Creek	GC
Gwynn Falls	GF	Little Contentnea	LC
Saint Mary's A	SM	Mantua	Ma
Southeast Creek	SC	Middle Creek	MC
Upper Patuxent	UP	Middle River	MiR
Ahoskie	Ah	Pamunkey	Pa
Buffalo Creek	BC	Repaupo	Re
Chickahominy	Ch	White Deer Creek	WDC
Christian Creek	ChC	Wisconisco	Wi
Clearfield Creek	ClC		

14.3 Partial Order Analysis, Based on Level 1

14.3.1 Hasse Diagram

X: the set of 21 watersheds
IB: the set of five indicators of level 1 ([0,1]-normalized data)
Orientation: The larger the values of the indicators, the better the environmental health.

Once again five indicators are used as proxies for the abstract principle "environmental health" and the Hasse diagram (Fig. 14.1) shows how the watersheds can be positioned with respect to these five indicators.

Figure 14.1 shows the following:

- There are six levels: Strolling up the Hasse diagram, we find watersheds of increasing better state with respect to the abstract principle of environmental health.
- The incomparabilities tell us that a certain state with respect to the environmental health is realized by profiles (Chapter 3) crisscrossing each other.
- There is a least element, BR, having values with respect to all five indicators which are less than those of any other watershed.
- Shape: Approximately rectangular, the disparity in the values of the five indicators does not strongly vary with the levels.

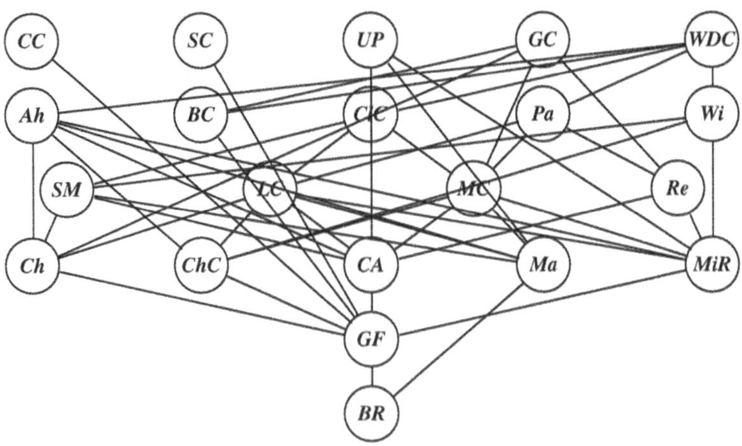

Fig. 14.1 Hasse diagram of (*X*, IB)

The Hasse diagram of Fig. 14.1 also supports some comparative decisions:

- A crude evaluation follows from the membership of watersheds to one of these order theoretical levels.
- There are some chains having at least four elements, allowing to order the watersheds uniquely without the use of LSI. For example, BR < GF < CA < LC < CC < GC, or BR < Ma < MC < CC < WDC. A list of all paths between two endpoints can be obtained by PyHasse.

The indicators of level 1 have different impact on the Hasse diagram as can be obtained from a sensitivity study (Chapter 4). For level 1 indicators, the following sequence (ordered for decreasing importance for a Hasse diagram) is found: IMP >> FOR > CORFOR > LDI ≅ MPAT.

CAM = 0.5. Therefore, any new indicator added or any deletion of an indicator may remarkably change the partial order (see Chapter 4).

14.3.2 Antagonism

Let X be the set of watersheds and $X_{res} := X - \{GF, BR\}$, then {CC, SC} and $X_{res} = \{UP, GC, WDC, Ah, BC, ClC, Pa, Wi, SM, LC, MC, Re, Ch, ChC, CA, Ma, MiR\} = X' \cup \{Ma\}$ are separated subsets (Chapter 5). By the tools provided by WHASSE, we find that IMP and CORFOR explain the separation at 94.1%. The complete separation (100%) is obtained if indicator FOR is included. Hence AIB = {FOR, IMP, CORFOR}. The scatter plot based on the 94.1 approximation is shown in Fig. 14.2.

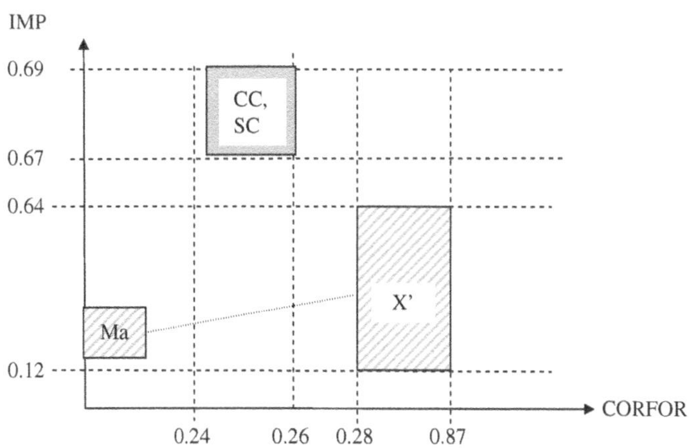

Fig. 14.2 Scatter plot explaining 94.1% antagonism between {SC,CC} and X_{res}. Watershed Ma belongs to X_{res} (indicated by a *broken line*)

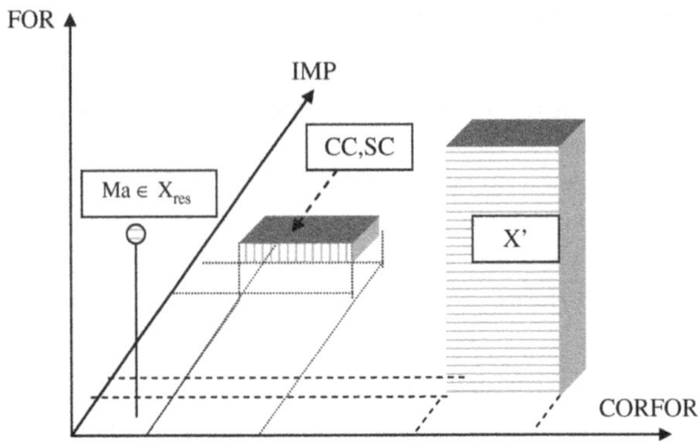

Fig. 14.3 3D schematic view on the results of the antagonism study

As one can see in Fig. 14.2, the separation {CC, SC} from X_{res} is not complete, because Ma $<_{\{\text{CORFOR, IMP}\}}$CC and Ma $<_{\{\text{CORFOR, IMP}\}}$SC. The third indicator FOR does the job of a complete separation. FOR(CC) < FOR(Ma) as well as FOR(SC) < FOR(Ma). Figure 14.3 summarizes schematically the results of the antagonism study.

We see from Fig. 14.3 that the range of FOR(X_{res}-{Ma}) includes that of {CC, SC}. This is consistent with the finding of Section 5.5.3.

14.4 Partial Order Point of View, Level 2 Indicators

The Hasse diagram of (X, $\text{IB}_{\text{level2}}$)

Object set X: 21 watersheds as before
$\text{IB}_{\text{level2}}$: Seven indicators of level 2.
Orientation: The larger the value, the better the state of the watersheds with respect to environmental health.

The Hasse diagram can be inspected in Fig. 14.4.

One may expect that the higher number of level 2 indicators leads to more contradictions in the data. This is indeed the case: Instead of six levels in the case of level 1 indicators, there are now only three. Furthermore, we see the following:

- ISO = {BC, ClC}
- WDC, GF, and GC are articulation points. Deletion of any of the corresponding rows from the data matrix generates at least one more isolated element. Deletion of WDC from the data matrix would lead to four more components in the Hasse diagram.

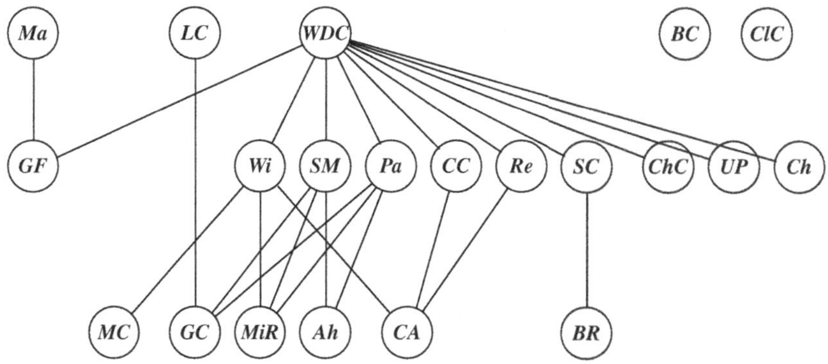

Fig. 14.4 Hasse diagram of $(X, \text{IB}_{\text{level2}})$

- MAX = {Ma, LC, WDC, BC, ClC}. The only maximal element which is also found through level 1 indicators is WDC.
- The proximity analysis between $(X, \text{IB}_{\text{level1}})$ and $(X, \text{IB}_{\text{level2}})$ (Chapter 10) renders fraction (isotone) = 0.08, fraction (indifferent) = 0.92, fractions of antitone, weak isotone, and equivalent = 0. We conclude that level 2 indicators do not contradict those of level 1. However, they strongly reveal different information about the watersheds.

14.4.1 Attribute-Related Sensitivity

Figure 14.5 shows the result of the sensitivity analysis.

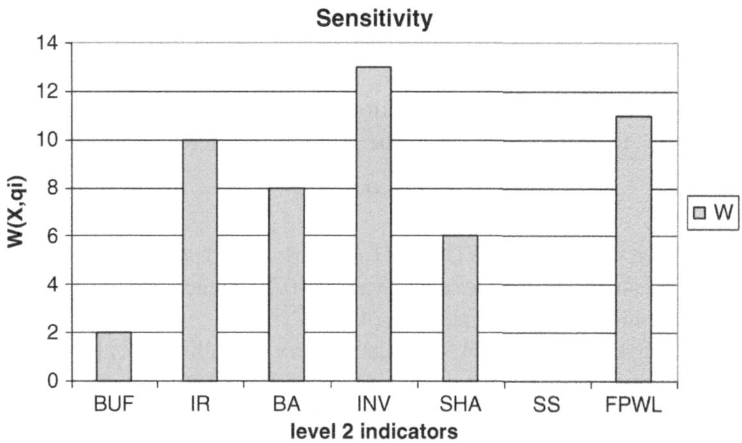

Fig. 14.5 Attribute-related sensitivity, level 2 indicators. The most important indicator is INV and the least one is SS

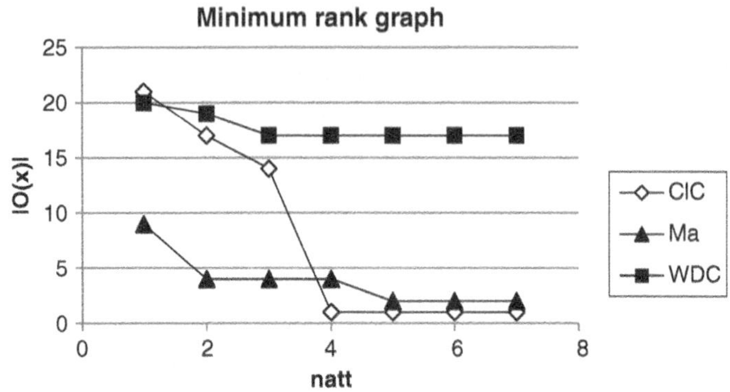

Fig. 14.6 Minimum rank graph of ClC, WDC and Ma in $(X, \mathrm{IB}_{\mathrm{Level2}})$ (see Chapter 4)

14.4.2 Minimum Rank Graph

We take ClC, WDC, and MA (which are maximal elements of $(X, \mathrm{IB}_{\mathrm{level2}})$ and determine their minimum rank graphs (Fig. 14.6).

In Fig. 14.6, we see the following:

- WDC has a slightly worse position than ClC but is pretty invariant, whereas ClC moves down through adding indicators.
- ClC has a steep gradient when the fourth indicator is added.
- The watershed Ma is in a middle position if only the fourth indicator, INV, is considered. All the other additional indicators affect Ma only slightly.

For a closer interpretation, we show the data profiles of ClC, WDC, and Ma in Fig. 14.7.

We see that each of the three watersheds has at least one indicator, where the watershed is better than the other two. In the case of indicator 4 of level 2, ClC is slightly better than WDC; however, the numerical difference is too small to be visualized.

WDC: Three indicators of WDC are 1 or nearly 1, inclusive of the most important indicator INV and the lowest value is 0.72. Hence adding the indicators has little influence on the position of WDC.

ClC: Adding the indicator BA to the data matrix must eliminate all successors of ClC, because BA(ClC) is near 0 (note: normalized data). All other watersheds have better values. Better values in the remaining indicators of ClC cannot increase the number of successors.

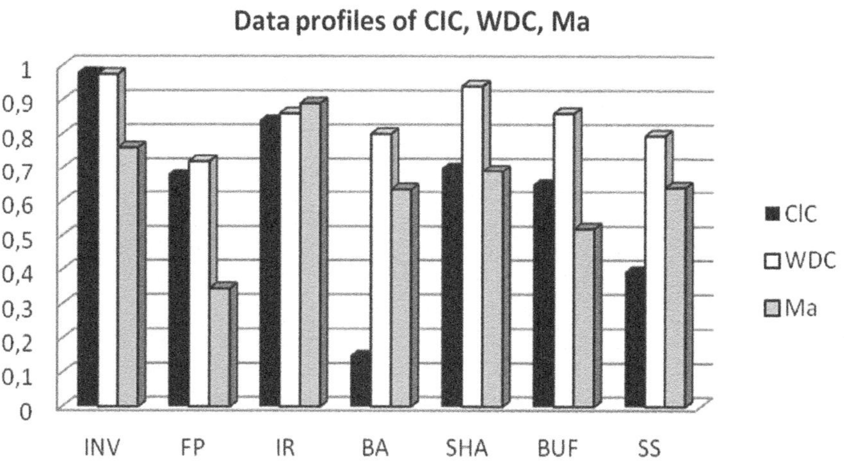

Fig. 14.7 Data profiles (normalized) of three maximal elements in $(X, \mathrm{IB}_{\mathrm{level2}})$, the level 2 indicators are ordered by $W(q_i)$

Ma: This watershed is a maximal element because of the good value of indicator IR. With respect to the indicator INV, the watershed Ma has only a medium to fair value.

Hence the minimum rank graph starts at rather low values. Adding the next important indicator FP excludes many successors, because Ma has here its lowest value. Therefore, a strong negative slope appears. As in the case of CIC, the better values in the remaining indicators cannot increase the number of successors.

14.5 Analysis Including the Level 3 Indicators

14.5.1 Hasse Diagrams

The Hasse diagram for the level 3 indicators is shown in Fig. 14.8.

Figure 14.8 shows the important role of the indicator NO_3 for the Hasse diagram.

14.5.2 Indicator NO_3 vs Biological Indicators FIBI and BIBI

Figure 14.8 motivates to study in more detail the role of NO_3 vs the biological indicators. Hereto we define

$$\mathrm{IBI} := 0.5^*(\mathrm{BIBI} + \mathrm{FIBI}) \text{ and } \varphi := g^*\mathrm{IBI} + (1 - g)^*\mathrm{NO_3} \qquad (14.4)$$

We perform the stability analysis (Fig. 14.9).

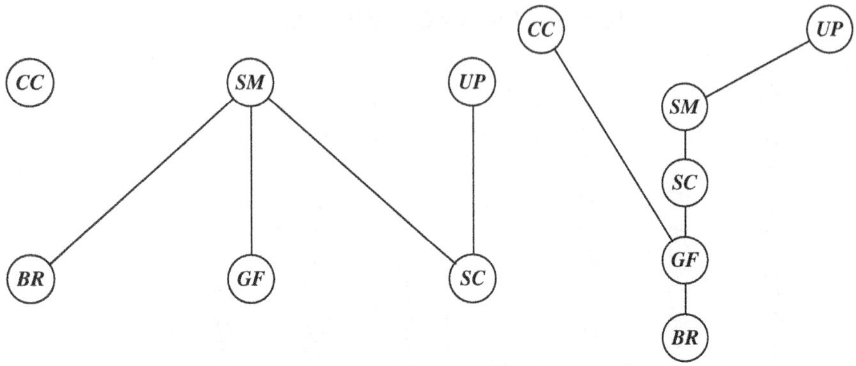

Fig. 14.8 (*LHS*) Hasse diagram for level 3 indicators; (*RHS*) FIBI and BIBI

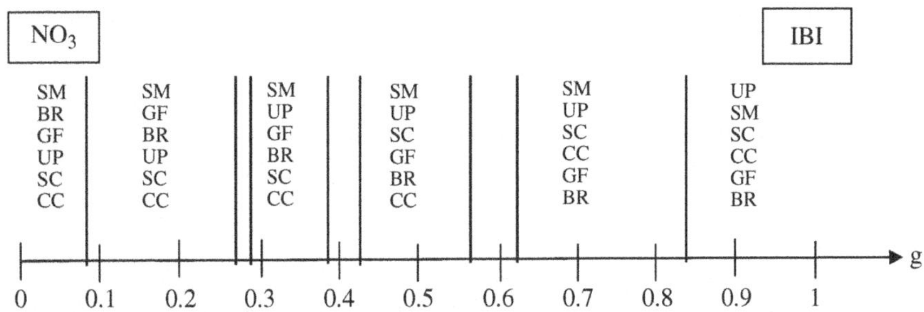

Fig. 14.9 Stability plot for the study of six watersheds and level 3 indicators and the composite indicator: $\varphi = g^*(0.5^*\text{BIBI} + 0.5^*\text{FIBI}) + (1 - g)^*\text{NO}_3$. *Vertical linear orders* given with enough space between two subsequent g_c values

In Fig. 14.9, the results of METEOR and stability analysis (see Chapter 7) are shown. We identify eight crucial weights. The stability fields together with the linear orders are displayed. With $g = 0$ (LHS), the linear order due to indicator NO_3 is obtained and with $g = 1$ (RHS), that of indicator IBI is obtained. One can see that

- the high height in the linear orders of watershed SM is rather stable; only if the weight g is larger than 0.84, it changes its position with watershed UP.
- the watershed CC has the lowest position until $g \approx 0.6$ but remains in the lower part of the ranking.
- the watershed SC has height = 2 for $0 \leq g \leq 0.39$. For all larger values of g, the watershed SC remains in the height position 4. The range of g values around 0.39 is a hot spot for SC.
- watershed GF is pretty sensitive to the amount how far NO_3 is mixed with IBI.

- there are two stability fields which are rather large, one between $g^* \approx 0.1$ and $g^* \approx 0.3$ and another between 0.6 and 0.85. If the indicator NO_3 is to be included, then the ranking of the watersheds does not actually depend on weights taken from these two ranges.

14.6 Proximity Analysis of Level 1, 2, and 3 Indicators on the Basis of Six Watersheds

We conclude the partial order analysis of the wetlands with the focus on comparing the three sets of indicators on the basis of six watersheds. What we want to know is, which set of indicators is a better proxy for level 3 indicators when a comparative analysis is our focus. Therefore we analyze the following:

- level 3 vs level 2
- level 3 vs level 1
- level 1 vs level 2

We perform for all indicators a discretization ($K = 3$, $\min_i$ and $\max_i$ values taken from the data matrix). The resulting three Hasse diagrams were compared by means of the proximity analysis (Chapter 10). The results are shown in Fig. 14.10.

We see the following:

1. There is no contribution to antitone
2. There are no weak isotone contributions
3. Dominating is the frequency of indifferent matchings
4. Focusing on how well level 3 indicators are modeled by level 2 or level 1 indicators, the degree of isotone between level 3 and level 1 is 10, whereas that between level 3 and level 2 is only 2.

We conclude the following:

1. The indicators of the three levels do not contradict each other.
2. The indicators are sharp enough so that there do not appear combinations like ($\cong$, <) (see Section 10.6). Therefore, the number of weak isotone equals 0.
3. Any indicator scheme has its own scientific value. Therefore, the objects are likely to be incomparable. Hence the contribution of "indifferent" is pretty high.
4. Taking into account that the results are based on only six watersheds and on a specific discretization scheme, we hypothesize that level 1 indicators are better suitable to be used as proxies for level 3 indicators compared to level 2 indicators.

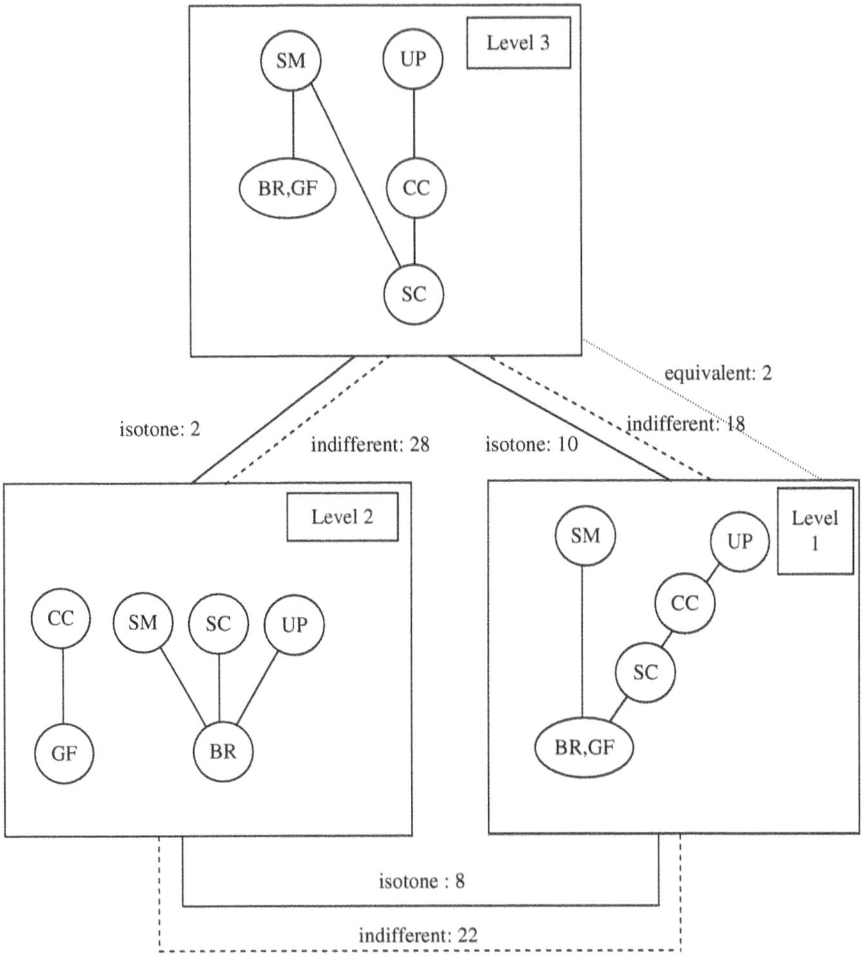

Fig. 14.10 Proximity analysis of the partial orders obtained from the three-level indicator systems for six watersheds

14.7 Analysis of LSI and SWR

14.7.1 Where Are We?

We have studied the Hasse diagrams and got an impression about the positions of the watersheds depending on the set of indicators without crunching the 5, 7, or 3 indicators into a composite indicator. All the three Hasse diagrams (level 1, level 2, and level 3) allow some comparison of the watersheds. Furthermore, we analyzed the indicator NO_3 vs. IBI as if we want to construct a composite indicator based on NO_3 and IBI, without having an idea about the weights. The order theoretical answer is to construct stability fields and hot spots in order to identify ranges of the weights, on the one hand, where some freedom in selecting the numerical value is and, on the other hand, where a slight variation will change the linear order of the watersheds.

However, the question is: Can we provide an alternative to the linear or the weak order a composite indicator provides? Here we do not want to be repetitive with apply methods explained in Chapter 10. Instead we will examine what the partial order tool POSAC (Chapter 3) has to offer to us.

14.7.2 Analysis with POSAC

As example, we take a closer look at the index SWR: We compare the weights given by the experts with weights which we develop from the data matrix itself. The tools we are applying is POSAC (see Chapter 3) and the concordance method to find the loadings, i.e., how far the original indicators contribute to the latent order variables of POSAC.

In this section we are closely following Patil (2001).

14.7.2.1 Loadings

As shown in Section 3.5, POSAC finds two latent order variables, LOV1 and LOV2 in short, and each object has a LOV1 and a LOV2 value corresponding to the POSAC diagram. We are interested in understanding the strength of the influence of the original indicators on the LOVs, the "loading." The loadings are computed for each indicator, and a loading gives a measure of similarity between the LOV and the data from a particular indicator. To allow for small deviations in the POSAC algorithm, we discretize both the LOVs and the original data into eight equidistant intervals. We compute a concordance value for each indicator and each of the both LOVs.

For the level 2 data set, 84.6% of the comparabilities are preserved by the two-dimensional POSAC model, and the two-dimensional POSAC diagram is in Fig. 14.11.

Table 14.3 shows the loadings concerning the level 2 indicators.

For level 2 the latent order variable LOV_1 is most impacted by indicators IR, which is the incision ratio, IR, followed by INV, which is invasive cover class, and SHA, the stream habitat assessment score. The latent order variable LOV_2 is most impacted by BUF, which is the buffer score of the watershed, and to a smaller extent by INV, SHA, and FPWL.

14.7.2.2 Derivation of Weights from the Data Matrix

Using the results of the analysis above on the loadings, we generate weights for the indicators which are solely based on the data matrix. Let I_i be one of the indicators and a_{ij} the loading for the jth LOV:

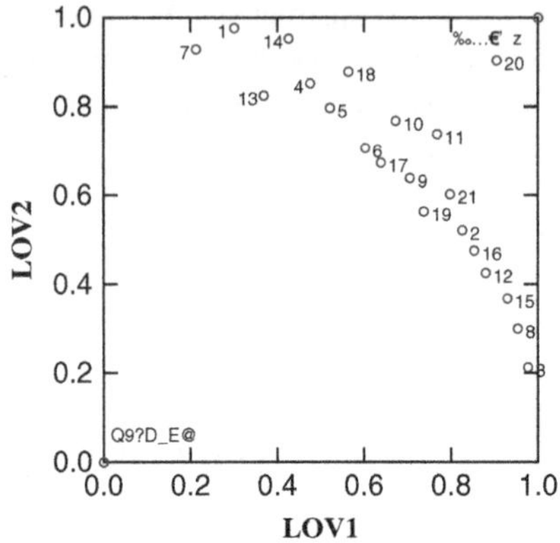

Fig. 14.11 POSAC Plot for level 2 data

Table 14.3 Loadings a_{i1}, a_{i2}, using concordance method for level 2 indicators

	LOV_1	LOV_2
BUF	0.380952	0.571429
IR	0.761905	0.333333
BA	0.428571	0.380952
INV	0.619048	0.476191
SHA	0.571429	0.476191
SS	0.333333	0.428571
FPWL	0.190476	0.476191

$$I_i = a_{i1}{}^*\text{LOV}_1 + a_{i2}{}^*\text{LOV}_2$$

We define

$$g_i = (a_{i1} + a_{i2})/\Sigma(a_{i1} + a_{i2}) \tag{14.5}$$

The quantity g_i is the final weight with which we combine the (normalized) I_i to a data-driven composite indicator (DDI):

$$\text{DDI} = \Sigma g_i{}^* I_i \tag{14.6}$$

Looking at the data-based weights from POSAC (Table 14.4), we see that the data-based index gives approximately the same amount of weight to all the indicators with a little less weight to stream stressor and FPWL stressor. When compared to the investigator-based SWR index, the POSAC-derived weights give less weight to the indicators IR, SHA, and SS than does SWR, since SWR gives all three of these indicators a weight of 0.25.

Table 14.4 Weights for level 2 indicators

Indicator	DDI (POSAC)	SWR
BUF	0.150	0.063
IR	0.154	0.250
BA	0.137	0.063
INV	0.169	0.063
SHA	0.159	0.250
SS	0.126	0.250
FPWL	0.106	0.063

14.8 Summary and Commentary

Considerable effort is expended in the assessment of the quality of watersheds. Three levels of indicators are defined, where level 1 indicators are the cheapest and the level 3 indicators the most expensive.

We performed some partial order analyses to see how the wetlands can be compared under the abstract principle of "environmental health," without applying a composite indicator. In doing this, we study the system of order relations and consequently it is of interest to see how this system of order relations, displayed in Hasse diagrams, changes if we delete indicators from the data matrix. We found which indicators are important and saw that IMP (of the level 1 indicators) is very important, whereas the sensitivity values of the indicators of level 2 are more spread out, albeit INV turned out to be the most important one.

A large part of this chapter is devoted to compare the different systems. As a main result, we see that there is some indication that the level 1 indicators seem to be better proxies for level 3 than level 2 indicators.

As far as the process of constructing composite indicators is considered, the POSAC method may be a good alternative and it may be an issue to discuss the weights of SWR because the order theoretical approach found a different set of weights.

References

Brooks, R.P., McKinney-Easterling, M., Brinson, M., Rheinhardt, R., Havens, K., O'Brien, D., Bishop, J., Rubbo, J., Armstrong, B. and Hite, J. (2007). A Stream–Wetland–Riparian (SWR) index for assessing condition of aquatic ecosystems in small watersheds along the Atlantic Slope of the eastern U.S. (Manuscript).

Patil, G.P. (2001). Penn state environmetrics and ecometrics, cross-disciplinary classroom notes. University Park, PA: Center for statistical Ecology and Environmental Statistics, Penn State University.

Chapter 15
Case Study: Environmental Performance Index (EPI) (Human and Environmental Health)

15.1 Motivation

In the EPI study, 16 indicators were introduced to analyze nations with respect to the human health and ecosystem vitality. Once again, indicators are used as proxies of an abstract principle and partial order shows how nations are ordered following these proxies.

Data for 102 countries are available. However, in our study, we concentrate ourselves on 18 European and 10 ASEAN nations.

Our first issue is to see how the 16 indicators work as proxy for environmental stressors affecting human health. For this purpose, we selected 18 European and 10 ASEAN nations, discretized the indicators, and examined the corresponding two Hasse diagrams. Although the Hasse diagram concerning the European nations has many more comparabilities compared to that of the ASEAN nations, both Hasse diagrams are not considered as a good starting point for further analysis. Therefore, we changed our focus on what we can learn about the different logical interrelationships among the indicators. A proximity analysis is possible by which a similarity of ASEAN nations to those of Europe with 16 indicators can be established. As a result, we find that Japan and two more ASEAN nations are similar to European nations, although there are different climatic, sociological, economical, and environmental conditions.

Furthermore, a formal concept analysis (Chapter 8) based on six superindicators (defined by the EPI study) leads to a network of associations and implications and it was of interest to compare the network induced by European nations with that induced by ASEAN nations.

We found that a good value in biodiversity implies good values in water and natural resources in the ASEAN network, whereas in the European network, good values in sustainable energy were implied.

R. Brüggemann, G.P. Patil, *Ranking and Prioritization for Multi-indicator Systems*, Environmental and Ecological Statistics 5, DOI 10.1007/978-1-4419-8477-7_15,

15.2 Data Matrix and Aim of the Study

The environmental performance index (EPI) aims at two major goals in environmental protection: (1) the reduction of environmental stressors for the improvement of human health and (2) the support of ecosystem vitality and better management of our natural resources (Esty et al., 2006).

The first goal is covered by definition and quantification of 16 indicators (Table 15.1).

The second goal is covered by the definition of six categories (six superindicators in our sense) that are "representative of policies that support ecosystem vitality and resource management" (Esty et al., 2006). We will consider these six superindicators in later parts of this chapter. There are 102 countries for which we have data for all 16 indicators. Raw data were collected by the investigators for each country for each indicator and were then scaled in a range [0, 100]. The data matrix 102 × 16 for the EPI can be found in the appendix (Table A.18). The EPI study is an excellent study performed over several years by experts in all relevant scientific fields. It is not our aim to present better or more detailed results but to demonstrate where and how partial order can be helpful. Therefore, we restrict ourselves to 18 nations of the European Union and 10 nations of the ASEAN group (see Tables A.19, A.20, and A.21). ASEAN is an association of southeast Asian nations. In order to compare with the results in the foregoing sections, we repeat now some of the steps for the nations of ASEAN (where due to EPI three nations were additionally considered: China, Japan, and South Korea, see EPI study). Because of data gaps,

Table 15.1 Indicators and their classes in the EPI study

Indicator	Acronym	Code
Child mortality	CM	I_1
Drinking water	DW	I_2
Adequate sanitation	AS	I_3
Indoor air pollution	IA	I_4
Urban particulates	UP	I_5
Regional ozone	RO	I_6
Nitrogen loading	NL	I_7
Water consumption	WC	I_8
Wilderness protection	WP	I_9
Ecoregion protection	EP	I_{10}
Timber harvest rate	TH	I_{11}
Overfishing	OF	I_{12}
Agricultural subsidies	AC	I_{13}
Energy efficiency	EE	I_{14}
CO_2 per GDP	CG	I_{15}
Renewable energy	RE	I_{16}

Table 15.2 European and ASEAN nations

European nations				ASEAN nations	
Belgium	BEL	Poland	POL	Malaysia	MYS
Bulgaria	BGR	Portugal	PRT	Japan	JPN
Denmark	DNK	Romania	ROU	South Korea	KOR
Germany	DEU	Sweden	SWE	Philippines	PHL
Finland	FIN	Slovenia	SVN	Viet Nam	VNM
France	FRA	Spain	ESP	Thailand	THA
Greece	GRC	United Kingdom	GBR	Indonesia	IDN
Ireland	IRE	Cyprus	CYP	Myanmar	MMR
Italy	ITA			China	CHN
Netherlands	NLD			Cambodia	KHM

LAOS could not be considered. Nevertheless, in the following, we refer to ASEAN nations (Table 15.2).

15.3 Partial Order Analysis

Hasse diagrams of (X_{Eu}, IB) and (X_{As}, IB):

- The object set X_{Eu} consists of 18 European nations, while that of X_{As} consists of 10 ASEAN nations.
- The information base (IB) consists of 16 indicators.
- The orientation: The larger the indicator value, the better the nation.

Table 15.2 shows the European and ASEAN nations.

As in Chapter 6, we apply a discretization (discretization scheme: $K = 3$, min and max values taken from the two matrices). In Fig. 15.1, the two Hasse diagrams are shown. We see that in (X_{Eu}, IB), more comparabilities (30) appear and the degree of comparability (number of comparable pairs/$(0.5^*n^*(n-1))$, n being the number of objects of the Hasse diagram) is 0.196. In (X_{As}, IB), only two comparabilities appear and the degree of comparability is only 0.044. Obviously the degree of disparity among indicator values of the European nations is remarkably smaller than that of the ASEAN nations.

The few comparabilities in both diagrams result from (i) the large number of indicators and (ii) from low correlation of them. Hence there is a need for enriching the partial orders by stepwise aggregation as a future task.

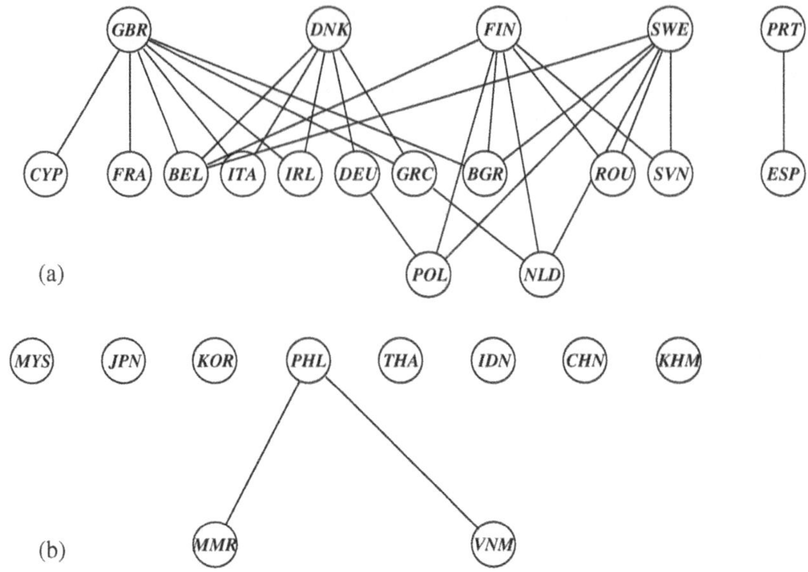

Fig. 15.1 Hasse diagrams of $(X_{\text{Eu}}, \text{IB})$ (**a**) and $(X_{\text{As}}, \text{IB})$ (**b**)

15.4 Comparison of 16 Indicators on the Basis of European and ASEAN Nations

15.4.1 Partial Order Analysis: European Nations

15.4.1.1 Transposed Data Matrices

One may ask how well any indicator out of the set of 16 is presented by the nations of the EU. That means that the 18 × 16 data matrix has to be transposed where now the 16 indicators are considered as objects and the nations are the attributes. Reading such a transposed matrix, let us take the row for UP, urban particulation, for the first seven nations:

	BEL	BGR	CYP	DEU	DNK	ESP	FIN
UP	87.1	67.5	67.8	91.3	90.9	78.4	92.5

From this part of the transposed data matrix, we learn that UP is best realized in Finland (FIN) and then in Germany (DEU). The worst realization is found in Bulgaria.

Now let us take two other rows:

	BEL	BGR	CYP	DEU	DNK	ESP	FIN
WC	9.0	33.3	100.0	70.9	95.9	32.3	99.2
WP	0.3	7.5	24.1	1.0	11.9	18.5	24.1

These two rows tell us that (within the set of seven nations – BEL to FIN) the indicator WP gets worse values, indicating that wilderness protection (WP) has smaller values in those nations, whereas water consumption (WC) has got larger values.

In Fig. 15.2, we see as to how far the 16 indicators (we take the original values of EPI) can be compared on the basis of their values for 18 European nations.

There are some chains containing four indicators, like WP < RO < UP < IA. In all 18 nations of the EU, IA is better than UP, UP better than RO, and RO better than WP. Such a chain (or better, the set of maximal chains) may be a characteristic for the subset of nations selected. In other subsets taken out of the 102 nations, such chains may not occur.

15.4.2 Partial Order Analysis: ASEAN Nations

Figure 15.3 shows the Hasse diagram of indicators.

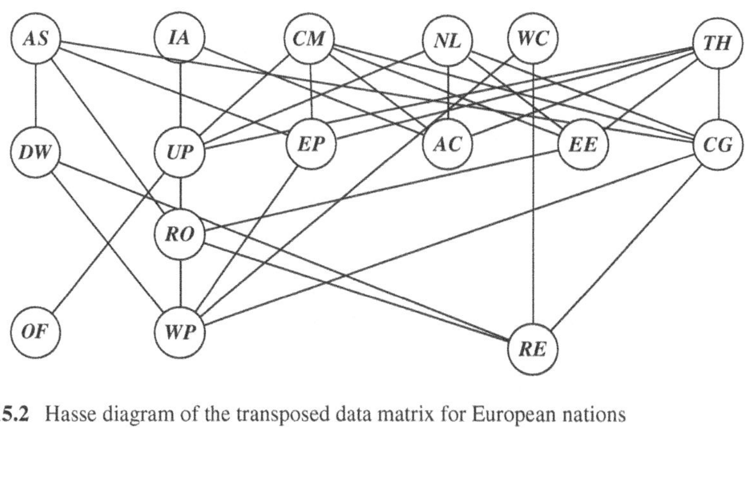

Fig. 15.2 Hasse diagram of the transposed data matrix for European nations

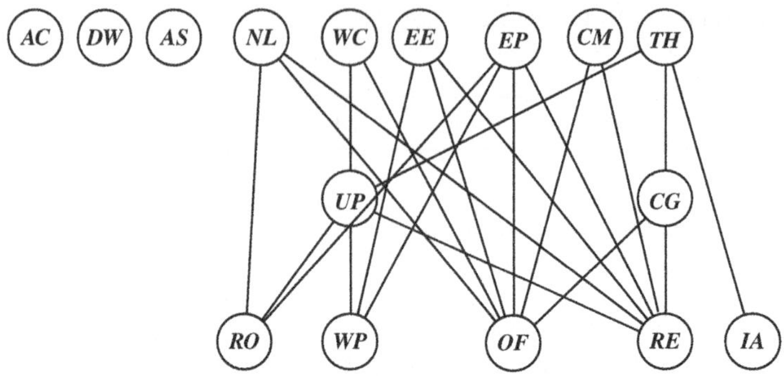

Fig. 15.3 Hasse diagram indicator values realized by different ASEAN nations

15.4.3 Comparison of Indicator Partial Orders for European and ASEAN Nations

In comparison to the poset found for the nations of the EU, we see that

- the Hasse diagram of European nations has four levels, whereas the Hasse diagram of ASEAN nations has only three levels.
- The ASEAN poset has isolated elements, like AC, DW, and AS: Some nations realize one attribute very good, but there are some others which at the same time do not have that good status.
- There is in both posets a chain of length 3 (i.e., it contains three indicators) with the same indicators: RE < CG < TH. Renewable energy (RE) is simultaneously worst for all European nations and also for ASEAN nations, CO_2 per GDP (CG) is better, and timber harvest (TH) is at the same time the best.
- There is no indicator pair *x*, *y* such that $x <_{\text{EU}} y$ but $x >_{\text{ASEAN}} y$ (see also the proximity analysis), where EU abbreviates European.
- From the six maximal elements of the European nations poset (AS, IA, CM, NL, WC, TH) there are four in common with those of the ASEAN nations: NL, WC, CM, TH and if we count isolated elements as maximal ones, then AS also belongs to the common group. Only IA (indoor air pollution) is an exception. It is a minimal element in ASEAN, showing the general need of improving the air pollution in ASEAN nations.
- From $V = 29$ (*V*, count of comparabilities (see Chapter 7 (Eq. 7.11))) in ASEAN, 20 order relations are realized in EU, hence the partial order based on EU is not an enrichment of that based on ASEAN nations.

Taking OF (overfishing indicator) as an example, OF $<_{\text{ASEAN}} x$, $x =$ WC, EE, EP, CG, CM, NL, TH. In EU, the indicator OF has not that bad state. See Figs. 15.3 and 15.4.

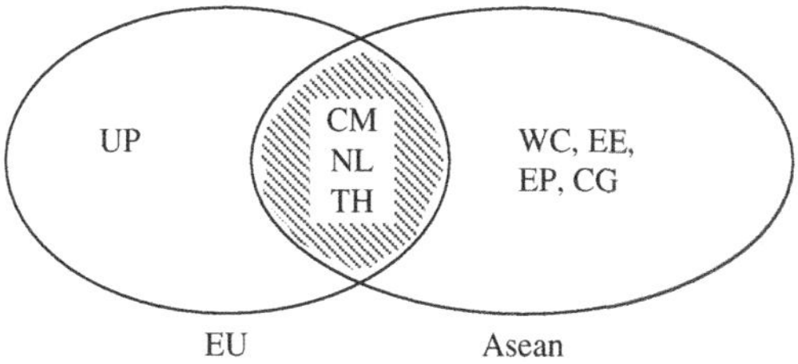

Fig. 15.4 Indicators comparable better than OF. Comparison of EU and ASEAN. There are three indicators in common: child mortality (CM), nitrogen loading (NL), and timber harvest rate (TM)

15.4.4 Proximity and Distance Analysis

15.4.4.1 Proximity

As described in Chapter 10, we perform a proximity analysis by counting the B_i classes. The result is shown in Fig. 15.5.

The fraction of common order relations is low as "isotone" counts only to less than 20%. We note that there is no contribution to "antitone," which confirms what we already found out by inspection of the Hasse diagrams.

15.4.4.2 Distance

Here is X the set of indicators and we have the following information bases:

EU: $= \mathrm{IB}_1$: set of European nations and
ASEAN the set of the ASEAN nations considered before.

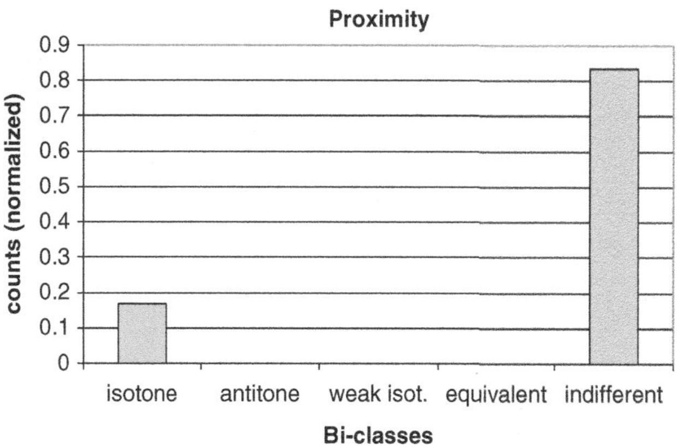

Fig. 15.5 Proximity analysis of the Hasse diagrams of Figs. 15.2 and 15.3

As further information bases, we introduce different unions of IB_1 with IB_2 as follows:

(1) "EU + JPN": = $IB_1 \cup \{JPN\}$
(2) "EU + MYS" = $IB_1 \cup \{MYS\}$
(3) "EU + PHL" = $IB_1 \cup \{PHL\}$
(4) "EU + 3" = $IB_1 \cup \{JPN, MYS, PHL\}$
(5) "EUASEAN" = $IB_1 \cup$ ASEAN

IB_2 in (1) is {JPN}, in (2) {MYS}, ..., in (5) ASEAN. The quantity $W(X, IB_1, IB_2)$ is a measure of the distance of the posets based on IB_1 to that based on IB_2 (Chapters 4 and 10). IB_1 is selected to be permanently EU. The information base IB_2 varies according to the list above, i.e., there are five scenarios for IB_2. Figure 15.6 shows the result.

Figure 15.6 shows that JPN, MYS, and PHL and all three together have only a slight impact on the order relations among the indicators found by the (rich and highly developed) EU nations, indicating intrinsic similarities of JPN, MYS, and PHL with the nations of the EU. However the residual group of nations of ASEAN influences the order relations, because more and more comparabilities are broken by the newly added columns referring to the nations. For instance, within EU nations, we find that RE < RO, RE < DW, and DW < AS. However, by adding ASEAN nations to the data matrix, these comparabilities will disappear.

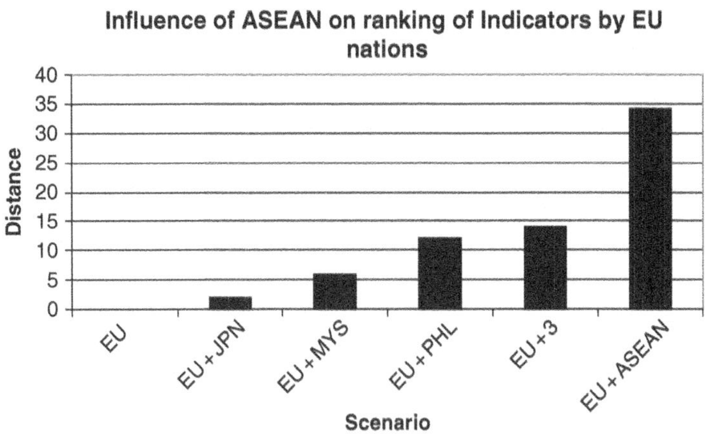

Fig. 15.6 Increasing distance $W(X, IB_1, IB_2)$. IB_2 includes different ASEAN nations as described above

15.5 Associations and Implications by Formal Concept Analysis for EU and ASEAN (Superindicators)

15.5.1 Superindicators

The scientists of the EPI study had a clear hierarchical approach in mind:

- A basic approach of 16 indicators, which allows a detailed analysis
- A coarsening by aggregation of contextually similar indicators to superindicators

The superindicators (SI_j, $j=1,\ldots,6$) are as follows:

- Environmental health, EH
- Air quality, AQ
- Water resources, WR
- Biodiversity and habitat, BH
- Productive natural resources, NR, and
- Sustainable energy, SE

Table 15.3 shows the assignment to superindicators; bold literals indicate the six superindicators and the dashed cells indicate which of the 16 indicators contribute to the superindicator.

For construction of the superindicators, we apply the weighting schemes as shown in Table 15.4. For more explanation, we refer to the EPI study.

Table 15.3 Superindicators "$SI_1,\ldots,SI_6$"

Indicator	Acronym	Code	**EH**	**AQ**	**WR**	**BH**	**NR**	**SE**
Child mortality	CM	I_1	■					
Drinking water	DW	I_2	■					
Adequate sanitation	AS	I_3	■					
Indoor air pollution	IA	I_4	■					
Urban particulates	UP	I_5	■	■				
Regional ozone	RO	I_6		■				
Nitrogen loading	NL	I_7			■			
Water consumption	WC	I_8			■	■		
Wilderness protection	WP	I_9				■		
Ecoregion protection	EP	I_{10}				■		
Timber harvest rate	TH	I_{11}				■	■	
Overfishing	OF	I_{12}					■	
Agricultural subsidies	AC	I_{13}					■	
Energy efficiency	EE	I_{14}						■
CO_2 per GDP	CG	I_{15}						■
Renewable energy	RE	I_{16}						■

Table 15.4 Weights according to EPI

Superindicator	Original indicator	Weight
EH	UP	0.13
	IA	0.22
	DW	0.22
	AS	0.22
	CM	0.21
AQ	UP	0.5
	RO	0.5
WR	NL	0.5
	WC	0.5
BH	WP	0.39
	EP	0.39
	TH	0.15
	WC	0.07
NR	TH	0.33
	OF	0.33
	AC	0.33
SE	EE	0.43
	RE	0.1
	CG	0.47

For example, EH is obtained as follows:

$$\mathrm{EH} = 0.13 * \mathrm{UP} + 0.22 * \mathrm{IA} + 0.22 * \mathrm{DW} + 0.22 * \mathrm{AS} + 0.21 * \mathrm{CM} \tag{15.1}$$

whereas AQ is simply:

$$\mathrm{AQ} = 0.5 * (\mathrm{UP} + \mathrm{RO}) \tag{15.2}$$

15.5.2 Context Table

We define

$$c_{ij} = \begin{cases} 1, \text{ if } \mathrm{SI}_j(x_i) > \text{mean of } \mathrm{SI}_j(x_i) \\ 0, \qquad \text{else} \end{cases} \tag{15.3}$$

$x \in$ EU or $x \in$ ASEAN. By c_{ij}, one-valued contexts were defined (Tables 15.5 and 15.6).

In Table 15.7, the mean values of EU and ASEAN are given.

15.5.3 Formal Concept Lattice

Figure 15.7 shows the lattice representation of the two mono-valued context tables.

Table 15.5 Mono-valued contexts of EU (representants of equivalence classes), cEH, cAQ, following Eq. (15.3)

	cEH	cAQ	cWR	cBH	cNR	cSE
BEL	1	1	0	0	1	1
BGR	0	0	0	0	1	0
CYP	0	0	1	1	0	1
DEU	1	1	0	0	0	1
DNK	1	1	1	1	1	1
ESP	1	0	0	1	0	1
FRA	1	1	1	1	0	1
GRC	1	0	1	0	1	1
IRL	1	1	1	0	1	1
NLD	1	0	0	0	1	1
POL	1	0	1	0	0	0
PRT	1	0	1	1	1	1
SVN	1	1	1	0	0	1

Equivalence classes: {DNK, FIN, GBR, SWE}, {ITA, ESP}, {ROU, BGR}

Table 15.6 Mono-valued contexts of ASEAN (representants of equivalence classes)

	cEH	cAQ	cWR	cBH	cNR	cSE
CHN	0	0	0	1	1	0
IDN	0	0	1	1	1	0
JPN	1	1	1	1	0	1
KHM	0	1	1	1	1	1
KOR	1	1	0	0	0	0
MMR	0	0	1	0	1	1
MYS	1	1	1	1	1	0
VNM	0	0	1	0	1	0

Equivalence classes: {PHL, KHM}, {THA, KOR}

Table 15.7 Mean values (columnwise) of EU and ASEAN

	EH	AQ	WR	BH	NR	SE
EU	95.0	56.0	86.0	40.5	63.6	71.9
ASEAN	63.9	46.5	91.8	61.3	63.8	71.6

Note that the lattices in Fig. 15.7 contain only representatives of the object set and of the attribute set. Furthermore, the marked lines indicate that a graphical editing may improve the layout. Here we do not take care of that. Furthermore, it may be helpful to consider the empty circles like a crossroad to differentiate them from other crossings in the diagram.

We see that more concepts are found for European nations than for the ASEAN nations due to the larger cardinality of the object set. Furthermore, we realize that

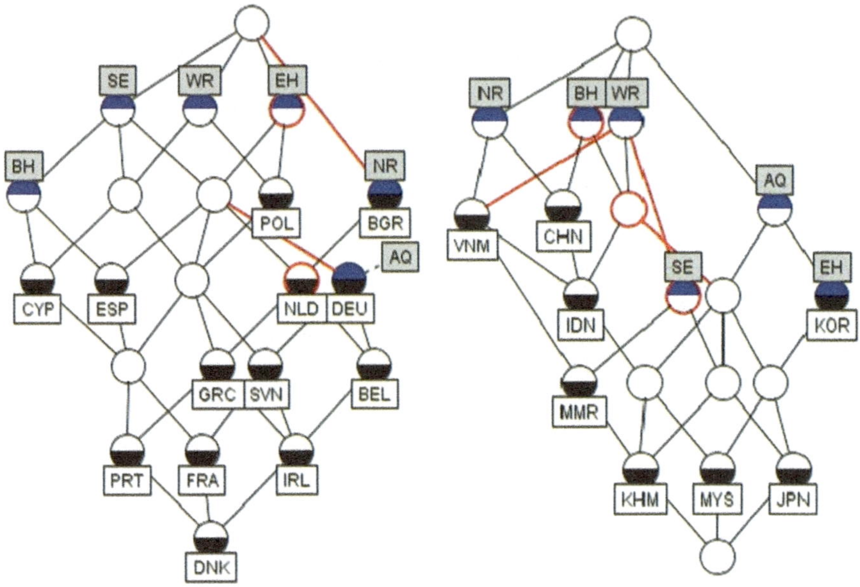

Fig. 15.7 The lattices of EU (*LHS*) and ASEAN (*RHS*)

the lattice of European nations has some more comparabilities among the concepts compared to that of the ASEAN ones; in fact the relation of number of cover relations to number of concepts is around 2 for nations of EU, whereas it is 1.75 for those of ASEAN. This observation is consistent with our remark at the beginning of Section 15.4.3.

We give two examples on how to read the lattice:

EU: AQ is a property pretty good for FRA, IRL, BEL, DNK, DEU, SVN
ASEAN: AQ is a property pretty good for KOR, KHM, MYS, JPN

Noting that ASEAN encompasses 8, whereas EU encompasses 18 nations, the proportion of nations having pretty good air quality, AQ, is larger in ASEAN than in EU.

Let us now look for the two indicators of resources NR and WR which are labels for the corresponding two concepts. NR and WR are covering a concept which is in the lattice of EU in the third level (counted from the bottom) of seven levels, whereas in ASEAN this concept is in the fifth level of seven levels. In the EU, only 4 of 19 nations have pretty good values simultaneously in both indicators, whereas this is the case for 5 out of 8 nations of ASEAN.

15.5.4 Network of Associations and Implications

In Table 15.8, we summarize the associations (see Chapter 8). The associations are thought of as being written as premise, PR, which implies the conclusion, CON, by the extent of association (EoA). For example, PR of the property WR has the objects {POL, SVN, GRC, IRL, DNK, CYP, FRA, PRT} and the conclusion (property SE) has the object set {BEL, CYP, DEU, DNK, ESP, FRA, GRC, IRL, NLD, PRT, SVN}. The intersection of both sets is {SVN, GRC, IRL, DNK, CYP, FRA, PRT} which is a proper subset of PR: $|PR \cap CON| = 7$, however $|PR| = 8$. Hence $EoA = 0.875$ or 88%.

Table 15.8 shows that in EU most often environmental health (EH) and sustainable energy (SE) are implied, whereas in ASEAN mainly the resource aspect is implied (water resources, WR).

Table 15.8 Associations and implications derived for EU and ASEAN

EU			ASEAN		
Premise	Conclusion	EoA	Premise	Conclusion	EoA
AQ	EH, SE	100	BH	WR	80
BH	SE	100	BH	NR	80
SE	EH	91	SE	WR	100
WR	SE	88	WR	NR	83
WR	EH	88	NR	WR	83
NR	EH, SE	86	EH	AQ	100

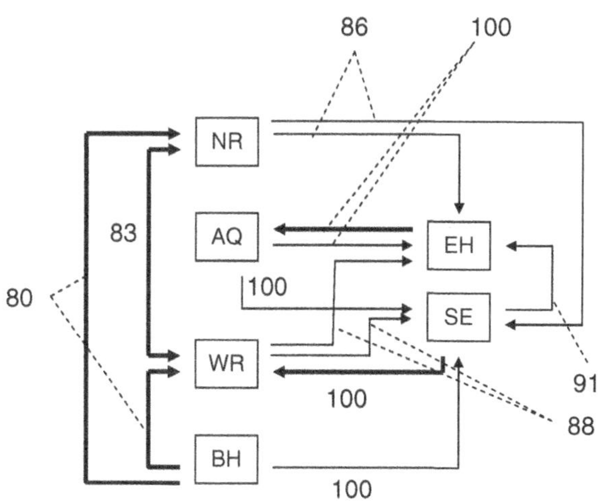

Fig. 15.8 Network of European "⟶" and ASEAN "➡" implications and associations

In EU, the conclusions refer to technical-oriented superindicators. We may therefore hypothesize that good standards in technical aspects in EU imply good standards in other technical aspects. Figure 15.8 renders a graphical presentation of Table 15.8.

Figure 15.8 tells us that if a nation achieves a "good" value in BH (biodiversity and habitat), then in ASEAN it is also true that a good value with respect to water resources (WR) and natural resources (NR) is obtained. In EU, however, this implies a good value in sustainable energy (SE). In ASEAN, natural and water resources are closely coupled, one aspect implies the other. This close coupling of resources is not found in EU. The arrow from the vertex SE to the vertex EH in the network (Fig. 15.8) is only realized in EU. Instead, in ASEAN, SE (sustainable energy) implies water resources. Indeed, as already commented above, WR is most often implied (three times) in ASEAN, whereas environmental health is most often implied in EU as it is the end point (sink) of four implications.

15.6 Summary and Commentary

The focus of this chapter is not the ranking of the nations or of a subset of nations, because the partial orders, even after classification of indicator values in discrete scores, were poor. In Chapter 7, we discussed how we can enrich the partial order. Instead of an application of METEOR which remains an interesting task for the future, we turned to analyzing the interrelationships among the 16 indicators and among the 6 superindicators.

In detail, we examined the role of indicators when different regions of the world are considered. Many order relations found for indicators in ASEAN are reproduced in EU, such as RO < UP and WP < WC. However, in ASEAN, indicators cannot be often ordered. Indicators are incomparable, because one indicator got large values by some nations and low values by some others, whereas the reverse happens for another indicator. This situation appears slightly more often in ASEAN than in EU. There is a larger disparity in the values of the indicator in ASEAN.

Formal concept analysis can help give more insights into this kind of comparison: In order not to get too large line diagrams, we concentrated on the six superindicators and tried to find out which associations and implications we will find for both regions. We found pretty different association structures. Here we were able to show only the first few steps. One obvious extension would be to analyze multivalued contexts, to find out which role a common mean value taken for both regions would play, how robust the association network is, and many other interesting questions.

Reference

Esty, D.C., Levy, M.A., Srebotnjak, T., De Sherbinin, A., Kim, C.H. and Anderson, B. (2006). Pilot 2006 environmental performance index. New Haven, CT: Yale Center for Environmental Law and Policy.

Chapter 16
Partial Order and Related Disciplines

16.1 Partial Order and Mathematics

It is always hard to try a positioning. Nevertheless, it may help interested readers to find their way through the jungle of concepts, relations, and equations of this text.

Certainly, partial order has to do with graph theory in discrete mathematics, as its visualization is a digraph and questions like connectivity or identification of articulation points and of separated subsets are typical of graph theory; see, e.g., Wagner and Bodendiek (1989) and Patil and Taillie (2004). There is also a connection to the network domain, as partial order constitutes a directed graph, which is one of the characteristics of networks. In our applications here, there is always a matrix, which quantifies the multi-indicator system, the data matrix. With or without the interim step of deriving the rank matrix, we arrive at a partial order. Once, however, the poset is derived, it may be analyzed as a mathematical object on its own right. So the comparative structure is not only inherent in the rank matrix, but other matrices can be found, which describe the order relation in different ways. Such matrices together with their arithmetic are realizations of incidence algebra; see Stanley (1986). So we have one example of relations to algebra. Another relation to algebra is the algebra of posets, i.e., how to combine them or how to find simpler graphs whose combination by different well-defined operations leads back to the original digraph (Neggers and Kim, 1998). The dismantling of an empirical poset finds its limits as to how far we can find an interpretation of the resulting simpler digraphs. Recently, an important step was done by partitioning the attribute set, construction of the posets induced by the indicators' subsets, and by an appropriate recombination of the posets. This procedure allows us to consider preferences among the attributes (Rademaker et al., 2008). Another relation to algebra can be established, when we realize that formal concept analysis is a powerful tool based on partial order. Concepts, being ordered by inclusion and forming a lattice, can be related to each other by two algebraic operations. Finally, formal concept analysis can be analyzed in terms of universal algebra.

The study of linear extensions and their properties, see, e.g., Habib et al. (1988) and Syslo (1985), is a field of combinatorics in discrete mathematics (see also Chapter 18), which also is important in applications of partial order analyzed in this monograph.

R. Brüggemann, G.P. Patil, *Ranking and Prioritization for Multi-indicator Systems*, Environmental and Ecological Statistics 5, DOI 10.1007/978-1-4419-8477-7_16,

16.2 Partial Order and Statistics

Welzl et al. (2002) have characterized the analysis of a data matrix with concepts of variance, distance, and order. This monograph is dedicated to partial order analysis (PoA) concerned with extracting ordinal information from the data matrix, when the aim of the ranking within a multi-indicator system is known and the indicators are appropriately oriented (Chapter 3). With statistical data processing of the day, we are confronted with three major questions:

Table 16.1 Comparison of partial order analysis (PoA), principal component analysis (PCA), and cluster analysis (CA)

Method	Advantage	Disadvantage	Remark
Partial order analysis (PoA)	Comparison of objects is the central topic. One of the most important tools of PoA is to provide a linear order of the objects without the need of a weighting of the indicators	We miss significance tests	An important concept is the ordinal modeling (Chapter 6). Its aim is to extract that information from the data matrix which is relevant for comparisons. However, we still miss theoretical guidance
Principal component analysis (PCA)	Insight into the structure of data matrix. Visualization techniques like biplots. Test statistics available. Weights can be constructed with which superindicators ("pillars") can be constructed	No direct access to order. Assumes linear models	Techniques are available to extend ordination technique to nonlinear models
Cluster analysis (CA)	Powerful access to group items due to their similarity. The items may be objects or attributes of the data matrix	Methodological artifacts, like the chain effect in single linkage methods	Reordering can be introduced and visualized as within any partitioning, there is freedom to order the classes of objects according to the partial order relations among them; see Mucha (2002)

1. How do we assess significance of partial order results when there is uncertainty in the data?
2. What kind of relation between partial order methods and multivariate statistics tools can be established?
3. How can we find good exploration and visualization techniques beyond Hasse diagram?

Ad 1: Assessing the significance of partial order results is done by simulations and can be a good topic for future research in partial order; see in that context Sørensen et al. (1998, 2000, 2009), Saltelli et al. (2008), Saltelli and Annoni (2010), and Annoni et al. (2012).

Ad 2: The second question may be answered by checking what the standard methods of multivariate statistics offer (Table 16.1).

Ad 3: Partially, this question is answered by application of statistical techniques (Table 16.1); however, the background of this question is "data mining" which is more closely discussed in Section 16.4.

16.3 Partial Order and Fuzzy Concepts

In Chapter 6, we applied the concept "ordinal modeling" because the order relations should not be overburdened by small data differences, which nevertheless are ordinal interpreted. One possibility is to introduce fuzzy concepts into partial order analysis. There are several possibilities:

(a) Instead of a hierarchical clustering, we may use a fuzzy cluster concept. This at least avoids the hard decision of whether or not an object belongs to a cluster. After an appropriate selection of a cluster center, partial order is applied to the cluster centers as fictitious objects; see Luther et al. (2000).

(b) In the Kosko approach, the crisscrossing of data profiles is replaced by a fuzzy subsethood. We have described this procedure and shown applications in this monograph (Chapters 6 and 11). Is the Kosko measure the ideal measure to obtain a fuzzy subsethood? What can be said about its relation to the mutual probabilities, derived from linear extensions? Could we find better measures than the Kosko measure which sums the indicator values? How to find optimal α-cuts (optimal with respect to what)? The question of α-cuts is discussed by Annoni et al. (2008). There, however, is still a need for theoretical work.

(c) An interesting alternative is provided by Fattore (2008), who does not use the Kosko measure but the height of an object in the set of linear extensions as a fuzzy membership function. This attractive method needs further attention, especially in its theoretical implications. It does not, however, directly contribute to "ordinal modeling."

16.4 Partial Order and Data Mining

16.4.1 Overview

We come back to some of the aforementioned points: There is a limit at present in the graphical presentation of partial order. Hasse diagrams are a wonderful visualization tool for working with posets with few elements. Alternatively, one may look for other visualization techniques, POSAC (Chapter 3), Bertin strategy, RRR, as well as the elimination of endmembers (EoE), and the use of dominance diagrams (Chapter 5).

16.4.2 POSAC

The idea is to project the m-dimensional attribute space due to m attributes of the information base into a two-dimensional plane spanned by two latent order variables LOV(1) and LOV(2). The projection is done by keeping at maximum the comparabilities found in the m-dimensional property space. The scatter plot allows an inspection of the whole object set and is – in principle – not restricted by the number of objects. The interpretation of the latent variables is sometimes difficult, and the computational methods lead to approximate solutions. By partial order dimension analysis, it can be checked as to whether a two-dimensional representation is intrinsically possible. However, there are still computational problems to be mastered.

16.4.3 Bertin Strategy

The starting point of Bertin strategy is the multicoordinate approach: The ranks of objects and the labels of the attributes represent the rows and columns, resp., of the Bertin matrix. An iterative procedure of row and column permutations is applied until the matrix gets as far as possible a blocked form (see http://en.wikipedia.org/wiki/Jacques_Bertin). The homogeneity of the block matrices is checked in order to maximize the homogeneity within the blocks and to minimize it among the block matrices. The complexity of this procedure corresponds to that of traveling sales man problem, hence heuristic approaches (cluster analysis) are to be applied. According to Welzl et al. (2002) there is, however, still need of statistical tests.

16.4.4 Rank Range Run (RRR) and Elimination of Endmembers (EoE)

The RRR approach was introduced by Myers et al. (2006). The main steps in rank range run (RRR) are the following:

1. Assign ranks to each of the attributes.
2. Order the objects according to their minimum rank.
3. If there are equal minimum ranks, take the maximum rank as an ordering property; if the maximal rank is equal, then take the median.
4. Each object is represented by a vertical line according to its minimum and maximum rank values.
5. Locate the objects along the horizontal axis by following the order of Step 3.
6. Mark the median of the ranks for each object.

Depending on how the orientation is selected (rank = 1 for the best or the worst value) the graphical display gives an overview about the ordinal properties with a focus on the whole set and with less focus on a single object. The length of any line associated with an object is associated with a degree of inequality. Here we stress that this approach does not depend on the representation by a graph, like the Hasse diagrams, and is suitable for data mining. Elimination of endmembers in RRR can be seen as a purification process; see Myers et al. (2006): One may ask oneself as to which elimination of an object with the highest rank gives the most reduction in the rank range (EoE gets positive values) and which object with minimum rank would give the most reduction in the rank range (EoE gets negative values). One may plot the EoE values vs the rank range run. This kind of analysis helps to identify attributes whose improvement would give a high effect on the overall status of an object or attributes whose status is responsible for the bad evaluation of some objects. For an example, see Newlin and Patil (2010).

Graphical analysis tools based on partial order concepts can be further developed, mainly based on the dominance relation (Chapter 5) and the local partial order approach (Chapter 9); see Myers and Patil (2010).

16.5 Partial Order and Network Analysis

Network is a topic in the systems analysis research because the analysis of networks as an abstract concept can deliver important results in several fields, such as

- Biology: food webs, biochemical networks
- Sociology: social networks
- Chemistry: reaction networks inclusive of biochemical networks
- Engineering: electrical networks
- Information technology: dependency networks of, e.g., compilers
- Urban drinking water systems
- River networks
- Transportation networks
- Bridge networks
- Implication networks as provided by the formal concept analysis (see Chapters 8, 13 and 15).

Even partial order can be considered as networks as comparative evaluation networks.

(a) What can network analysis learn from partial order approach and (b) what tools of network analysis can be helpful for partial order theory?

(a) Networks are vertex/node and directed edge evaluated graphs. So they fall into the general domain of graph theory. An obvious introduction of partial order is possible by considering the set of all subgraphs of a given graph and to order them by the (graph theoretical) inclusion relation. In chemistry, this conceptualization of molecular graphs and subgraphs as posets made an important contribution to the discovery of the relationships of chemical properties with molecular graphs obtained from molecules. See Klein (1986) in this context and Klein and Bytautas (2000) and Ivanciuc et al. (2005, 2006a, b) for the extended concepts like reaction graphs and substitution graphs.

   Another way to analyze a number of networks by partial order methods comes when networks are to be compared, i.e., when the set of networks is a poset. Then according to the aim of the comparative study, the indicators are obtained from the characterization of networks by network invariants, such as diameter, number of nodes, eccentricity, and centrality. In this case, networks are considered as objects described by multiple indicators. We have not seen this promising approach in the network analysis literature so far.

   Partial order finds application in network analysis when the set of vertices can be partitioned into two classes. In that case a Galois lattice provides useful tools (Wasserman and Faust, 2009).

(b) A powerful use of network concepts comes into play with well-known software graphviz to which PyHasse has an interface. The software graphviz resulted from network analysis and its graphical representation. The software graphviz (Gansner et al., 2009) uses many theoretical results concerning directed graphs and allows the user to draw Hasse diagrams under different options, such as

   - Rank separation,
   - Merging parallel connecting lines,
   - Aggregation of objects to clusters, and
   - Constrain rank assignments (subgraphs may get their own location for sources and sinks).

References

Annoni, P., Fattore, M. and Bruggemann, R. (2008). Analyzing the structure of poverty by fuzzy partial order. In J. Owsinski and R. Bruggemann (Eds.), Multicriteria ordering and ranking: Partial orders, ambiguities and applied issues (pp. 107–124). Warsaw: Systems Research Institute Polish Academy of Sciences.

Annoni, P., Fattore, M. and Bruggemann, R. (2012). A multi-criteria fuzzy approach for analyzing poverty structure. Statistica & Applicazioni, accepted.

Bertin strategy. http://en.wikipedia.org/wiki/Jacques_Bertin.

Fattore, M. (2008). Hasse diagrams, poset theory and fuzzy poverty measures. Riv. Int. Sci. Soc., 1, 63–75.

Gansner, E.R., Koutsofios, E. and North, S. (2009). Drawing graphs with *dot*. http://www.graphviz.org/pdf/dotguide.pdf.

Habib, M., Moehring, R.H. and Steiner, G. (1988). Computing the bump number is easy. Order, 5, 107–129.

Ivanciuc, T., Ivanciuc, O. and Klein, D.J. (2005). Posetic quantitative superstructure/activity relationships (QSSARs) for chlorobenzenes. J. Chem. Inf. Model., 45, 870–879.

Ivanciuc, T., Ivanciuc, O. and Klein, D.J. (2006a). Modeling the bioconcentration factors and bioaccumulation factors of polychlorinated biphenyls with posetic quantitative super-structure/activity relationships (QSSAR). Mol. Divers., 10, 133–145.

Ivanciuc, T., Ivanciuc, O. and Klein, D.J. (2006b). Prediction of environmental properties for chlorophenols with posetic quantitative super-structure/property relationships (QSSPR). Int. J. Mol. Sci., 7, 358–374.

Klein, D.J. (1986). Chemical graph-theoretic cluster expansions. Int. J. Quant. Chem., 20, 153–171.

Klein, D.J. and Bytautas, L. (2000). Directed reaction graphs as posets. Match, 42, 261–290.

Luther, B., Bruggemann, R. and Pudenz, S. (2000). An approach to combine cluster analysis with order theoretical tools in problems of environmental pollution. Match, 42, 119–143.

Mucha, H. (2002). Clustering techniques accompanied by matrix reordering techniques. In K. Voigt and G. Welzl (Eds.), Order theoretical tools in environmental sciences – order theory (Hasse diagram technique) meets multivariate statistics (pp. 129–140). Aachen: Shaker-Verlag.

Myers, W.L. and Patil, G.P. (2010). Partial order and rank range runs for compositional complexes in landscape ecology and image analysis, with applications to restoration, remediation, and enhancement. Environ. Ecol. Stat., 17, 411–436.

Myers, W.L., Patil, G.P. and Cai, Y. (2006). Exploring patterns of habitat diversity across landscapes using partial ordering. In R. Bruggemann and L. Carlsen (Eds.), Partial order in environmental sciences and chemistry (pp. 309–325). Berlin: Springer.

Neggers, J. and Kim, H.S. (1998). Basic posets. Singapore: World Scientific Publishing.

Newlin, J.T. and Patil, G.P. (2010). Application of partial order to bridge engineering, stream channel assessment, and infra structure management. Environ. Ecol. Stat., 17, 437–454.

Patil, G.P. and Taillie, C. (2004). Multiple indicators, partially ordered sets, and linear extensions: Multi-criterion ranking and prioritization. Environ. Ecol. Stat., 11, 199–228.

Rademaker, M., De Baets, B. and De Meyer, H. (2008). New operations for informative combinations of two partial orders with illustrations on pollution data. Comb. Chem. High Throughput Screen., 11(9), 745–755.

Saltelli, A. and Annoni, P. (2010). How to avoid a perfunctory sensitivity analysis. Environ. Model. Softw., 25, 1508–1517.

Saltelli, A., Ratto, M., Andres, T., Campolongo, F., Cariboni, J., Gatelli, D., et al. (2008). Global sensitivity analysis – The primer. Chichester: Wiley.

Sørensen, P.B., Bruggemann, R., Thomsen, M., Gyldenkaerne, S. and Kjaer, C. (2009). How to guide and assess risk reduction using risk characterization indicators. Am. J. Appl. Sci., 6(6), 1255–1263.

Sørensen, P.B., Mogensen, B.B., Carlsen, L. and Thomsen, M. (2000). The influence on partial order ranking from input parameter uncertainty – Definition of a robustness parameter. Chemosphere, 41, 595–600.

Sørensen, P.B., Mogensen, B.B., Gyldenkaerne, S. and Rasmussen, A.G. (1998). Pesticide leaching assessment method for ranking both single substances and scenarios of multiple substance use. Chemosphere, 36(10), 2251–2276.

Stanley, R.P. (1986). Enumerative combinatorics (Vol. I). Monterey: Wadsworth and Brooks/Cole.

Syslo, M.M. (1985). A graph-theoretic approach to the jump-number problem. In I. Rival (Ed.), Graphs and order (pp. 185–215). Dordrecht: D. Reidel Publishing Company.

Wagner, K. and Bodendiek, R. (1989). Graphentheorie I: Anwendungen auf Toplogie, Gruppentheorie und Verbandstheorie. Mannheim: BI Wissenschaftsverlag.

Wasserman, S. and Faust, K. (2009). Social network analysis – Methods and applications. Cambridge: Cambridge University Press.

Welzl, G., Voigt, K. and Bruggemann, R. (2002). Order theory meets statistics – Environmental statistics. In K. Voigt and G. Welzl (Eds.), Order theoretical tools in environmental sciences – order theory (Hasse diagram technique) meets multivariate statistics (pp. 41–54). Aachen: Shaker-Verlag.

Chapter 17
Partial Order and Software

17.1 Software Available

Halfon (2006) reviews available software. We summarize and update the review for the convenience of the reader:

RANA, Pavan (2003)
DART, Manganaro et al. (2008)
PRORANK, Pudenz (2005) and Voigt et al. (2006)
CORRELATION, Sørensen et al. (2005)
WHASSE, Bruggemann et al. (1999)
POSAC, Shye (1994) and Borg and Shye (1995); see also http://ca.huji.ac.il/bf/hudap-Info.pdf
POSET, Patil et al. (2009, personal communication (POSET-ranking))
PyHasse, Bruggemann et al. (2008a, b), Bruggemann and Voigt (2009), and Voigt et al. (2008a, b)
VB-RAPID, Joshi et al. (2010)

If formal concept analysis is included then the list above can be extended; see the home page: http://www.upriss.org.uk/fca/fcasoftware.html:

TOSCANA, see Vogt and Wille (1995a, b)
CONIMP-variants, see Burmeister (1997)
CONEXP1.3, see Yevtushenko (2000), http://sourceforge.net/projects/conexp

17.2 Brief Characterization of Some of the Software

Some software packages may be presented briefly. The selection is subjective and does not reflect any quality or importance.

PRORANK (programming language: JAVA): Still under development, intends to include multivariate statistics as far as possible. It already has tools to edit the graphics and to handle subsets of objects and indicators. In comparison with the software WHASSE, data handling is greatly facilitated.

R. Brüggemann, G.P. Patil, *Ranking and Prioritization for Multi-indicator Systems*, Environmental and Ecological Statistics 5, DOI 10.1007/978-1-4419-8477-7_17,

CORRELATION (programming language: DELPHI): The very idea is to examine two partial orders and how far a "correlation" can be found on the basis of these two posets.

WHASSE (programming language: DELPHI): Includes down sets, antagonism, object selection wizards, matrix W, linear extensions and applications to calculate rank frequency distributions, averaged ranks and mutual probabilities, and CAM (called P(IB)). WHASSE is professionally programmed, has a well-developed graphical user interface, and can be delivered as a stand-alone package, i.e., it is not necessary to use Internet for installing the software.

DART (programming language C++): Includes multivariate procedures like PCA and KMEANS clustering and several functions to provide linear orders and also has some facilities for posetic approaches.

POSAC: In SYSTAT.

POSET (programming language: C++): Development at Penn State Center for Statistical Ecology and Environmental Statistics. It provides linear ranks on the basis of linear extensions.

PyHasse (programming language: PYTHON): Major software used in the monograph. Therefore, we describe PyHasse in more detail later (Section 17.3).

VB-RAPID (VISUAL BASIC): Developed by Joshi et al. (2010). It is described in more detail in Section 17.4.

17.3 PyHasse

17.3.1 Overview

PyHasse is based on the free downloadable PYTHON programming software, version 2.6. PYTHON programs can be used on different platforms and under different operating systems; there are many specific and powerful free downloadable libraries available.

Graphical user interfaces (GUIs) can be programmed by Tkinter, which is available together with PYTHON and is based on Tk/Tcl. PYTHON supports testing and can be considered as an "experimental software," allowing the programmer to quickly gain experience in programming work and, more important, to test and efficiently program new theoretical tools.

17.3.2 General Principles of PyHasse

First of all, PyHasse should be considered as a test version. It actually consists of more than 30 programs (called "modules") and is still pretty dynamically under development. An overview with status of March 2009 can be found in Bruggemann and Voigt (2009).

The modules are independently written programs, so new ideas can be easily programmed without having to take care of already used variable names. All modules are related to two libraries, written by Bruggemann, which contain basic procedures and basic classes of object-oriented programming: rmod2 and raioop2. Some modules have interfaces by which results can be interchanged.

One of the modules is "pyhassemenue7," the central platform from where general information can be obtained (for example a tutorial) and from where actual interesting modules can be selected.

The appearance of the modules (i.e., their user interfaces) is similar as far as possible. Each module has a "help" function. This help function informs about

- aim of the module,
- prerequisites (especially how to handle Excel® data files as input),
- usage (or steps),
- known bugs or difficulties, and
- recommended example files (provided with the PyHasse software).

In many cases, there is also an "about" button, which informs about the status of the module and gives background information, for example, about important literature.

17.3.3 List of Modules

In PyHasse, three types of modules are available:

M: Basic PyHasse Analysis Tool
D: Simple versions of decision support systems
H: Supporting modules (interfaces, tutorial writers) (Table 17.1)

Table 17.1 PyHasse modules, alphabetically sorted (status November 2009)

	Name	Main tasks	Class	Remark
1	antag2.py	Which pair of attributes leads to the maximal Sep(X_1, X_2)	M	
2	avrank4.py	Canonical order based on lattice theoretical method. Module avrank4.py is mainly based on the free software lcell of Wienand (2005, 2006). See also Morton et al. (2006, 2009)	M	For a broader background, see also Chapter 9
3	avs6.py	Changes of attribute values: Which consequences	M	Will be replaced in the near future by pooc
4	cap6.py	Comparative acquisition profile	M	
5	concord2.py	Concordance analysis	H	
6	covi2.py	Reads interactively cover information, generates a Hasse diagram, and translates it into graphviz format	H	

Table 17.1 (continued)

	Name	Main tasks	Class	Remark
7	covreader4	Reads information from an external cover matrix	H	
8	dahp4	The weights for super-attributes are found by the AHP procedure of Saaty (1994)	M	A comparison with weights obtained from other methods is of interest; however, we leave it for future work
9	dds8.py	Calculation of dominance diagrams	M	
10	Disco2.py	Discordance–concordance analysis	D	
11	discretiz1.py	Performs a discretization, transformed data matrix is available for mainHD16	H	
12	fuzzyHD12.py	Fuzzy partial order analysis	M	
13	genlinext1.py	If the number of objects is less than 10, then the averaged ranks and the height frequency matrix are calculated very fast. Height frequency plots for selected objects are available	H	
14	graphviz1.py	Reads information from cover matrix (available from, e.g., mainHD16 and provides the Hasse diagram in graphviz format)	H	
15	hdgt4	Some graph theoretical information of the Hasse diagram. Provides averaged ranks by extended local partial order model version (Bruggemann and Carlsen, 2011)	M	
16	HDsimpl1	Quick access to the Hasse diagram from a data matrix	H	
17	hpor1.py	Hierarchical partial order analysis. Based on averaged ranks form of groups of attributes; Carlsen (2008)	M	
18	interval4.py	Analysis by m^2-order and inclusion order of the intervals	M	
19	linagg6.py	Monte Carlo Simulation of the rank of an index, randomly selecting the weights	M	

Table 17.1 (continued)

	Name	Main tasks	Class	Remark
20	linext_play2.py	Reads in linear extensions and calculates their intersection	H	
21	LPOMstruct1.py	Reads in characteristics of a Hasse diagram and calculates the average heights	H	
22	mainHD19.py	Hasse diagram, down sets, up sets, intervals, minimum spanning trees, linear extensions after Bubley Dyer, LPOM, chain statistics	M	The most important tool
23	mutprobavrk.py	Reads in characteristics of a Hasse diagram and calculates mutual ranking probabilities	H	
24	optimsim5.py	Which attribute subset makes a partial order most similar to a given one	M	Will be replaced in the near future
25	oreste6.py	If preferences of $a > b$, vs $b > a$ are known then a graphical characterization of the decision situation is given	D	
26	owa3.py	Aggregation to superindicators applying fuzzy concepts; Yager (1993)	M	
27	palg4.py	Application of p-algorithm	M	
28	pir3.py	Information about PyHasse texts	H	
29	pooc3	Attribute-related sensitivity	M	Will be upgraded in the near future
30	POTanalysis1	Module mainHD19 is simplified to fit into pyhassemenue7	H	
31	prom6	PROMETHEE (simplified)	D	
32	pyHasse_progr1.py	Information about PyHasse modules	H	
33	pyhassemenue7.py	Information platform and access to the modules of PyHasse	H	
34	randomdm2.py	Generates random data matrices	H	
35	sensi11.py	Attribute-related sensitivity analysis	M	
36	sep3.py	Calculates which set of attributes is common for X_1 and X_2 such that for all $x \in X_1, y \in X_2, x > y$; common for X_1 and X_2, such that for all $x \in X_1, y \in X_2, x < y$; common for X_1 and X_2, such that for all $x \in X_1, y \in X_2, x = y$	M	sepanal2.py with many more tools replaced sep3.py (July 2010)

Table 17.1 (continued)

	Name	Main tasks	Class	Remark
37	simi4.py	Proximity analysis of two partial orders, test for inclusion of two partial orders, set of edges corresponding to the symmetric difference of any two partial orders	M	In testing phase
38	stability3.py	Calculates stability fields and hot spots	M	
39	zetareader1	Reads in an external zeta matrix, calculation of mutual probability after De Loof et al. (2008a)	H	

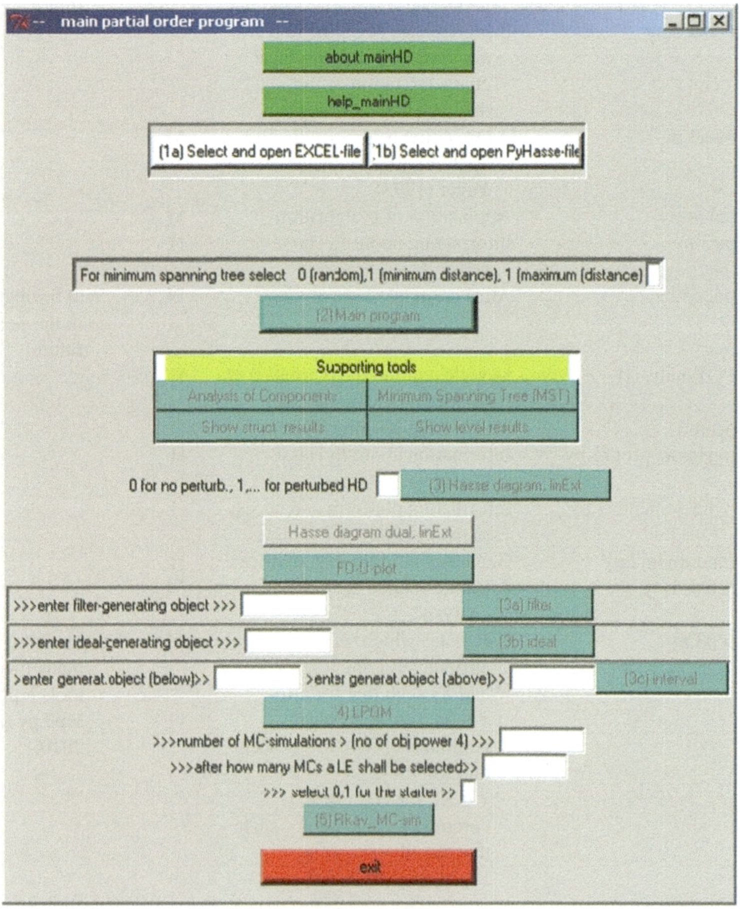

Fig. 17.1 Graphical user interface of mainHD19.py

The module mainHD19 is the main working module and can be used to analyze transformed data matrices of the modules discretiz1.py and palg4.py. Additionally mainHD19 provides data formats such that the graph theoretical program graphviz (see http://4webmaster.de/wiki/Graphviz-Tutorial) can be applied to obtain readable directed graphs. The user interface of mainHD19.py is shown in Fig. 17.1.

There are four areas in the graphical user interface:

1. informal part and the access to different data
2. characteristics of a poset can be obtained as well as the Hasse diagrams
3. navigation within a Hasse diagram
4. linear or weak orders by LPOM or Bubley Dyer algorithm

Some buttons are only activated if the needed information is provided.

Table 17.2 lists the use of PyHasse in the theoretical part of the monograph.

Table 17.2 Use of PyHasse in the theory part of the monograph

Sections	Figures	Topic	PyHasse module	Remark
4.2.5		Sensitivity measures	sensi11.py	
4.4.1		Stability and related graphs	snsi11.py	
5.2	Figure 5.3	Incomparabilities related to levels	mainHD16.py	Now (30 July 2010): mainHD19.py
5.4.2		Antagonistic attributes	antag2.py	Only analysis for pairs of attributes
5.5	Figure 5.20	Dominance	dds.8	
6.3		Discretization	discretiz1.py	
6.4		Fuzzy partial order	fuzzyHD12.py	
6.5		p-algorithm	palg4.py	
7.2.5	Figure 7.7	MC simulation	linagg6.py	
7.3		m^2 order, inclusion order	interval4.py	Now (30 July 2010) interval7.py
7.4.2		Comparability acquisition profile	cap6.py	
7.5		Stability fields	stability3.py	
9.3.3		Local partial order model	mainHD16.py	LPOMstruct1.py: interactive program
9.4		Bubley Dyer algorithm	mainHD19.py	
9.6		Lattice method	avrank4.py	
9.8.2	Figure 9.8	Mutual probability	mutprobavrk1.py	Interactive program
10.4		Concordance analysis	concord2.py	
10.6		Proximity analysis	simi4.py	Now (30 July 2010): simi5.py

17.4 RAPID

17.4.1 Standards

Under the auspices of the USNSF project for digital governance and hot spot geoinformatics for monitoring, etiology, early warning, and sustainable management and development at the Penn State Center for Statistical Ecology and Environmental Statistics, G.P. Patil, Principal Investigator, effort has been in progress for methodology and software development for ranking and prioritization information delivery (RAPID).

The software "RAPID" has been under development to clearly encompass features of some well-known programs and more, such as

- WHASSE
- POSET
- POSAC
- PyHasse

17.4.1.1 Steps of Developing RAPID

RAPID is developed in several steps. RAPID0 provides the Hasse diagram and basic tools to analyze it. RAPID1 will contain additional features arising from the partial order context.

Of most importance is that a tool of getting linear or weak orders out of a poset is available. The general concept is explained in Fig. 17.2.

There are several crucial steps:

a) The starter for the Monte Carlo Markov chain calculation (MCMC) after Bubley Dyer,
b) Sampling of the final subset of linear extensions, and
c) Defining conditions in the decision mark.

Especially (c) still uses some heuristics.

The programming language is VISUAL BASIC at present.

17.4.2 Modules and Facilities of VB-RAPID

In contrast to PyHasse, VB-RAPID 1 consists of one single program and the access to different tools of partial order follows by menus and submenus. The main menus are

File: Open and save data
Functions: Basic information about the data matrix

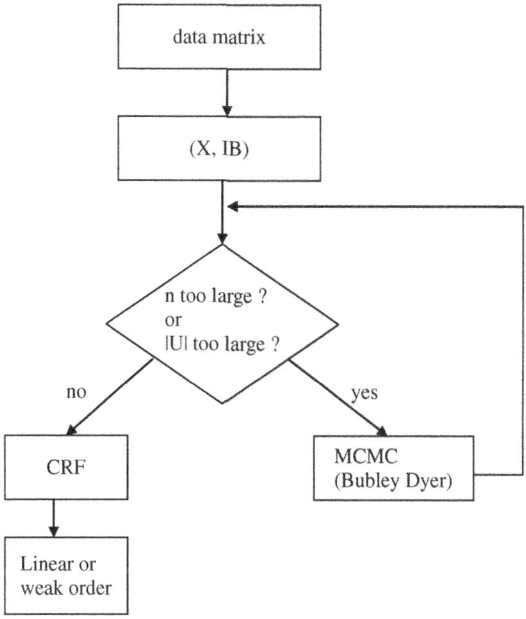

Fig. 17.2 RAPID-ranking, a combination of the Bubley Dyer and the cumulative rank frequency (CRF) algorithm; see Chapter 9

HASSE Diagram: Hasse diagram in two possible orientations
Results: Access to partial order tools (see below)
Help: Context specific help texts written in HTML

The menu "Results" pops up to the following submenu:

1. Level population
2. Cover matrix
3. Down sets and up sets
4. Intervals
5. Maximal, minimal, and isolated elements
6. Structural details (predecessors, successors, and incomparable elements)
7. Sensitivity, based on the matrix W (W(X,IB(i),IB(j)))
8. LPOM
9. D-matrix (which we did not consider in the monograph)
10. Minimum rank graph
11. Articulation points
12. Bubley Dyer simulation (combined with CRF)

Information in (3)–(5), (6), (8), (9), (11) is rendered in textual form, all others display a graphic additionally, like, e.g., in (12) height probability graphs.

In contrast to PyHasse, VB-RAPID provides a graphical editor (menu HASSE Diagram), by which the number of crossings can be manually reduced.

References

Borg, I. and Shye, S. (1995). Facet theory – Form and content. Thousand Oaks, CA: Sage.

Bruggemann, R. and Carlsen, L. (2011). An improved estimation of averaged ranks of partial orders. Match Commun. Math. Comput. Chem., 65, 383–414.

Bruggemann, R. and Voigt, K. (2009). Analysis of partial orders in environmental systems applying the new software PyHasse. In W. Jochen and F. Michael (Eds.), Simulation in Umwelt- und Geowissenschaften, Workshop Potsdam 2009 (pp. 43–55). Aachen: Shaker Verlag.

Bruggemann, R., Restrepo, G. and Voigt, K. (2008a). Towards a new and advanced partial order program: PyHasse. In J. Owsinski and R. Bruggemann (Eds.), Multicriteria ordering and ranking: Partial orders, ambiguities and applied issues (pp. 11–33). Warsaw: Systems Research Institute Polish Academy of Sciences.

Bruggemann, R., Bucherl, C., Pudenz, S. and Steinberg, C. (1999). Application of the concept of partial order on comparative evaluation of environmental chemicals. Acta Hydrochim. Hydrobiol., 27(3), 170–178.

Bruggemann, R., Voigt, K., Restrepo, G. and Simon, U. (2008b). The concept of stability fields and hot spots in ranking of environmental chemicals. Environ. Model. Softw., 23, 1000–1012.

Burmeister, P. (1997). Program CONIMP4, Technische Hochschule Darmstadt, Arbeitsgruppe 1, Fachbereich 4 (Mathematik) WWW-Adresse. http://www.mathematik.th-darmstadt.de/ags/ag1.

Carlsen, L. (2008). Hierarchical partial order ranking. Environ. Pollut., 155, 247–253.

De Loof, K., De Baets, B. and De Meyer, H. (2008a). Properties of mutual rank probabilities in partially ordered sets. In J. Owsinski and R. Bruggemann (Eds.), Multicriteria ordering and ranking: Partial orders, ambiguities and applied issues (pp. 146–165). Warsaw: Systems Research Institute Polish Academy of Sciences.

Formal Concept Analysis. Home page: http://www.upriss.org.uk/fca/fcasoftware.html.

graphviz. See http://4webmaster.de/wiki/Graphviz-Tutorial.

graphviz, download. e.g.: http://www.graphviz.org/Download.php.

Halfon, E. (2006). Hasse diagrams and software development. In R. Bruggemann and L. Carlsen (Eds.), Partial order in environmental sciences and chemistry (pp. 385–392). Berlin: Springer.

Joshi, S., Bruggemann, R., Patil, G.P. and Koli, R. (2010). VB-RAPID, user manual.

Manganaro, A., Ballabio, D., Consonni, V., Mauri, A., Pavan, M. and Todeschini, R. (2008). The DART (Decision Analysis by Ranking Techniques) software. In M. Pavan and R. Todeschini (Eds.), Scientific data ranking methods – theory and applications, Data handling in Science and Technology (pp. 193–208, Vol. 27). Elsevier.

Morton, J., Pachter, L., Shiu, A., Sturmfels, B. and Wienand, O. (2006). Geometry of rank tests (pp. 1–9). http://arvix.org/abs/math/0605173.

Morton, J., Pachter, L., Shiu, A., Sturmfels, B. and Wienand, O. (2009). Convex rank tests and semigraphoids. SIAM J. Discr. Math. 23, 1117–1134.

Pavan, M. (2003). Total and partial ranking methods in chemical sciences. University of Milan, Bicocca, pp. 1–277. (Cycle XVI, Tutor: Prof. Todeschini).

POSAC. See http://ca.huji.ac.il/bf/hudap-Info.pdf

Pudenz, S. (2005). ProRank – software for partial order ranking. Match – Commun. Math. Comput. Chem., 54(3), 611–622.

Saaty, T.L. (1994). How to make a decision: The analytical hierarchy process. Interfaces, 24, 19–43.

Shye, S. (1994). Facet theory. In T. Husen and T.N. Postlethwaite (Eds.), International encyclopedia of education (pp. 2213–2219). Oxford: Pergamon Press.

Software conexp1.3. http://sourceforge.net/projects/conexp/files/conexp/1.3/conexp-1.3.zip/download.

Sørensen, P.B., Bruggemann, R., Thomsen, M. and Lerche, D. (2005). Applications of multidimensional rank-correlation. Match – Commun. Math. Comput. Chem., 54(3), 643–670.

Vogt, F. and Wille, R. (1995a). TOSCANA – A graphical tool for analyzing and exploring data. Knowl. Org., 22, 78–81.

Vogt, F. and Wille, R. (1995b). TOSCANA – A graphical tool for analyzing and exploring data. In R. Tamassia and I.G. Tollis (Eds.), Graph drawing (pp. 226–233). Berlin: Springer.

Voigt, K., Bruggemann, R. and Pudenz, S. (2006). A multi-criteria evaluation of environmental databases using the Hasse diagram technique (ProRank) software. Environ. Model. Softw., 21, 1587–1597.

Voigt, K., Bruggemann, R., Schramm, K. and Kirchner, M. (2008a). PYHASSE: A new software tool for partially ordered sets, example: Ranking of contaminated regions in the alps. In A. Moeller, B. Page, and M. Schreiber (Eds.), Environmental informatics and industrial ecology, 22nd international conference on informatics for environmental protection, Lueneburg, Sept. 10–12, 2008 (pp. 631–636). Aachen: Shaker Verlag.

Voigt, K., Bruggemann, R., Schramm, K. and Kirchner, M. (2008b). PYHASSE: A new software for partially ordered sets. Ranking soil against needles. In J. Owsinski and R. Bruggemann (Eds.), Multicriteria ordering and ranking: Partial orders, ambiguities and applied issues (pp. 37–45). Warsaw: Systems Research Institute Polish Academy of Sciences.

Wienand, O. (2005). http://bio.math.berkeley.edu/ranktests/lcell/index.html

Wienand. O. (2006). http://adsabs.harvard.edu/abs/2006math......5173M

Yager, R.R. (1993). Families of OWA operators. Fuzzy Sets Syst., 59, 125–148.

Yevtushenko, S.A. (2000). System of data analysis 'concept explorer'. Proceedings of the 7th National Conference on Artificial Intelligence, Russia, K II-2000, K-II, pp. 127–134.

Chapter 18
Ranking and Prioritization with Partial Order for Multi-indicator Systems – An Integrative View with a Look Forward

18.1 Looking Back

We started with "Why prioritization, why ranking." We showed that the comparability is a concept, which is suitable for performing prioritization or ranking. When we use computational support, concepts like "comparability" must be formalized. Partial order fits best into the powerful evaluation and utilization of multi-indicator systems.

In Table 18.1, we summarize some published partial order material.

In Chapter 1, we showed examples, where ranking is needed, and posed questions, such as

(1) How do rankings depend on weighting schemes?
(2) Can we provide tools to perform rankings without subjectivism?
(3) Can we give alternatives to ranking by composite indicators?

The monograph has been designed to answer these questions and more.

Now that we are at the end of this monograph, what have been our answers?

(1) We relate the maximal ranking interval of an object due to a composite indicator with partial order characteristics.
(2) Yes, we can. The Hasse diagram allows to identify chains. Objects which are in a chain can be compared without subjectivism, because all attributes uniquely rank one object of the chain higher than another one.
(3) The theoretical approach is to determine from the set of linear extensions the averaged ranks. This is a task of high computational complexity (Pruesse and Ruskey, 1994). Besides the lattice theoretical method (Chapter 9), we have provided alternatives. One promising alternative is the use of the "local partial order model" (LPOM), which is approximate in nature but simple in its application.

R. Brüggemann, G.P. Patil, *Ranking and Prioritization for Multi-indicator Systems*, Environmental and Ecological Statistics 5, DOI 10.1007/978-1-4419-8477-7_18,

Table 18.1 Partial order applications

Set of objects	Main result	References
Regions of Baden-Wuerttemberg, Germany	Identification of pollution pattern which may be caused by former mining activities	Bruggemann et al. (1999)
Sediment sites in Lake Ontario	A classification concerning the loading pattern causing hazards for drinking water and bathing activity	Bruggemann et al. (2001)
European countries	Which services are considered as sufficient and which not	Annoni and Bruggemann (2009)
Web pages	Which Web pages inform best about drinking water quality and why	Voigt and Welzl (2002)
Chemical compounds	How properties of chemicals can be estimated from their position in a partially ordered set	Ivanciuc et al. (2006a, b)
Management strategies	Which strategy is most favorable and why	Simon et al. (2005)
High production volume chemicals	Which chemical should first be examined more closely by simulation models	Lerche et al. (2002)
Regions in Italy	Poverty is a multidimensional problem. Which economical criteria are of most concern	Annoni et al. (2008)
Creeks in southeast of Berlin, Germany	Which creeks should be kept although their maintenance is cost intensive	Bruggemann et al. (2002)
Refrigerants	Which new chemical substances can best replace refrigerants which pose a risk to the environment	Restrepo et al. (2008)
Strategies dismantling nuclear reactors	Which strategy is the best	Van de Walle et al. (1995)
Countries in the world	Human–environment interface based rankings of the countries using land, air, and water indicators at national levels	Patil and Taillie (2004)
Bridges at stream crossings in Pennsylvania, USA	Rankings and prioritizations of bridges and indicators	Newlin and Patil (2010)
Pennsylvania wide 635 square mile hexagonal cells	Rank range runs and endmember eliminations for restoration	Myers and Patil (2010)

As almost everywhere, there is no answer which does not have its "but." So let us take a closer look.

(1) If there is no need to discuss weights then the ranking interval is of no interest.
(2) If there are few chains or if the length of the chains is short, then chains are not helpful. We encountered such a case in the EPI study, see Chapter 15. By METEOR, however, an enrichment is possible for which we need to find weights.
(3) Linear or weak orders based on the combinatorial analysis of the linear extensions depend solely on the partial order implicit in a data matrix. Different data matrices can generate the same partial order, so long as they have a common rank matrix.

However, such linear orders are useful as a means to revisit the weights, or the data matrix itself.

Chapter 2: We introduced the axioms of partial order and discussed the issue of equivalence classes. We arrived at the central instrument for displaying partial order, the Hasse diagram, and presented basic characteristics of partial order, like chains, antichains, maximal and minimal elements, which can be nicely viewed on a Hasse diagram.

Chapter 3: The set of linear extensions is introduced as an important tool. Many partial order concepts are based on linear extensions. We introduced POSAC and showed how the concept of partial order dimension can be helpful.

How can we study complex Hasse diagrams? This issue is of much importance because real-life studies provide us with partial orders whose Hasse diagrams contain a messy system of lines. We introduced down sets and up sets as order theoretical "zooms." We also established a relation between maximum ranking intervals and partial order.

Chapter 4: Here we render tools for discussing the attributes forming the columns of a data matrix: If we deleted one column from the data matrix or added a new column to the data matrix, what is the effect on the Hasse diagram? We developed several tools in the context of attribute-related sensitivity and provided graphs allowing us a view on the evolution of partial order as a function of the canonical sequence of attributes.

Chapter 5: The intricate interplay between attribute values and the Hasse diagram is the main focus of this chapter. Down sets and up sets help us to find relations between the position of an object in a Hasse diagram and properties of the data matrix. The relations supporting properties of the data matrix $\Leftrightarrow$ properties of the partial order are the leading ideas in this chapter and we arrive at the concepts of separability, antagonism, and dominance degree. Separability is a genuine outcome of partial order. Incomparability is not a hindrance to obtain a linear order but a consequence of the data matrix. Once separated object sets are identified, the antagonism is an important concept to see which attributes are responsible for the separation.

Chapter 6: The ordinal character of Hasse diagrams requires a suitable ordinal interpretation of data, even if there may be a loss of small accuracy. A reasonable data manipulation which allows an approximate interpretable Hasse diagram needs to be acceptable. The leading idea is that of order-preserving map: Transformation of data matrices is a legitimate way to explore the data matrix. If the order of objects is the central point, it is clear that the transformation should not change the orders among the objects, i.e., the transformation of the data matrix should be order preserving. An order-preserving transformation will lead to a new poset which is an enrichment of the original one. Clearly, the requirement for order-preserving transformations is not sufficient, since we want to do an ordinal modeling which keeps all "relevant" information to the maximal extent. We discuss several methods, such as, equidistant classification, the p-algorithm, and the fuzzy partial order approach.

Thinking of attribute values as ordinal information implies the question about the changes in a partial order as a result in a change of an attribute value. Correspondingly, the partial order depends not only on the design of the data matrix (in terms of the selection of attributes, their values, and the set of objects) but also on the values of any entry and we call this analysis the attribute value related sensitivity analysis.

Chapter 7: In Chapter 6, we discussed methods to get clearer Hasse diagrams by object-oriented manipulations. In Chapter 7, however, the focus is on manipulations concerning the attributes. We revisit the calculation of an index, observe that the set of linear extensions is more general than any composite indicator. Furthermore, we introduce METEOR and its variants to obtain stability fields and hot spots in the space of weights. Stability fields in the space of weights are useful because they show us where we have some flexibility in selecting numerical values for weights, and where not. When we accept stepwise introduction of weights of linearly aggregated and normalized attributes, then there is also the need of finding the best cumulative aggregation strategy, i.e., that one which enriches the partial order most efficiently. Hence we introduce a method to find out the best aggregation strategy, the method of "comparative acquisition profile" (CAP).

Chapter 8: Whereas in Chapter 6 the objects and in Chapter 7 the attributes are in the focus, Chapter 8 provides a unifying approach: It provides an analysis which takes a symmetric view on the data matrix, the formal concept analysis. An attractive outcome of formal concept analysis is the automatic generation of associations and implications among attributes. How are attributes and their values related with each other given the set of objects of the actual study? We cannot apply this attractive method everywhere, because it needs on the one hand a discretization and suitable scaling, and on the other hand, its lattice diagram becomes very large and very complex.

Chapter 9: How do we get linear orders? This is the main topic in this chapter. We start with the simple concept of levels, discuss local partial order model, give a brief description of the Bubley Dyer algorithm and the lattice theoretical method and of the procedure used in VB-RAPID. One may not always be interested in finding a linear or weak order for all objects. Instead sometimes it is of interest how two incomparable objects rank relatively to each other. An appropriate concept is the mutual probability and we render an estimation method. We are aware that this method is approximate and not applicable for all partial orders because the estimation formula is based on certain structural restrictions of the poset.

Chapter 10: The monograph discusses alternate methods of getting linear orders. Clearly we want to compare them with the index calculations. Accordingly, the focus of this chapter is on how we can compare linear orders or more generally partial orders. Here we introduce concordance analysis, discuss the intersection of posets as a method to compare them, and introduce the concept of proximity of partial orders. For example, it is applied in the study of the Environmental Health Performance Indicator (EPI).

Chapter 11: With Chapter 10, the first part of the monograph is finished. In Chapter 11, we provide real-life examples to illustrate theoretical concepts. For example, we are applying fuzzy partial order to the problem of evaluation of biomanipulation of lakes (Kasprzak et al. 1988) (Section 11.10).

Chapters 12–15: The remaining chapters (Chapters 12, 13, 14, and 15) dwell on real-life case studies, where concepts discussed in former chapters are applied.

18.2 Looking in Between

With progress in sciences and computational advances, the world is not getting simpler, but more and more complex. We are more and more able to describe factors which may be important for characterizing management options. One may even apply complex simulation models to obtain indicators, as briefly discussed in Sections 11.7 and 11.8. Clearly, management will be more and more confronted with multi-indicator systems. Simon et al. (2005), for example, discuss a system of 108 indicators in order to rank nine water management options. These indicators are partially based on mathematical simulation models.

In multi-indicator systems, indicators are carefully invented and quantified, requiring a high degree of sophistication and effort. Most often the indicators are simply combined into a composite indicator. Even if considerable effort is put into the task of finding suitable weights, there are disadvantages:

- Loss of information due to the weighted average. All the efforts and insights put in single indicators get intertwined.
- Subjectivity in the weights.
- Contextual overlap, if several indicators have some aspects in common (see Chapter 12, where the aspect "health" appears three times in the final indicators of the UNICEF study).

Can we do better? What research do we need to let partial order provide essential guidance for handling multi-indicator systems?

Although somewhat repetitive, it may be useful first to summarize the guidance partial orders provide (Table 18.2).

Table 18.2 Multi-indicator system and partial order guidance

Multi-indicator system	Partial order guidance
Role of the attributes of a data matrix. Statistical analysis	Ambiguity graph, attribute-related sensitivity.
Discussion of the results due to a composite indicator	Minimum rank graph and other variants, antagonism, chains, down sets, and up sets. Establish linear or weak orders on the basis of partial order.
Comparing the results of a composite indicator, depending on subjective weights. Performing robustness tests	Attribute value related sensitivity, dominance diagrams, "leading" indicators by search for latent order variables and their relation to the original set of indicators.

Ideally, after the construction of the data matrix, consistent with the aim of the ranking, we should be able to answer:

(1) Whether the loss of information due to a composite indicator is "low," "medium," or "high?" A measure for the loss of information (information seen as a range of values corresponding to the multi-indicator system) can be the rank range of each object.
(2) Whether the partial order can deliver a linear order with only few ties in relation to the total number of order relations?
(3) Whether the ranking based on composite indicator is deviating from the canonical order taken from partial order?
(4) For which object subsets the deviation is strong?
(5) What are then the main reasons for deviations, in terms of weights, attributes, and attribute values?
(6) How to evaluate the findings in (5) above and start an iteration cycle to reduce the deviations?

These six issues are closely related. Software tools should extract satisfactory answers. At the moment, however, it is up to the user to combine appropriately the results of the software tools and to evaluate them. The development of such a software needs computational effort, but also much scientific research on partial order theory.

18.3 Looking Forward

18.3.1 Conceptual Developments

18.3.1.1 Mathematical Concepts of Partial Order

The mathematical study of partial order in its own right provides many concepts which are also useful for applications in multi-indicator systems. For example, we may wish to have a closer look at concepts like the jump and bump numbers which are characteristics of linear extensions and turn out to be useful in queuing problems; see Habib et al. (1988). Do they provide a useful weighting system for linear extensions (Patil and Taillie, 2004)? Bump numbers of linear extensions help identify where chains of the partial order are preserved. Can we extract useful guidance for multi-indicator systems? We think, yes.

If a data matrix consists of data with (white) noise, then depending on the number of attributes, noise will tend to increase the number of incomparabilities. Incomparable pairs are differently represented in linear extensions. Some linear extensions preserve more the chains (bump number is high and correspondingly the jump number is low) whereas some others locate incomparable objects somewhere in the linear order (jump number is high, the bump number is low). Therefore, one may suppress those linear extensions which take to a high degree into account the incomparabilities. In other words, an appropriate weighting scheme for linear extensions based on jump or bump numbers can reduce the effect of noise in the data matrix.

18.3.1.2 Linear Orders and Comparison of Linear Orders

Linear or weak order derived from partial order is an essential component for guidance with a multi-indicator system. Therefore the task is to make optimal use of what is known in the scientific literature in the context of canonical order. For example:

(a) An alternative to get linear order may be to get good estimates of the mutual ranking probabilities, see De Loof et al. (2008a) and from them the linear order (De Loof, 2010).
(b) It is attractive to extend the local partial order model. The crucial point is to classify the incomparable elements in a suitable manner. The LPOM concept for example considers all elements incomparable to an actually selected element x as isolated, with the consequence of many artificial ties, whereas in Bruggemann et al. (2005) and Bruggemann and Carlsen (2011), the elements incomparable to x are differently handled.

18.3.2 Partial Order Concepts vs Composite Indicator

When we obtain linear or weak orders from posets, the comparison with a composite indicator based ranking may reveal discrepancies. It is then of interest to identify subsets of objects or subsets of attributes where either the discrepancies are above a certain limit or below. In any case, we need a systematic procedure which

- identifies the discrepancies,
- make a suggestion for limits when a discrepancy is to be considered as large or small,
- identifies object sets of high/low discrepancy, and
- suggests indicators which are mainly responsible for large/low discrepancies.

Table 18.3 Comparability knowledge discovery

Chapters	Concepts	CI	Non-CI	Ordinal Exploration
2, 3, 6	Partial order and Hasse diagram: Chains and antichains	Yes	No	Yes
3	$\Delta h^{\max}(U)$	Yes	Yes	No
4	Sensitivity analysis	Yes	Yes	Yes
4	Cumulative ambiguity graph	Yes	Yes	Yes
5	Separated subsets	No	No	Yes
5	Antagonism	No	Yes	Yes
5	Dominance	No	Yes	Yes
7	Stability fields	Yes	Yes	No
8	Implications	No	Yes	Yes
9	Canonical orders	Yes	Yes	No
10	Proximity	Yes	Yes	Yes

Here it may be useful to summarize the interplay of partial order techniques and the weights if a composite indicator is already known or not (Table 18.3). In this table, we will consider three basic cases:

Header "CI": Composite indicator is known. Partial order as a tool to get more insights into the aggregation procedure to obtain a composite indicator.

Header "non-CI": Composite indicator is not known. Alternatives to crunch a multi-indicator system by means of databased weights into an index. Indicators serve as proxies for a certain abstract but unknown principle.

Header "Ordinal Exploration": Exploration of ordinal dependencies of a data matrix. A linear (or weak) order is not the primary aim.

The column CI describes how different tools support the known composite indicator, i.e., it is clarified how and how much the ordinal analysis of the data matrix justify the construction of the composite indicator

(a) with respect to the weighting scheme and
(b) with respect to the elected functional form (linear or not).

In case of the composite indicator as a linear function, the analysis reduces to an analysis of the weights. For example, in the first row and third column of Table 18.3, the identification of a chain tells us how many objects are not crucially ordered by the order due to the composite indicator. In the case of the second row but the fourth column, $\Delta h^{\max}(U(x))$ tells us how changing the weights affects the position of objects.

The sensitivity analysis throws light on the collection of the indicators and how much influence the removal of an indicator will have on the poset. Stability fields: A representation of sensitivity and invariance of rankings with respect to weights.

Ranking without weights (canonical order) enables us to examine the reasonableness of composite indicators. Proximity: Different multi-indicator systems having the same object set can be ordinally compared.

18.3.3 Computational Advances and Needs for the Future

Posets are "in good hands" if their mathematical behavior is to be analyzed, because of the increased interest in studying posetic structures in pure mathematics. So, instead of claiming the need of further mathematical research, it is rather the task of the users of posets to make optimal use of the rich knowledge about posets in the mathematical literature (see also Section 16.1). However, even if the mathematical concept turned out to be useful in practical data analytical work, the application may be difficult because of many simple but tedious calculations. Hence, the application of mathematical knowledge for empirical posets requires software which is accessible and understandable by the average trained user and not only by computational experts of the corresponding field. The PyHasse software is a trial to overcome this kind of gap between mathematical development and practical applications. However, we see PyHasse certainly as a preliminary experimental software which can be the starting point for professionally written software.

It is also important that preferences of stakeholders and experts are integrated in the formulation of the framework for the partial order, see Bruggemann et al. (2007) and Rademaker et al. (2008). In this context, the conceptualization behind METEOR (Chapter 7) may be a good example for the incorporation of the preferences of stakeholders and experts:

(1) METEOR includes valuable knowledge about mutual preferences between two indicators and does not require knowledge of weights for the whole set of indicators at once.
(2) Each aggregation enriches the partial order, thus more or longer chains are found (Section 11.8).

So we see METEOR and its further development as a main methodological step toward an efficient help for stakeholders and decision makers.

For further software-oriented development of METEOR, we first have to check whether or not a composite indicator is known.

18.3.3.1 Composite Indicator as a Linear Function Is Known

In that case, we are restricted in the flexibility of selecting weights of the stepwise aggregation, because finally the known set of weights must be obtained. The methodology of CAP (see Chapter 7) fits into this restriction. Within PyHasse (Chapter 17), the CAP methodology is included, and there is also a sequence of aggregations under the guidance of pairwise Spearman correlation.

Independent of the sequence of aggregations, we ask as to how to interpret steep slopes in the CAP graph in terms of the object set. How stable is such a steep slope if we remove or insert objects from and into the data matrix?

18.3.3.2 Composite Indicator Is Not Known

In such a case, weights are uncertain. Here the methodology of stability fields and hot spots in the space of weights applies.

Separability

Separability and related concepts, such as antagonism, are a consequence of applying product order. When object subsets are contextually defined, one may ask about their separation, i.e., ask about their separability degree. If this separability degree is large enough, it is of interest to find the reasons for the separation in terms of the attributes and their values. Corresponding software tools (PyHasse) are under development, however, they still need much effort.

18.3.4 Statistical Significance

We urgently need within the methodology of PoA a quantification of what may be considered as noise and what as significant. What is the significance of a result of matrix W, how sure we are that a maximal element is a maximal element, how significant is an order relation like a < b. To answer these kinds of questions, we have to develop not only a series of well-designed simulation experiments, but also practical guidance applicable even when the multi-indicator system and the object set are large.

18.3.5 Contextual Work

The conceptual work mentioned in Sections 18.2 and 18.3 needs a steady control and verification by case studies. The development of guidance for multi-indicator systems cannot be performed on the basis of pure theoretical work. We need new case studies and also continuing analysis of available case studies. Some ideas follow.

18.3.5.1 Poverty

The available procedures in poverty study are unsatisfactory, since they are based on crude aggregation tools (weighted means), where ordinal variables are treated as they were real numbers (Annoni et al., 2011). Poset theory provides evaluation algorithms that are data driven and do not aggregate ordinal variables, see Fattore

(2008). He derives from the mutual probability a fuzzy membership function assessing the degree of poverty. The problem of poverty is thus translated into the fuzzy framework. Some issues and research questions follow:

- How to define a fuzzy poverty membership function taking into account that the number of linear extensions can be untractable?
- How is the degree of deprivation of an individual assessed?
- Material deprivation changes over time. We need new tools to evaluate the intensity and the structure of material deprivation dynamics.
- Posets arising from material deprivation data are huge. Thus we come back to the problem of data mining in the context of partial order.

18.3.5.2 Bridge Sites

The formal concept analysis was restricted to the "bad alignment bridges." We obtained a network of implications which could be verified by engineers. It will be of interest to examine as to how far this network of implications refers to other states of bridge sites and compare these implication networks. An interesting approach which, however, needs a close cooperation with the engineers is an analysis of the subsets according to the channel types. What can be said about the dominances among such subsets?

18.3.5.3 EPI Index

The EPI index and its data matrix is still a challenge. An important question, for example, can be as to how stable the association networks are when objects are deleted from or added to the data matrix. Furthermore, these association networks depend on the context table. What is the influence of different scaling models? Finally, the association networks among the indicators require an analysis in terms of network concepts.

References

Annoni, P. and Bruggemann, R. (2009). Exploring partial order of European countries. Soc. Indicators Res., 92, 471–487.

Annoni, P., Fattore, M. and Bruggemann, R. (2008). Analyzing the structure of poverty by fuzzy partial order. In J. Owsinski and R. Bruggemann (Eds.), Multicriteria ordering and ranking: Partial orders, ambiguities and applied issues (pp. 107–124). Warsaw: Systems Research Institute Polish Academy of Sciences.

Annoni, P., Bruggemann, R. and Saltelli, A. (2011). Partial order investigation of multiple indicator systems using variance – based sensitivity analysis. Environ. Model. Softw., 26, 950–958.

Bruggemann, R., Bucherl, C., Pudenz, S. and Steinberg, C. (1999). Application of the concept of partial order on comparative evaluation of environmental chemicals. Acta Hydrochim. Hydrobiol., 27(3), 170–178.

Bruggemann, R. and Carlsen, L. (2011). An improved estimation of averaged ranks of partial orders. Match Commun. Math. Comput. Chem., 65, 383–414.

Bruggemann, R., Fredrich, F., Wolter, C., Pudenz, S. and Steinberg, C. (2002). Partielle ordnungen: Ein hilfsmittel zur beschreibung von artengemeinschaften. In A. Gnauck (Ed.), Theorie und modellierung von oekosystemen, Workshop Koelpinsee 2000 (pp. 173–200). Aachen: Shaker-Verlag.

Bruggemann, R., Halfon, E., Welzl, G., Voigt, K. and Steinberg, C. (2001). Applying the concept of partially ordered sets on the ranking of near-shore sediments by a battery of tests. J. Chem. Inf. Comput. Sci., 41(4), 918–925.

Bruggemann, R., Simon, U. and Mey, S. (2005). Estimation of averaged ranks by extended local partial order models. Match – Commun. Math. Comput. Chem., 54(3), 489–518.

Bruggemann, R., Voigt, K., Sørensen, P.B. and De Baets, B. (2007). Partial order concepts in ranking environmental chemicals. In O. Hryniewicz, J. Studzinski, and A. Szediw (Eds.), Environmental informatics and systems research, volume 2: Workshop and application papers (pp. 169–175). Aachen: Shaker Verlag.

De Loof, K., De Baets, B. and De Meyer, H. (2008). Properties of mutual rank probabilities in partially ordered sets. In J. Owsinski and R. Bruggemann (Eds.), Multicriteria ordering and ranking: Partial orders, ambiguities and applied issues (pp. 146–165). Warsaw: Systems Research Institute Polish Academy of Sciences.

De Loof, K., De Baets, B. and De Meyer, H. (2010). Counting linear extension majority cycles in partially ordered sets on up to 13 elements. Comput. Math. Appl., 59, 1541–1547.

Fattore, M. (2008). Hasse diagrams, poset theory and fuzzy poverty measures. Riv. Int. Sci. Soc., 1, 63–75.

Habib, M., Moehring, R.H. and Steiner, G. (1988). Computing the bump number is easy. Order, 5, 107–129.

Ivanciuc, T., Ivanciuc, O. and Klein, D.J. (2006a). Modeling the bioconcentration factors and bioaccumulation factors of polychlorinated biphenyls with posetic quantitative super-structure/activity relationships (QSSAR). Mol. Divers., 10, 133–145.

Ivanciuc, T., Ivanciuc, O. and Klein, D.J. (2006b). Prediction of environmental properties for chlorophenols with posetic quantitative super-structure/property relationships (QSSPR). Int. J. Mol. Sci., 7, 358–374.

Kasprzak, P., Benndorf, J., Koschel, R. and Recknagel, F. (1988). Applicability of the food-web manipulation in the restoration program of a hypertrophic stratified lake: Model studies for Lake Haussee (Feldberg, GDR). Limnologica, 19, 87–95.

Lerche, D., Bruggemann, R., Sorensen, P.B., Carlsen, L. and Nielsen, O.J. (2002). A comparison of partial order technique with three methods of multicriteria analysis for ranking of chemical substances. J. Chem. Inf. Comput. Sci., 42, 1086–1098.

Myers, W.L. and Patil, G.P. (2010). Partial order and rank range runs for compositional complexes in landscape ecology and image analysis, with applications to restoration, remediation, and enhancement. Environ. Ecol. Stat., 17, 411–436.

Newlin, J.T. and Patil, G.P. (2010). Application of partial order to bridge engineering, stream channel assessment, and infra structure management. Environ. Ecol. Stat., 17, 437–454.

Patil, G.P. and Taillie, C. (2004). Multiple indicators, partially ordered sets, and linear extensions: Multi-criterion ranking and prioritization. Environ. Ecol. Stat., 11, 199–228.

Pruesse, G. and Ruskey, F. (1994). Generating linear extensions fast. SIAM J. Comput., 23(2), 373–386.

Rademaker, M., De Baets, B. and De Meyer, H. (2008). New operations for informative combinations of two partial orders with illustrations on pollution data. Comb. Chem. High Throughput Screen., 11(9), 745–755.

Restrepo, G., Bruggemann, R., Weckert, M., Gerstmann, S. and Frank, H. (2008). Ranking patterns, an application to refrigerants. Match – Commun. Math. Comput. Chem., 59, 555–584.

Simon, U., Bruggemann, R., Mey, S. and Pudenz, S. (2005). METEOR – application of a decision support tool based on discrete mathematics. Match – Commun. Math. Comput. Chem., 54(3), 623–642.

Van de Walle, B., De Baets, B. and Kersebaum, K.C. (1995). Fuzzy multi-criteria analysis of cutting techniques in a nuclear dismantling project. Fuzzy Sets Syst., 74, 115–126.

Voigt, K. and Welzl, G. (2002). Drinking water analysis systems in German cities: An evaluation approach combining Hasse diagram technique with multivariate statistical methods. In K. Voigt and G. Welzl (Eds.), Order theoretical tools in environmental sciences – order theory (Hasse diagram technique) meets multivariate statistics (pp. 113–127). Aachen: Shaker-Verlag.

Appendix

Glossary

$\sigma(q_i)$: Normalized sensitivity measure $= 2^*W(X, \text{IB}, \{q_i\})/(n^*(n-1))$, n is the number of objects

$\Gamma(x)$: $= \Sigma g_i{}^* q_i(x) : q_i$ the columns of the data matrix, columnwise normalized, the attributes (indicators) characterizing the objects

Γ: an aggregation function, a function based on the attributes of the information base. It is a weak positive monotone function of the attributes

ζ matrix: A convenient way to code a partial order. Given a partial order $(X, \leq)$ with $|X| = n$, ζ matrix is an $n \times$ n matrix, one row for each element and one column for each element of X. The cell in the row corresponding to an element a and in the column corresponding to an element b of X is 1 if $a \leq b$ and zero otherwise

(X, IB): objects partially ordered on the basis of the information base IB

$|A|$: number of elements in the set A

Aggregation: Technique to reduce the number of attributes. Mostly by weighted sums

AIB(X_1, X_2): set of antagonistic indicators with Sep(X_1, X_2) = 1

AIB: AIB set of antagonistic indicators.

Antichain: Given a partial order $(X, \leq)$, if a subset $X' \subset X$ is such that for no $(x, y) \in X' \times X'\, x \perp y$ holds, then this subset, equipped with the partial order relation, is an antichain.

Articulation point: element whose elimination increases the number of components in the graph

Attributes: Properties of objects that are relevant or helpful in prioritization. Synonyms: indicators. Denoted by $q, q_1, q_2, \ldots$. Properties are ordinal measurements/observations

Axioms of partial order

- if $x \leq y$ and $y \leq x$, then $x = y$ (anti-symmetry)
- if $x \leq y$ and $y \leq z$, then $x \leq z$ (transitivity)
- $x \leq x$ (reflexivity)

R. Brüggemann, G.P. Patil, *Ranking and Prioritization for Multi-indicator Systems*, Environmental and Ecological Statistics 5, DOI 10.1007/978-1-4419-8477-7,

Behavior classes B_i: Comparison of two posets by counting appropriately the matchings $(<, <)$, $(<, >)$. etc. The symbol like $(<, <)$ is a shorthand notation of $(x <_{\mathrm{IB1}} y)$ and $(x <_{\mathrm{IB2}} y)$

Break: by an additional indicator, $x \perp y$ is changing to $x \parallel y$

$\mathrm{CAM}_{\text{object set}} = U_{\text{object set}}/[n^*(n-1)]$

$\mathrm{CAM}_{\text{quotient set}} = U_{\text{quotient set}}/[n_K{}^*(n_{K-1})]$

Canonical order: ranking purely based on the data matrix and the assumption that all linear extensions are equally probable

CAP: Comparative acquisition profile. Method to evaluate aggregation strategies

Chain: If a subset $X' \subset X$ is such that for all $(x, y) \in X' \times X'$ a complete order can be found, then X' together with the partial order relation is a chain

Comparability: Given the data matrix for (X, IB), where $\mathrm{IB} = \{q_1, q_2, \ldots, q_m\}$, objects x and y are comparable if either $x \leq y$ or $y \leq x$

Complete, total, or linear order: A partial order $(X, \leq)$, where $X = \{x_1, x_2, \ldots, x_n\}$ such that $x_1 \leq x_2 \leq \ldots \leq x_n$

Concept: A pair of object set X and property set Q such that $X' = Q$ and $Q' = X$

Concordance analysis: Comparison of two families of ordered subsets

Context table: Table representing $g(x) = q$: $x \in X$, $q \in Q$, x has the property q or q belongs to x

Component: weak connected subposets of a poset

CRF: Cumulative rank frequency

$$d_{\text{coinc}} = 1 - 2^* \, |U_X| \, / \left(n^* \, (n-1)\right)$$

Data matrix: A matrix with n rows and m columns. The cell in the ith row and the jth column is the value $q_i(j)$ of the jth attribute q_j for the object no i

Derivation operator: Relates an object set to its property set or the property set to its object set. $X_i' = \{q \in Q : g(x) = q$, for all $x \in X_i\}$, $Q_i' = \{x \in X : g(x) = q$, for all $q \in Q_i\}$. Instead of the prime as operator, we use the sign d

Discretization scheme: Selection of $\min_i$, $\max_i$, and of $K(q_i)$

Discretization:

$$I(q_i) = [\min_x(q_i(x), \max_x(q_i(x))], \; x \in X$$

The interval $I(q_i)$ is subdivided in $K(q_i)$ subintervals having the same lengths $I_k(q_i)$

$$I(q_i) = \bigcup I_k(q_i), \; k = 1, \ldots, K(q_i), \;\; I_k(q_i) = \min_i + \frac{\max_i - \min_i}{K(q_i)} \cdot [k-1, k),$$

If $k = K(q_i)$, then the closed interval is to be taken.

$$\mathrm{Dom}(X_1, X_2) + \mathrm{Dom}(X_2, X_1) + \mathrm{Sep}(X_1, X_2) = 1$$

$$\mathrm{Dom}(X_1, X_2) := \left|\{(\mathrm{x}, \mathrm{y}) \in X_1{}^* X_2, x \geq y\}\right| / \left(|X_1|^* \, |X_2|\right)$$

$$\mathrm{Dom}(X_2, X_1) := \left|\left\{(x,y) \in X_1{}^*X_2, x \leq y\right\}\right| / \left(|X_1|^*\,|X_2|\right)$$

Elements: members of a set. If the set-theoretical background is important, then objects are considered as elements of a certain set

Equivalence relation $\Re$: A binary relation among objects which is symmetric, reflexive, and transitive. The most often used equivalence relation is the equality of two vectors $q(x)$ and $q(y)$

Equivalent classes: If $q(x) = q(y)$, then x is equivalent to y. The set of all elements, which are mutually equivalent, is called an equivalence class

Equivalent objects $x \cong y$: Given $(X, \{q_1, q_2, \ldots, q_\mathrm{m}\})$, x and y in X are equivalent if $q_i(x) = q_i(y)$, for $i = 1, 2, \ldots, m$

$F(x)$: Principal up set generated by x. $F(x) = \{y \text{ in } X \mid x \leq y\}$. Synonymously, order filter

Greatest element: If there is only one maximal element

Hasse diagram: Visual representation of a partially ordered set

Hasse diagram technique: abbreviation HDT, understood as partial orders derived from data matrices

hav(x): Average height of x in X over LE(X)

Height of a poset: number of elements in the maximum of maximal chain

$h_\mathrm{le}(x)$: Height of an object x in a linear extension le of (X, $\leq$) is the number of elements y such that $y \leq x$ in the linear extension

I_Γ: The rank of a linear or a weak order induced by the index is considered as attribute value

$I(x, y)$: Order interval generated by the pair x, y. $I(x, y) = \{z : \in X, x \leq z \leq y, x, y$ included$\}$. Instead of $I(x, y)$, one also uses $[x, y]$

$\mathrm{IB}(i) = \mathrm{IB} - \{q_i\}$

$\mathrm{IB}^{(k)}$: IB with k attributes

IB: Information base, the set of attributes $\{q_1, q_2, \ldots, q_m\}$

IB_i: any information base

Incomparability: Notion that $x \,||\, y$

Index: An aggregation function that is just a weighted sum of normalized attributes. Synonymously used, composite indicator

Indicators: Attributes

I_poset : The rank of a linear or a weak order derived by partial order is considered as attribute value

Isolated element x: element x for which there is no other element z for which $z > x$ and no other element y for which $y < x$

Isolated elements are maximal and minimal elements at the same time

Kosko measure: $\mathrm{SH}(a, b) = \Sigma \min(q_i(a), q_i(b)) / \Sigma\, q_i(a)$

LE(X): The set of all linear extensions of a poset X

Least element: If there is only one minimal element

Length of a poset, lg: number of cover relations in the maximum of maximal chains

Level 1 object: Given (X, IB), x in X is a level 1 object in the Hasse diagram if there is no y in X such that $y \leq x$

Level: elements in the same vertical position of a Hasse diagram

Level number: Count of levels, starting with the bottom level

Linear extension: Given a partial order $(X, \leq)$, a linear order which preserves the orders of $(X, \leq)$, equivalent

Linear extension: Given a partial order $(X, \leq)$, permutation of X that is order preserving

LOV(.): Latent order variable

LPOM: Local partial order model

m: number of attributes in the data matrix

matrix W: see W matrix

METEOR: method of evaluation by order theory. CAP and stability field and hot spot identification in the space of weights are tools of METEOR

Maximal element x of a chain: An element x for which there is no other element z for which $z > x$

Minimal element x of a chain: An element x for which there is no other element z for which $z < x$

m^r orders: Orders derived by Eq. (2.3) applied on rows of the data matrix which are ordered for increasing values. m^2: min and max values, m^3: min, median, and max values

mutual probability probm$(x > y)$: Count of frequencies how often $x > y$ in the set of linear extensions divided by the total number of linear extensions

$$N(X_1, X_2) = |X_1|^*|X_2|, X_1 \cap X_2 = \varnothing$$

n: number of objects to be prioritized

Navigation: Methods how to identify objects and why they are in positions, where they are. Equations (5.8) and (5.9) are mostly used

O_Γ: Order induced by the index Γ

O<x>: Order induced by <x>. For example, $O_{\text{hav\_LPOM}}$ is the order induced by averaged heights calculated through the local partial order model

$O(x)$: principal down set (often called principal order ideal), generated by x. $O(x) = \{y \text{ in } X \mid y \leq x\}$

$O(x, \text{IB})$: principal order ideal generated by x. $O(x) = \{y \text{ in } X|y \leq x\}$, where X is the poset induced by (X, IB)

Objects: Entities to be prioritized or ranked in order of importance. Object sets denoted by X, X_1, X_2

O_{poset}: Order induced by canonical order

Order preserving map: A map g: $X_1 \rightarrow X_2$ such that $x \leq_1 y$ implies $g(x) \leq_2 g(y)$, given two partial orders $(X_1, \leq_1)$ and $(X_2, \leq_2)$ are order preserving with respect to $\leq_1$ and $\leq_2$

Orientation: A decision about the meaning of high and low values of attributes for the ranking aim

$P(x)$: $P(x) = F(x) - \{x\}$, the predecessors of x

p-algorithm: Transformation of the data matrix

Partial order: A pair $(X, \leq)$ with a set X and a binary relation "$\leq$" over X which is reflexive, antisymmetric, and transitive

Poset: Set with a partial order

Poset ranking: Monte Carlo Markov chain (MCMC) method combined with cumulative rank frequency (CRF) technique

Principal down set: synonym, principal order ideal induced by one element x

Prioritization: Ranking entities in order of importance

probm($x > y$), mutual probability that $x > y$: If $x||y$ in the poset, then pm($x > y$) = (number of linear extensions of poset X with height of x greater than that of y)/|LE(X)|

proper maximal element x: An element for which there $z \neq x$ with $z < x$, but no element $z' \neq x$ for which $z' > x$

proper minimal element x: An element for which there $\mathrm{z} \neq \mathrm{x}$ with $\mathrm{z} > \mathrm{x}$, but no element $\mathrm{z}' \neq \mathrm{x}$ for which $\mathrm{z}' < \mathrm{x}$

property: special case that $q_i(x) = 0$ or 1. If $q_i(x) = 1$, then x "has the ith property"

$q(x) \leq q(y)$: Given (X, IB) and x, y in X, $q(x) \leq q(y)$ if and only if $q_i(x) \leq q_i(y)$, for all q_i in IB

$q_i(x)$: value of the ith attribute for object x

RAPID ranking: Software realization of poset ranking

Quotient set: The set of equivalence classes under a certain equivalence relation, $X/_{\mathfrak{R}}$, $\mathfrak{R}$ often being $\cong$

$S(x)$: $S(x) = \mathrm{O}(x) - \{x\}$, the "successors" of x

Scores: $q_i(x)$ transformed by discretization to $s_i(x)$

$\mathrm{Sep}(X_1, X_2) = |U(X_1, X_2)|\, / N(X_1, X_2)$

$\mathrm{Sep}(X_1, X_2)\!: = |U(X_1, X_2)|\, |\{(x, y) \in X_1{}^*X_2, x||y\}|\, /(|X_1|^*|X_2|)$, then $\mathrm{Sep}(X_1, X_2, \mathrm{IB}) = |U(X_1, X_2, \mathrm{IB})|/N(X_1, X_2)$

Separated object sets X_1, X_2 with $X_1 \cap X_2 = \varnothing$: if for all $x \in X_1$ and for all $y \in X_2$ is valid: $x \mid\mid y$

Set-theoretical representation of (X, IB): a set of ordered pairs $(x, y) \in X^2$ such that $x \leq y$

SH: Subsethood relation

Shape (of a Hasse diagram): visual impression of a Hasse diagram as rectangular or triangular

Superindicator: weighted sum of some indicators

SW: Swamp: Subset of unimportant object set after p-algorithm

Symmetric difference Δ: A and B are sets: $A \ \Delta\ B = A \cup B - A \cap B$

$U(x)\!: = \{y \in X, y||x \text{ in } (X, \mathrm{IB})\}$

$U(X_1, X_2) = \{(x, y)\!: x||y, x \in X_1, y \in X_2, X_1 \cap X_2\}$

$U(X_1, X_2, \mathrm{IB}) = \{(x, y)\!: x||_{\mathrm{IB}}\ y, x \in X_1, y \in X_2, X_1 \cap X_2\}$

$U_{X/\cong}\!: = \{(x, y), x, y$ representants of equivalence classes with $x \mid\mid y\}$

$U_X\!: = \{(x, y), x, y \in X \text{ with } x \mid\mid y\}$

$V = |\{(x, y) \in (X, \mathrm{IB})\}|$

$W(X' \subseteq X, \mathrm{IB}, \mathrm{IB} - \{q_i\})$: sensitivity of a single indicator q_i

$W(x \in X', \mathrm{IB}', \mathrm{IB}'')$: distance measure between $O(x, \mathrm{IB}')$ and $O(x, \mathrm{IB}'') = \left|O(x, \mathrm{IB}')\Delta O(x, \mathrm{IB}'')\right|$

$W(X', \mathrm{IB}', \mathrm{IB}'')$: distance between (X', IB') and $(X', \mathrm{IB}'') = \Sigma\ W(x \in X', \mathrm{IB}', \mathrm{IB}'')$, summed over x in X'

W matrix: $W(X, \mathrm{IB}(i), \mathrm{IB}(j))$ is an entry of the W matrix

Weak order: A linear order of the quotient set; there are equivalence set with more than 1 element (sequence like $a > b = c > d > \ldots$)

Weight vector: A vector of numbers g_i, where $1 \geq g_i \geq 0$ and $\Sigma g_i = 1$. Weights are needed to formulate an index:

Width of a poset: maximum set of mutually incomparable elements

Width: Number of elements in the maximum antichain

W matrix: $W(X, \mathrm{IB}_i, \mathrm{IB}_j)$

$x \leq y$: Given (X, IB) and x and y in X, $x \leq y$ if and only if $q(x) \leq q(y)$

$x < y$: Given $(X, \{q_1, q_2, \ldots, q_m\})$ and x and y in X, $x \leq y$ with $q_i(x) < q_1(y)$ for some i

$x \perp y$: x and y are comparable, without indicating whether $x < y$ or $x > y$

$x \mid\mid y$: Given a partial order $(X, \leq)$),and x and y in X, $x||y$ if and only if neither $x \leq y$ nor $y \leq x$ holds. For (X, IB), $x||y$ if and only if x and y are incomparable

Some Abbreviations Appearing in the Case Studies

ASC: Atlantic slope consortium
EPI: environmental performance index
HD: Hasse diagram
HDT: Hasse diagram technique
HEI: Human environment interface index
HPVC: high production volume chemicals
METEOR: method of evaluation by order theory
PAH: polycondensated aromatic hydrocarbons
PCB: polychlorinated biphenyls
PoA: partial order analysis
POT: partial order theory
QSAR: quantitative structure activity relationships (chemistry)
QSPR: quantitative structure property relationships
VOC: volatile organic chemicals
wwtp: wastewater treatment plant
DPSIR: indicator system of OECD, driving forces, pressures, states, impacts, responses

Tables of the First 11 Chapters

Table A.1 Illustrative example, data matrix (Chapter 6)

	q_1	q_2
a	4.00E − 01	3.00E − 01
b	3.10E + 00	4.00E + 00
c	2.50E + 00	2.10E + 00
d	1.30E + 00	1.40E + 00
e	1.40E + 00	4.90E + 00
f	3.00E + 00	2.90E + 00
g	3.40E + 00	3.00E + 00
h	5.00E + 00	5.00E + 00
i	5.01E + 00	4.80E + 00
j	6.30E + 00	2.00E + 00

Table A.2 Total concentrations of Pb, Cd, and Zn in the epiphytic mosses (mg/kg dry mass) (Chapter 7)

Id	Pb	Cd	Zn
6	11	0.2	31
8	20	0.4	55
7	14	0.3	41
17	13	0.3	63
9	17	0.3	45
16	13	0.4	51
22	14	0.3	41
14	12	0.6	41
5	14	0.4	45
29	9	0.4	29

Data are rounded. "Id" is the identifier for the regions

Table A.3 Data matrix (normalized) of pollution in Baden-Wuerttemberg (Germany)

Regions	Pbnorm	Cdnorm	Znnorm	Snorm
6	0.41964	0.14286	0.00963	0.38043
8	0.64286	0.14286	0.00788	0.38043
7	0.50893	0.19048	0.00876	0.33967
17	0.24107	0.11905	0.01576	0.39946
9	0.01339	0.45238	0.72855	0.0625
16	0.41964	0.2619	0.01226	0.31793
22	0.41964	0.04762	0.00876	0.48913
18	0.19643	1	0.00876	1
30	0.33036	0.16667	0.00788	0.34239
23	0.46429	0.07143	0.02102	0.44837
15	0.375	0.21429	0.00525	0.3587
14	0.41964	0.38095	0.01401	0.40217

Table A.3 (continued)

Regions	Pbnorm	Cdnorm	Znnorm	Snorm
5	0.46429	0.21429	0.01226	0.44565
28	0.375	0.09524	0.01401	0.3587
39	0.41964	0.21429	0.01751	0.37772
40	0.28571	0.11905	0.01401	0.38587
29	0.24107	0.30952	0.00788	0.36141
41	0.28571	0.38095	0.01839	0.40489
42	0.28571	0.21429	0.01313	0.36413
27	0.01786	0.2619	0.00701	0.33967
38	0.73214	0.40476	0.01401	0.37228
49	0.33036	0.2381	0.01664	0.36141
37	0.24107	0.2619	0.01313	0.33424
47	0.46429	0.2381	0.00613	0.35326
48	1	0.97619	0.01313	0.33967
51	0.33036	0.30952	0.0035	0.35054
4	0.33036	0.02381	0.00701	0.3913
3	0.33036	0.30952	0.01138	0.36957
13	0.05357	0.40476	1	0
26	0.33036	0.09524	0.00088	0.34511
36	0.50893	0.09524	0.01138	0.33152
46	0.33036	0.19048	0.01313	0.36141
50	0.59821	0.28571	0.00963	0.375
53	0.41964	0.2619	0.01576	0.38043
45	0.64286	0.38095	0.02364	0.38859
54	0.28571	0.21429	0.00701	0.38043
59	0.55357	0.28571	0.00701	0.30435
60	0.41964	0.45238	0.01226	0.49185
58	0.41964	0.2381	0.00876	0.44293
57	0.73214	0.33333	0.01839	0.40761
35	0.00893	0.54762	0.61471	0.4375
34	0.03571	0.90476	0.81611	0.01359
33	0.04464	0.59524	0.68476	0.04891
25	0.375	0.19048	0.01489	0.30163
12	0.04464	0.52381	0.78109	0.30163
21	0	0.54762	0.71103	0.07337
11	0.375	0.16667	0.00788	0.37228
2	0.28571	0.30952	0.00788	0.38587
1	0.41964	0.07143	0.00263	0.32337
10	0.41964	0.04762	0.00963	0.38859
20	0.64286	0.30952	0.01226	0.375
24	0.73214	0.40476	0.01839	0.37772
31	0.46429	0.33333	0.00876	0.37772
32	0.50893	0.04762	0.01489	0.39946
19	0.33036	0	0	1
43	0.19643	0.2381	0.01839	1
44	0.33036	0.16667	0.01751	0.39402
52	0.86607	0.52381	0.01576	1
56	0.41964	0.2381	0.01401	0.44022

Table A.4 Baden-Wuerttemberg: Equivalence classes and their pollution profile

Equivalent classes (we omit "{" and "}")	Pattern of pollution	Count of objects in each equivalence class
1, **6**, 7, 8, 10, 11, 15.16, 20, 25, 28, 36, 39, 47, 50, 53, 59	1000	17
2, 3, 26, 27, 29, **30**, 37, 40, 42, 46, 49, 51, 54	0000	13
4, **17**, 19, 43, 44	0001	5
9, 12, 13, 21, 33	0120	5
5, **22**, 23, 32, 56, 58	1101	6
14, 60	1101	2
52, **57**	2101	2
24, **38**	2100	2
31, **45**	1100	2
48	2200	1
34	0220	1
35	0111	1
41	0101	1
18	0201	1

Objects used as representatives (see Chapter 2) are in bold letters

Table A.5 HEI data matrix

Country	Country ID	Land index	Air index	Water index	HEI
Antigua and Barbuda	AB	0.5	0.941	0.93	0.79
Afghanistan	AF	0.5	0.999	0.125	0.541
Algeria	AG	0.5	0.958	0.905	0.788
Albania	AL	0.485	0.994	0.94	0.806
Angola	AN	0.495	0.994	0.41	0.633
Austria	AS	0.505	0.905	1	0.803
Australia	AU	0.498	0.787	1	0.761
Azerbaijan	AZ	0.508	0.94	0.795	0.748
Bangladesh	BA	0.506	0.998	0.725	0.743
Brunei Darussalam	BD	0.49	0.795	1	0.762
Burkina Faso	BF	0.497	0.999	0.355	0.617
Belgium	BG	0.498	0.848	1	0.782
Bahamas	BH	0.5	0.929	0.985	0.805
Burundi	BI	0.47	1	0.83	0.766
Belize	BL	0.418	0.98	0.71	0.702
Benin	BN	0.467	0.998	0.43	0.632
Botswana	BO	0.489	0.972	0.805	0.755
Barbados	BR	0.5	0.931	1	0.81
Bhutan	BT	0.5	0.998	0.66	0.719
Bulgaria	BU	0.51	0.926	1	0.812
Bolivia	BV	0.492	0.982	0.765	0.746
Brazil	BZ	0.486	0.979	0.815	0.76
Central A. Republic	CA	0.497	0.999	0.475	0.657
Cambodia	CB	0.483	0.999	0.235	0.572
Chad	CD	0.497	1	0.28	0.592

Table A.5 (continued)

Country	Country ID	Land index	Air index	Water index	HEI
D. R. of the Congo	CG	0.487	0.999	0.33	0.606
China	CH	0.51	0.971	0.575	0.685
Chile	CI	0.498	0.952	0.945	0.799
Cameroon	CM	0.475	0.999	0.685	0.72
Canada	CN	0.5	0.794	1	0.765
Colombia	CO	0.49	0.98	0.885	0.785
Costa Rica	CR	0.487	0.984	0.94	0.803
Comoros	CS	0.488	0.999	0.97	0.819
Cote d'Ivoire	CT	0.456	0.989	0.665	0.703
Cuba	CU	0.513	0.973	0.945	0.81
Cape Verde	CV	0.565	0.996	0.725	0.762
Cyprus	CY	0.53	0.91	1	0.813
Djibouti	DJ	0.5	0.993	0.955	0.816
Dominica	DM	0.472	0.986	0.9	0.786
Denmark	DN	0.501	0.866	1	0.789
Dominican Republic	DR	0.5	0.971	0.765	0.745
Ecuador	EC	0.474	0.975	0.855	0.768
Egypt	EG	0.5	0.981	0.975	0.819
Equatorial Guinea	EQ	0.48	0.994	0.485	0.653
El Salvador	ES	0.482	0.988	0.795	0.755
Finland	FI	0.501	0.852	1	0.784
Fiji	FJ	0.495	0.989	0.45	0.645
France	FR	0.506	0.918	1	0.808
Gambia	GA	0.524	0.998	0.495	0.672
Guinea-Bissau	GB	0.468	0.998	0.56	0.675
Germany	GE	0.5	0.872	1	0.791
Georgia	GG	0.5	0.988	0.895	0.794
Ghana	GH	0.472	0.997	0.725	0.731
Guinea	GI	0.493	0.998	0.53	0.674
Grenada	GN	0.5	0.977	0.96	0.812
Gabon	GO	0.498	0.972	0.695	0.721
Greece	GR	0.512	0.89	1	0.801
Guatemala	GU	0.474	0.989	0.865	0.776
Guyana	GY	0.488	0.977	0.905	0.79
Haiti	HA	0.487	0.998	0.37	0.618
Honduras	HO	0.472	0.99	0.815	0.759
Hungary	HU	0.504	0.933	0.99	0.809
Iceland	IC	0.5	0.893	1	0.798
Indonesia	ID	0.462	0.987	0.665	0.705
Ireland	IL	0.513	0.872	1	0.795
India	IN	0.501	0.987	0.56	0.683
Iraq	IQ	0.5	0.955	0.82	0.758
Iran (Islamic R. of)	IR	0.5	0.948	0.875	0.774
Israel	IS	0.513	0.881	1	0.798
Italy	IT	0.505	0.907	1	0.804
Jamaica	JM	0.474	0.949	0.955	0.793
Jordan	JO	0.5	0.974	0.975	0.816
Japan	JP	0.5	0.889	1	0.797
Kazakhstan	KA	0.504	0.911	0.95	0.788

Table A.5 (continued)

Country	Country ID	Land index	Air index	Water index	HEI
Kenya	KE	0.491	0.996	0.72	0.736
Kiribati	KI	0.5	0.997	0.48	0.659
Korea, D. P. R.	KO	0.5	0.886	0.995	0.794
Korea, Republic of	KR	0.497	0.907	0.775	0.726
Kuwait	KU	0.5	0.681	1	0.727
Kyrgyzstan	KY	0.506	0.984	0.885	0.792
Lao P. D. R.	LA	0.488	0.999	0.335	0.607
Lebanon	LE	0.499	0.94	0.995	0.811
Libyan A. Jamahiriya	LI	0.5	0.92	0.845	0.755
Madagascar	MA	0.489	0.999	0.445	0.644
Morocco	MC	0.5	0.986	0.74	0.742
Maldives	MD	0.5	0.986	0.78	0.755
Mexico	ME	0.483	0.954	0.81	0.749
Mali	ML	0.496	0.999	0.67	0.722
Mongolia	MO	0.498	0.965	0.45	0.638
Mauritania	MR	0.499	0.986	0.35	0.612
Mauritius	MT	0.497	0.982	0.995	0.825
Malawi	MW	0.46	0.999	0.665	0.708
Myanmar	MY	0.458	0.998	0.68	0.712
Mozambique	MZ	0.496	0.999	0.5	0.665
Namibia	NA	0.495	1	0.59	0.695
Nicaragua	NC	0.449	0.992	0.81	0.75
Niger	NG	0.497	0.999	0.395	0.63
Netherlands	NL	0.502	0.864	1	0.789
Norway	NO	0.505	0.89	1	0.798
Nepal	NP	0.472	0.998	0.58	0.683
Nigeria	NR	0.477	0.991	0.58	0.683
New Zealand	NZ	0.508	0.911	1	0.806
Oman	OM	0.5	0.9	0.655	0.685
Peru	PE	0.489	0.987	0.755	0.744
Papua New Guinea	PG	0.487	0.994	0.62	0.7
Philippines	PH	0.484	0.988	0.845	0.772
Pakistan	PK	0.497	0.992	0.76	0.75
Palau	PL	0.5	0.85	0.895	0.748
Panama	PN	0.463	0.975	0.91	0.783
Portugal	PO	0.533	0.934	1	0.822
Paraguay	PR	0.484	0.99	0.86	0.778
Qatar	QA	0.5	0.05	1	0.517
Republic of Moldova	RM	0.502	0.974	0.955	0.81
Rwanda	RW	0.468	0.999	0.245	0.571
Saudi Arabia	SA	0.5	0.835	0.975	0.77
Saint Lucia	SC	0.457	0.984	0.935	0.792
Sudan	SD	0.478	0.998	0.685	0.721
Senegal	SE	0.487	0.996	0.74	0.741
South Africa	SF	0.499	0.897	0.865	0.754
Singapore	SI	0.5	0.721	1	0.74
Saint Kitts and Nevis	SK	0.5	0.969	0.97	0.813
Sri Lanka	SL	0.472	0.995	0.855	0.774
Samoa	SM	0.453	0.991	0.99	0.811

Table A.5 (continued)

Country	Country ID	Land index	Air index	Water index	HEI
Solomon Islands	SN	0.492	0.995	0.525	0.671
Slovakia	SO	0.52	0.902	1	0.807
Spain	SP	0.509	0.92	1	0.81
Sierra Leone	SR	0.473	0.999	0.615	0.696
Suriname	SU	0.5	0.939	0.875	0.771
Saint V. and the Gren.	SV	0.487	0.983	0.945	0.805
Sweden	SW	0.5	0.923	1	0.808
Syrian A. Republic	SY	0.5	0.961	0.85	0.77
Switzerland	SZ	0.506	0.929	1	0.812
Tajikistan	TA	0.5	0.99	0.75	0.747
Thailand	TH	0.488	0.962	0.9	0.784
Tunisia	TN	0.5	0.972	0.82	0.764
Togo	TO	0.48	0.998	0.44	0.639
Turkey	TR	0.502	0.963	0.86	0.775
Trinidad and Tobago	TT	0.477	0.795	0.945	0.739
United Arab Emirates	UA	0.505	0.559	1	0.688
Uganda	UG	0.476	0.999	0.655	0.71
United Kingdom	UK	0.504	0.891	1	0.798
Ukraine	UN	0.503	0.927	0.985	0.805
Uruguay	UR	0.515	0.979	0.96	0.818
United States	US	0.502	0.764	1	0.755
U. R. of Tanzania	UT	0.494	0.999	0.79	0.761
Vanuatu	VA	0.503	0.996	0.94	0.813
Venezuela	VE	0.487	0.921	0.755	0.721
Viet Nam	VN	0.508	0.993	0.62	0.707
Yemen	YE	0.499	0.99	0.535	0.675
Zambia	ZA	0.439	0.998	0.71	0.716
Zimbabwe	ZI	0.456	0.985	0.725	0.722

Table A.6 Biological indicators discretized. 15 Italian regions (Val Baganza)

	VRI	HRA	VRA	Sro	SZ
a	2	2	2	1	0
b	2	1	2	1	0
c	2	0	2	1	1
d	1	2	0	0	0
e	2	1	2	0	0
f	1	1	2	0	0
g	2	1	1	2	2
h	2	1	2	1	0
i	2	1	0	1	1
j	1	2	1	0	0
k	2	2	1	1	0
l	1	1	0	0	0
m	0	1	0	0	0
n	1	2	0	0	0
o	2	1	0	0	0

Data: Case Studies

Table A.7 Child development: Ranks of 21 nations with respect to any of the six indicators[a]

		wb	hs	ed	fa	br	sub
		Material well-being	Health and safety	Educational well-being	Family and peer relationships	Behaviors and risks	Subjective well-being
Netherlands	Ne	10	2	6	3	3	1
Sweden	Sw	1	1	5	15	1	7
Denmark	Dk	4	4	8	9	6	12
Finland	Fi	3	3	4	17	7	11
Spain	Es	12	6	15	8	5	2
Switzerland	Su	5	9	14	4	12	6
Norway	No	2	8	11	10	13	8
Italy	It	14	5	20	1	10	10
Ireland	Ire	19	19	7	7	4	5
Belgium	Be	7	16	1	5	19	16
Germany	De	13	11	10	13	11	9
Canada	Ca	6	13	2	18	17	15
Greece	Gr	15	18	16	11	8	3
Poland	Pl	21	15	3	14	2	19
Czech Republic	Cz	11	10	9	19	9	17
France	Fr	9	7	18	12	14	18
Portugal	Pt	16	14	21	2	15	14
Austria	Au	8	20	19	16	16	4
Hungary	Hu	20	17	13	6	18	13
United States	US	17	21	12	20	20	
Unit. Kingdom	UK	18	12	17	21	21	20

[a]US: missing value for the attribute sub

Table A.8 Individual sensitivities (Section 12.9)

Nation	wb	hs	ed	fa	br	sub
Ne	5	0	0	2	0	0
Sw	0	0	2	7	0	1
Dk	0	0	1	2	0	4
Fi	0	0	1	3	0	1
Es	2	0	2	1	0	0
Su	0	1	4	1	0	1
No	0	1	1	2	0	1
It	0	0	3	0	0	0
Ire	1	0	0	0	0	0
Be	0	1	0	0	0	1
De	0	0	0	2	0	0
Ca	0	1	0	0	0	1
Gr	1	1	1	0	0	0
Pl	0	0	0	0	0	0
Cz	0	0	0	0	0	1
Fr	0	0	1	0	0	0
Pt	0	0	0	0	0	0
Au	0	0	0	1	0	0
Hu	0	0	0	0	0	0
US	0	1	0	0	0	0
UK	0	0	0	0	0	0

Table A.9 Results of attribute value sensitivity

Sub	$\|P\|$	$\|S\|$	$\|U\|$	ed	$\|P\|$	$\|S\|$	$\|U\|$	wb	$\|P\|$	$\|S\|$	$\|U\|$
10	0	3	17	14	0	3	17	18	0	3	17
11	0	3	17	15	0	3	17	17	0	3	17
12	0	4	16	16	0	3	17	16	0	3	17
13	0	5	15	17	0	3	17	15	0	3	17
14	0	5	15	18	0	3	17	14	0	3	17
15	0	5	15	19	0	3	17	13	0	2	18
16	0	5	15	20	0	4	16	12	1	1	18
17	0	5	15	21	0	4	16	11	1	1	18
18	0	6	14					10	1	1	18
19	0	7	13					9	1	1	18
20	0	7	13					8	1	1	18
21	0	7	13					7	1	1	18
								6	1	1	18
								5	1	1	18
								4	1	0	19
								3	1	0	19
								2	1	0	19
								1	1	0	19

Table A.10 Bridge: Basic data matrix

Bridge	I_1	I_2	I_3	I_4	I_5	I_6	I_7	I_8	I_9	I_{10}	I_{11}	I_{12}	I_{13}	Index
1	7	4	6	10	4	7	9	4	10	9	11	11	10	7.846154
2	7	3	5	9	2	8	11	1	6	5	11	10	10	6.769231
3	8	4	7	6	4	11	11	4	7	3	8	8	4	6.538462
4	9	10	8	11	8	11	8	4	11	7	10	9	9	8.846154
5	6	10	8	11	4	10	9	6	8	8	10	11	6	8.230769
6	1	1	4	6	2	8	11	2	4	3	5	6	10	4.846154
7	4	1	3	6	2	5	10	2	5	3	7	6	5	4.538462
14	5	6	9	4	4	9	7	3	3	4	4	4	7	5.307692
15	5	6	7	3	2	3	4	1	1	2	1	1	3	3
16	6	9	8	5	3	7	4	6	2	5	4	3	10	5.538462
17	1	9	7	1	2	3	3	1	1	2	1	1	10	3.230769
18	3	7	7	3	5	9	6	2	3	4	6	5	10	5.384615
19	6	6	7	5	2	3	6	6	5	6	5	6	5	5.230769
20	7	8	7	8	8	7	4	6	4	4	7	3	5	6
21	7	6	10	7	4	9	5	5	3	6	8	10	3	6.384615
22	5	7	7	2	3	5	6	7	1	6	1	4	5	4.538462
23	8	9	6	1	3	2	4	7	1	4	6	1	5	4.384615
24	6	8	7	3	2	7	7	8	3	4	8	7	10	6.153846
25	9	10	11	7	8	9	9	8	3	4	8	2	3	7
26	10	10	10	6	6	11	9	9	5	5	7	7	10	8.076923
27	5	8	7	6	7	9	8	8	3	2	7	8	3	6.230769
28	4	8	7	6	10	9	5	9	3	5	6	9	9	6.923077
29	10	10	8	6	10	10	6	10	4	2	6	7	9	7.538462
30	10	10	7	4	11	9	4	4	2	2	2	2	4	5.461538
31	5	11	9	8	10	8	8	5	8	11	11	11	7	8.615385
32	9	11	5	11	1	8	5	2	8	8	9	6	9	7.076923
33	6	9	8	5	6	6	8	6	3	5	9	6	8	6.538462
34	8	10	5	6	8	5	5	8	5	3	9	4	3	6.076923
35	8	11	8	9	10	10	9	8	4	8	5	6	6	7.846154

Table A.10 (continued)

Bridge	I_1	I_2	I_3	I_4	I_5	I_6	I_7	I_8	I_9	I_{10}	I_{11}	I_{12}	I_{13}	Index
36	2	4	5	5	4	4	6	7	3	4	3	4	2	4.076923
37	8	7	8	7	7	8	9	8	5	5	7	7	9	7.307692
38	10	10	9	7	6	5	8	11	6	8	5	9	2	7.384615
39	7	9	10	6	3	5	8	10	5	6	9	9	10	7.461538
40	9	10	9	3	3	4	6	10	2	4	4	3	4	5.461538
41	5	8	8	9	4	8	9	10	4	4	3	7	2	6.230769
42	8	11	10	11	11	10	10	9	8	10	9	11	5	9.461538
43	2	8	8	9	3	1	7	8	3	1	1	3	3	4.384615
44	3	4	3	6	4	7	8	1	1	5	2	5	1	3.846154
45	6	9	7	8	8	9	8	11	4	2	4	6	9	7
48	11	10	10	8	12	11	9	12	8	12	9	11	5	9.846154
49	10	10	10	8	12	9	9	10	7	8	9	11	6	9.153846
50	9	10	9	9	10	8	9	8	6	4	9	11	4	8.153846
51	7	9	9	7	10	8	10	10	5	3	7	5	5	7.307692
52	9	10	10	10	9	10	10	10	7	12	11	12	6	9.692308
53	9	10	10	9	12	11	9	10	8	8	8	9	5	9.076923
54	10	11	8	10	7	11	9	5	7	7	7	11	1	8
55	8	10	10	8	6	9	9	6	8	8	7	11	10	8.461538
56	7	10	6	10	8	11	2	7	10	10	7	12	5	8.076923
57	10	11	10	10	9	10	10	9	8	9	9	12	8	9.615385

Table A.11 *W* matrix based on the 13 indicators

W_{ij}	Case 0	Case 1	Case 2	Case 3	Case 4	Case 5	Case 6	Case 7	Case 8	Case 9	Case 10	Case 11	Case 12	Case 13
Case 0	0	6	4	7	11	9	6	25	32	1	18	7	4	85
Case 1	6	0	10	13	17	15	12	31	38	7	24	13	10	91
Case 2	4	10	0	11	15	13	10	29	36	5	22	11	8	89
Case 3	7	13	11	0	18	16	13	32	39	8	25	14	11	92
Case 4	11	17	15	18	0	20	17	36	43	12	29	18	15	96
Case 5	9	15	13	16	20	0	15	34	41	10	27	16	13	94
Case 6	6	12	10	13	17	15	0	31	38	7	24	13	10	91
Case 7	25	31	29	32	36	34	31	0	57	26	43	32	29	110
Case 8	32	38	36	39	43	41	38	57	0	33	50	39	36	117
Case 9	1	7	5	8	12	10	7	26	33	0	19	8	5	86
Case 10	18	24	22	25	29	27	24	43	50	19	0	25	22	103
Case 11	7	13	11	14	18	16	13	32	39	8	25	0	11	92
Case 12	4	10	8	11	15	13	10	29	36	5	22	11	0	89
Case 13	85	91	89	92	96	94	91	110	117	86	103	92	89	0

Table A.12 W matrix for four-indicator data set

W_{ij}	Case 0	Case 1	Case 2	Case 3	Case 4
Case 0	0	88	99	63	324
Case 1	88	0	187	151	412
Case 2	99	187	0	162	423
Case 3	63	151	162	0	387
Case 4	324	412	423	387	0

Table A.13 Bridge implications context table (in transposed form)

Bridge	I_1	I_2	I_3	I_4	I_5	I_6	I_7	I_8	I_9	I_{10}	I_{11}	I_{12}	I_{13}
15	1	0	0	0	0	0	0	0	0	0	0	0	1
21	1	0	1	1	1	1	0	0	1	1	1	1	1
25	1	1	1	1	1	1	1	1	1	1	1	0	1
27	1	1	0	0	1	1	1	1	1	0	1	1	1
34	1	1	0	0	1	0	0	1	1	0	1	0	1
36	0	0	0	0	1	0	0	0	1	1	0	0	0
38	1	1	1	1	1	0	1	1	1	1	1	1	0
41	1	1	1	1	1	1	1	1	1	1	0	1	0
43	0	1	1	1	0	0	0	1	1	0	0	0	1
44	0	0	0	0	1	1	1	0	0	1	0	1	0
54	1	1	1	1	1	1	1	0	1	1	1	1	0

Table A.14 Watershed: Level 1 indicators, normalized and correctly oriented (large values indicate a good status of the watershed)

	Level 1				
Watershed	Forest-shed_score	LDI-shed_score	IMP-shed_score	MPAT-shed_score	CORFOR-shed_score
Back River	0.140715	0.066475	0.022456	0.079241	0.070260
Cattail Creek	0.315800	0.660926	0.688812	0.296692	0.240528
Gwynn Falls	0.245400	0.154413	0.044251	0.182014	0.123783
Saint Mary's A	0.694700	0.760678	0.306705	0.633718	0.573722
Southeast Creek	0.323720	0.529329	0.665981	0.419773	0.262891
Upper Patuxent	0.385400	0.673689	0.644129	0.365625	0.400212
Ahoskie	0.701700	0.750497	0.471692	0.664144	0.724929
Buffalo Creek	0.303800	0.604162	0.560414	0.392625	0.653580
Chickahominy	0.446000	0.441737	0.122522	0.384063	0.366770
Christian Creek	0.299400	0.636326	0.445786	0.385581	0.315367
Clearfield Creek	0.741100	0.838575	0.553802	0.716695	0.613931
Conodoguinet A	0.317100	0.518752	0.203652	0.245001	0.282654
Grindle Creek	0.575100	0.679615	0.630803	0.541836	0.665654
Little Contentnea	0.585300	0.655572	0.511001	0.536146	0.542742
Mantua	0.368300	0.416782	0.138940	0.248248	0.119976
Middle Creek	0.428100	0.677209	0.538128	0.432322	0.579040
Middle River	0.308700	0.603747	0.338287	0.298532	0.278166
Pamunkey	0.618600	0.765106	0.599850	0.669773	0.589294
Repaupo	0.354800	0.624655	0.568231	0.379430	0.307367
White Deer Creek	0.945400	0.960655	0.615706	1.000000	0.865975
Wisconisco	0.845500	0.887929	0.479786	0.762334	0.719116

Table A.15 Watershed: Level 2 data. Normalized

	Level 2						
Watershed	BUF_SCORE	IR_SCORE	BA_SCORE	INV_ SCORE	SHA_SCORE	STRM_STRESS	FP_WLSTRES
Back River	0.604700	0.575100	0.428444	0.202500	0.521500	0.218750	0.703750
Cattail Creek	0.357850	0.796550	0.568842	0.652500	0.702250	0.410000	0.279000
Gwynn Falls	0.323200	0.767632	0.564050	0.682500	0.676500	0.311250	0.165000
Saint Mary's A	0.777400	0.689364	0.599000	0.837500	0.696667	0.635000	0.669000
Southeast Creek	0.770100	0.819450	0.581350	0.507500	0.610750	0.571250	0.706000
Upper Patuxent	0.682800	0.637450	0.725421	0.612500	0.812250	0.690000	0.542000
Ahoskie	0.562965	0.361736	0.519488	0.597500	0.477083	0.400000	0.588500
Buffalo Creek	0.352403	0.875346	0.581555	0.860000	0.631000	0.388750	0.244750
Chickahominy	0.583337	0.659803	0.643118	0.760000	0.543000	0.452500	0.498000
Christian Creek	0.094771	0.594500	0.247863	0.920000	0.704000	0.388750	0.466750
Clearfield Creek	0.646642	0.837002	0.155808	0.980000	0.703250	0.395000	0.678750
Conodoguinet A	0.323320	0.723568	0.363688	0.647368	0.692895	0.367105	0.214737
Grindle Creek	0.456235	0.335350	0.467854	0.590000	0.481353	0.447500	0.616250
Little Contentnea	0.519905	0.726832	0.628001	0.822500	0.687745	0.627500	0.743500
Mantua	0.522608	0.893311	0.635562	0.759375	0.687813	0.640625	0.345000
Middle Creek	0.361110	0.790042	0.451871	0.794737	0.670526	0.378947	0.262368
Middle River	0.190991	0.523930	0.266439	0.835000	0.618750	0.250000	0.306750
Pamunkey	0.701264	0.573006	0.703947	0.910000	0.671248	0.545000	0.676500
Repaupo	0.531330	0.848151	0.567568	0.670588	0.710882	0.758824	0.436765
White Deer Creek	0.859772	0.860582	0.801578	0.975000	0.936250	0.795000	0.720000
Wisconisco	0.580086	0.807446	0.524934	0.840000	0.716750	0.436250	0.429500

Table A.16 Six watersheds with level 3 data, not normalized and not correctly oriented

Watershed	Level 3		
	BIBI	FIBI	NO_3
Back River	1.515	2.215	1.318
Cattail Creek	3.756	3.268	4.332
Gwynn Falls	1.938	2.445	1.362
Saint Mary's A	2.858	3.875	0.196
Southeast Creek	2.687	3.444	3.008
Upper Patuxent	3.750	4.113	2.836

Table A.17 LSI and SWR indices

Watershed	Level 1 (LSI)	Level 2 (SWR)
Back River	0.086644	0.454389
Cattail Creek	0.419760	0.590053
Gwynn Falls	0.165877	0.547895
Saint Mary's A	0.610704	0.6578
Southeast Creek	0.420902	0.6608
Upper Patuxent	0.475743	0.703947
Ahoskie	0.669110	0.425078
Buffalo Creek	0.469730	0.634135
Chickahominy	0.367849	0.56638
Christian Creek	0.396977	0.522032
Clearfield Creek	0.700867	0.557112
Conodoguinet A	0.314043	0.55524
Grindle Creek	0.611351	0.415143
Little Contentnea	0.569343	0.704768
Mantua	0.276758	0.704304
Middle Creek	0.513816	0.582975
Middle River	0.356022	0.459299
Pamunkey	0.643537	0.62629
Repaupo	0.431547	0.717355
White Deer Creek	0.887110	0.864193
Wisconisco	0.756694	0.698257

Table A.18 EPI: Data matrix for the EPI study

ISO3Cod	#	I_1	I_2	I_3	I_4	I_5	I_6	I_7	I_8	I_9	I_{10}	I_{11}	I_{12}	I_{13}	I_{14}	I_{15}	I_{16}
AGO	1	0.0	9.7	14.9	0.0	18.3	84.1	94.0	90.0	10.6	56.8	100.0	66.7	100.0	87.4	77.8	9.7
ALB	2	91.0	94.6	86.6	85.0	0.0	28.8	99.5	100.0	0.3	0.7	100.0	66.7	100.0	78.7	80.4	41.0
ARE	3	99.0	96.4	100.0	100.0	51.4	25.6	100.0	24.1	0.0	100.0	100.0	33.3	100.0	0.0	73.7	0.0
ARG	4	97.7	89.2	78.1	100.0	56.6	69.6	86.9	55.9	10.0	69.4	100.0	50.0	93.1	81.3	88.7	13.8
AUS	5	98.8	100.0	100.0	100.0	93.9	0.0	78.0	16.6	14.0	71.5	100.0	83.3	100.0	69.4	81.7	3.7
BEL	6	98.3	93.6	100.0	100.0	87.1	31.0	97.5	9.0	0.3	2.0	100.0	33.3	88.6	70.0	92.3	0.7
BEN	7	36.6	42.2	17.3	12.0	73.7	84.2	98.8	100.0	69.8	100.0	100.0	16.7	100.0	92.4	85.2	0.1
BGD	8	78.8	54.9	36.8	4.0	2.5	11.4	98.8	83.9	14.1	36.6	0.0	16.7	100.0	96.3	85.7	1.8
BGR	9	96.6	100.0	100.0	94.0	67.5	30.2	98.2	33.3	7.5	27.2	100.0	50.0	82.6	43.4	19.6	2.5
BRA	10	91.9	80.1	69.6	73.0	83.7	44.3	99.6	95.8	15.6	58.7	100.0	50.0	92.8	80.1	90.7	37.0
CAN	11	98.9	100.0	100.0	100.0	91.2	21.2	99.8	97.0	9.9	76.5	100.0	66.7	55.0	47.4	85.3	25.9
CHL	12	98.3	91.0	90.3	85.0	60.7	66.7	97.6	69.9	47.5	76.9	100.0	0.0	88.9	78.3	82.4	23.8
CHN	13	94.1	58.5	31.9	70.0	44.7	0.0	35.0	64.3	41.2	84.3	98.7	0.0	100.0	77.3	36.0	6.3
CIV	14	17.8	71.1	27.1	7.0	61.4	91.0	99.4	96.6	46.1	79.7	100.0	33.3	100.0	90.1	80.8	16.6
CMR	15	23.4	33.2	36.8	23.0	46.9	88.0	99.2	100.0	20.8	61.8	100.0	33.3	100.0	97.3	84.4	38.6
COD	16	0.0	2.5	13.7	0.0	70.9	93.8	99.4	100.0	17.5	66.0	100.0	16.7	100.0	98.0	85.9	76.6
COG	17	61.7	2.5	0.0	0.0	42.8	100.0	99.7	100.0	28.8	79.9	100.0	50.0	100.0	89.2	81.9	22.9
COL	18	92.8	85.6	83.0	64.0	89.4	49.4	99.9	94.8	21.4	78.4	100.0	50.0	98.4	91.0	85.6	32.1
CRI	19	98.3	94.6	90.3	42.0	80.2	41.0	99.9	100.0	50.0	100.0	100.0	50.0	99.4	88.2	91.3	52.2
CUB	20	98.5	83.8	97.6	58.0	89.3	11.1	97.5	47.6	32.8	89.6	100.0	50.0	100.0	44.3	77.0	1.8
CYP	21	98.9	100.0	100.0	76.0	67.8	29.3	96.4	100.0	24.1	79.1	100.0	50.0	0.0	78.8	85.6	0.0
DEU	22	99.0	100.0	100.0	100.0	91.3	31.4	98.2	70.9	1.0	2.2	100.0	33.3	34.2	80.2	93.0	3.8
DNK	23	98.7	100.0	100.0	100.0	90.9	32.9	98.4	95.9	11.9	38.0	100.0	16.7	87.1	84.4	94.8	9.2
DOM	24	83.8	87.4	47.7	52.0	79.3	11.0	98.9	62.7	32.4	100.0	100.0	50.0	100.0	87.3	66.9	4.9
DZA	25	96.7	76.5	90.3	96.0	53.3	25.3	0.0	55.3	16.0	39.5	82.3	33.3	100.0	78.5	56.3	0.0
ECU	26	95.0	74.7	66.0	72.0	87.3	69.2	99.7	64.9	34.7	81.0	100.0	16.7	100.0	72.4	71.3	18.8
EGY	27	93.7	96.4	61.1	92.0	0.0	29.5	89.5	53.5	6.1	46.4	0.0	16.7	100.0	70.4	56.4	5.7
ESP	28	99.0	100.0	100.0	100.0	78.4	20.0	92.4	32.3	18.5	96.5	100.0	16.7	49.2	80.9	90.4	9.4
FIN	29	99.2	100.0	100.0	100.0	92.5	38.1	99.7	99.2	24.1	59.4	100.0	50.0	94.6	72.0	92.2	16.3

Table A.18 (continued)

ISO3Cod	#	I_1	I_2	I_3	I_4	I_5	I_6	I_7	I_8	I_9	I_{10}	I_{11}	I_{12}	I_{13}	I_{14}	I_{15}	I_{16}
FRA	30	99.1	100.0	100.0	100.0	95.2	27.7	98.6	84.7	7.1	70.4	100.0	33.3	5.5	79.0	95.1	5.7
GAB	31	61.0	76.5	22.2	66.0	92.2	100.0	99.9	100.0	5.0	100.0	100.0	66.7	100.0	87.8	84.5	25.4
GBR	32	98.9	100.0	100.0	100.0	93.6	29.6	99.2	84.7	28.9	68.7	100.0	50.0	64.9	83.2	89.6	1.2
GEO	33	97.2	56.7	79.3	29.0	37.4	29.0	98.8	87.2	4.3	23.6	100.0	66.7	100.0	58.9	58.8	52.7
GHA	34	58.3	62.1	48.9	5.0	83.4	91.1	98.9	100.0	8.6	69.9	85.9	16.7	100.0	95.4	82.4	36.7
GIN	35	32.3	11.6	0.0	1.0	58.2	81.0	99.0	100.0	13.8	95.6	100.0	50.0	100.0	100.0	93.2	19.9
GMB	36	43.8	67.5	42.9	2.0	41.0	68.8	99.2	100.0	0.5	10.7	67.2	33.3	100.0	100.0	86.6	0.0
GNB	37	0.0	26.0	19.8	5.0	45.8	77.5	99.8	100.0	21.4	44.0	100.0	83.3	100.0	86.2	75.0	0.0
GRC	38	98.8	100.0	100.0	100.0	73.4	28.4	97.9	91.9	4.1	11.5	100.0	33.3	85.3	80.9	84.6	4.3
GTM	39	86.9	91.0	52.6	27.0	65.2	0.0	99.8	100.0	53.2	67.7	100.0	50.0	100.0	92.5	86.7	17.4
HND	40	83.5	81.9	61.1	34.0	72.6	6.3	99.8	95.8	45.3	100.0	99.8	66.7	100.0	84.5	75.1	17.5
HTI	41	48.6	47.7	19.8	18.0	71.6	9.7	98.9	97.2	1.3	27.1	0.0	66.7	100.0	99.3	88.1	9.5
IDN	42	88.6	60.3	41.6	37.0	34.9	15.4	99.9	99.6	16.8	97.1	100.0	50.0	89.6	79.8	69.2	4.6
IND	43	67.1	74.7	14.9	19.0	43.9	12.9	96.5	38.8	11.5	57.1	69.6	16.7	100.0	87.8	45.6	5.3
IRL	44	98.8	100.0	100.0	100.0	91.0	29.6	99.2	100.0	3.5	10.7	92.8	33.3	91.4	90.1	90.5	1.9
IRN	45	94.4	87.4	80.5	98.0	56.4	5.8	91.0	53.7	11.9	63.3	100.0	50.0	100.0	52.4	29.8	1.7
ISL	46	99.1	100.0	100.0	100.0	92.3	30.7	100.0	98.3	14.4	93.7	100.0	0.0	0.0	41.2	94.1	71.4
ISR	47	99.0	100.0	100.0	100.0	70.2	28.9	92.2	0.0	27.8	54.6	100.0	16.7	0.0	82.7	86.5	0.1
ITA	48	98.9	89.4	100.0	100.0	83.8	26.7	93.0	67.7	12.2	62.6	100.0	33.3	35.7	85.6	91.5	6.8
JAM	49	94.3	87.4	75.7	53.0	68.5	26.9	99.8	100.0	65.0	100.0	99.5	66.7	100.0	42.5	52.0	1.3
JOR	50	96.9	83.8	91.5	90.0	52.3	28.8	91.7	0.0	16.3	96.1	80.8	33.3	0.0	62.9	52.7	0.2
JPN	51	98.9	100.0	100.0	100.0	83.5	21.8	99.8	89.7	26.7	100.0	100.0	0.0	0.0	80.8	95.0	6.2
KEN	52	46.5	31.4	36.8	15.0	75.8	98.2	94.9	74.7	18.5	69.9	97.4	16.7	100.0	87.5	77.4	26.2
KHM	53	49.9	0.0	0.0	0.0	58.3	54.8	99.8	100.0	56.1	100.0	100.0	33.3	100.0	100.0	97.3	6.8
KOR	54	98.4	85.6	100.0	100.0	76.8	17.4	99.2	82.3	8.8	39.5	100.0	16.7	0.4	67.5	83.6	0.7
LBN	55	96.0	100.0	97.6	91.0	75.2	29.0	96.8	81.7	0.0	7.0	79.8	50.0	100.0	64.3	70.9	4.5
LBR	56	1.8	31.4	10.0	17.0	78.0	95.1	99.9	100.0	15.3	22.9	100.0	66.7	100.0	97.7	84.1	0.0
LKA	57	97.4	60.3	89.1	11.0	40.4	64.9	96.6	69.8	32.4	70.7	77.2	16.7	100.0	95.5	85.4	15.4
MAR	58	91.5	63.9	52.6	89.0	86.3	22.6	0.0	13.1	2.4	97.2	100.0	16.7	97.0	89.7	77.8	2.1

Table A.18 (continued)

ISO3Cod	#	I_1	I_2	I_3	I_4	I_5	I_6	I_7	I_8	I_9	I_{10}	I_{11}	I_{12}	I_{13}	I_{14}	I_{15}	I_{16}
MDG	59	43.0	0.7	18.5	1.0	73.9	75.5	99.4	78.3	5.2	43.9	100.0	50.0	100.0	95.6	85.8	15.1
MEX	60	95.9	83.8	72.0	78.0	69.1	0.0	0.0	42.4	13.9	64.6	100.0	33.3	84.0	77.0	72.8	4.8
MMR	61	60.2	63.9	67.2	0.0	43.6	11.2	99.8	96.5	11.9	43.2	98.3	33.3	100.0	97.2	96.3	15.1
MOZ	62	8.1	0.0	11.2	13.0	74.2	75.1	98.0	75.4	13.6	36.4	100.0	66.7	100.0	73.7	91.7	92.3
MRT	63	33.4	20.6	29.5	31.0	26.8	35.1	0.0	71.1	0.2	2.9	0.0	66.7	100.0	69.2	43.8	0.8
MYS	64	97.1	91.0	95.1	71.0	90.0	69.6	100.0	98.6	30.2	97.8	100.0	33.3	100.0	65.7	69.2	2.6
NAM	65	64.9	63.9	14.9	17.0	69.2	69.1	78.4	5.0	35.5	99.3	100.0	50.0	100.0	89.7	89.5	28.8
NGA	66	0.0	27.8	24.6	33.0	33.2	78.7	98.2	91.5	15.8	42.0	88.6	16.7	100.0	77.9	73.3	8.4
NIC	67	89.9	65.7	58.7	27.0	77.5	23.5	99.9	100.0	46.9	75.0	100.0	66.7	100.0	91.9	65.0	14.0
NLD	68	98.3	100.0	100.0	100.0	80.8	31.0	97.0	55.9	4.3	14.2	100.0	33.3	68.1	73.5	93.3	1.3
NOR	69	98.9	100.0	100.0	100.0	92.4	33.2	99.9	100.0	8.0	28.0	100.0	0.0	0.0	62.2	93.3	60.4
NZL	70	98.6	94.6	100.0	100.0	95.1	72.2	99.7	97.9	54.7	78.0	100.0	33.3	51.0	65.8	88.9	35.3
OMN	71	97.8	62.1	86.6	100.0	32.2	24.1	100.0	31.5	11.1	50.0	100.0	66.7	100.0	61.3	66.9	0.0
PAK	72	62.1	81.9	44.1	24.0	0.0	16.4	36.7	39.1	6.0	46.5	0.0	33.3	100.0	81.1	64.9	14.0
PAN	73	93.8	83.8	66.0	63.0	69.2	48.0	99.9	95.3	58.1	100.0	100.0	33.3	100.0	66.1	84.8	14.4
PER	74	81.1	65.7	53.8	60.0	63.2	52.5	98.0	69.6	16.6	80.2	100.0	0.0	41.8	90.2	88.3	33.4
PHL	75	94.4	72.9	67.2	15.0	72.0	50.8	99.9	94.5	23.9	100.0	96.1	16.7	95.7	91.8	79.4	22.0
PNG	76	70.8	0.0	33.1	3.0	84.9	62.6	100.0	96.8	2.0	30.8	100.0	83.3	100.0	93.1	88.1	20.4
POL	77	98.4	100.0	100.0	93.0	76.1	31.8	97.6	89.8	2.0	18.6	100.0	16.7	48.0	73.3	49.4	0.7
PRT	78	98.2	100.0	100.0	100.0	83.0	17.2	96.6	81.8	11.7	76.0	99.2	16.7	91.4	83.4	89.0	16.4
ROU	79	95.9	22.4	40.4	91.0	54.6	30.5	72.6	68.5	18.6	25.2	100.0	50.0	47.6	67.3	37.2	9.7
RUS	80	95.3	92.8	84.2	99.0	88.8	22.4	99.7	96.2	10.6	90.9	100.0	50.0	100.0	12.8	20.0	6.1
SAU	81	96.0	81.9	87.8	100.0	31.7	28.7	99.5	5.7	14.9	100.0	100.0	66.7	100.0	28.5	44.7	0.0
SDN	82	49.2	44.0	19.8	0.0	0.0	49.9	89.1	80.5	6.0	48.4	97.6	50.0	100.0	97.9	87.1	9.8
SEN	83	46.5	49.5	41.6	21.0	41.5	64.3	28.3	75.6	22.0	100.0	99.5	16.7	100.0	90.6	82.8	0.0
SLE	84	0.0	22.4	25.8	8.0	62.5	88.4	99.9	100.0	11.5	77.9	97.7	50.0	100.0	92.5	82.5	0.0
SLV	85	91.7	67.5	55.0	35.0	76.4	8.6	99.6	100.0	0.5	12.2	48.4	50.0	100.0	91.7	85.6	29.7
SUR	86	94.7	85.6	91.5	31.0	71.0	76.4	99.9	100.0	16.2	100.0	100.0	83.3	100.0	0.0	32.3	39.3
SVN	87	98.2	100.0	100.0	100.0	81.9	30.4	99.0	100.0	0.0	4.3	100.0	0.0	11.5	73.9	85.0	10.8

Table A.18 (continued)

ISO3Cod	#	I_1	I_2	I_3	I_4	I_5	I_6	I_7	I_8	I_9	I_{10}	I_{11}	I_{12}	I_{13}	I_{14}	I_{15}	I_{16}
SWE	88	99.3	100.0	100.0	100.0	96.2	36.6	99.7	99.4	14.3	72.7	100.0	50.0	93.0	72.5	96.2	28.1
SYR	89	97.2	62.1	72.0	81.0	34.5	29.1	96.5	0.0	1.6	3.2	100.0	16.7	100.0	48.1	0.0	12.6
TGO	90	51.0	11.6	19.8	4.0	74.4	90.3	98.4	100.0	32.9	100.0	67.0	16.7	100.0	97.2	70.6	0.2
THA	91	95.0	72.9	98.8	28.0	53.0	42.1	99.6	84.0	34.8	77.2	72.4	0.0	64.5	79.1	72.4	3.2
TTO	92	95.0	83.8	100.0	100.0	89.9	58.9	99.8	100.0	7.4	18.7	100.0	66.7	100.0	0.0	7.3	0.0
TUN	93	97.1	67.5	75.7	71.0	73.3	24.8	65.0	5.1	0.3	4.1	20.3	50.0	79.3	86.6	81.4	0.3
TUR	94	92.3	87.4	79.3	89.0	68.6	29.5	97.4	74.6	4.5	25.6	100.0	16.7	89.2	78.9	74.3	10.8
TWN	95	92.2	100.0	100.0	100.0	63.1	31.6	99.6	100.0	29.9	86.9	100.0	0.0	14.1	75.6	81.5	1.8
TZA	96	33.4	51.3	34.3	4.0	80.6	91.9	97.0	80.2	38.2	99.4	100.0	16.7	100.0	92.3	84.1	37.9
UKR	97	97.9	96.4	98.8	89.0	82.1	31.1	74.6	55.8	6.6	47.8	100.0	33.3	100.0	8.1	0.0	1.7
USA	98	98.5	100.0	100.0	100.0	89.3	0.1	86.6	61.1	31.8	90.6	100.0	16.7	0.0	68.8	85.1	4.0
VEN	99	88.5	69.3	61.1	100.0	95.8	58.0	99.8	82.3	72.5	100.0	100.0	33.3	0.0	12.5	52.8	20.9
VNM	100	91.4	51.3	28.3	2.0	53.7	36.9	99.6	94.5	12.0	50.1	82.0	33.3	100.0	86.5	52.7	21.6
YEM	101	72.5	44.0	14.9	34.0	37.6	41.4	100.0	0.0	0.0	0.0	90.1	66.7	100.0	67.8	64.3	0.0
ZAF	102	68.1	76.5	59.9	72.0	89.9	67.3	66.5	0.0	11.5	76.9	84.2	33.3	27.6	64.6	54.6	0.2

Table A.19 Values for 16 indicators for 18 nations, belonging to the EU and for which complete data set was available (for the abbreviations of the nations, see Table 15.2)

	CM	DW	AS	IA	UP	RO	NL	WC	WP	EP	TH	OF	AC	EE	CG	RE
BEL	98.3	93.6	100	100	87.1	31	97.5	9	0.3	2	100	33.3	88.6	70	92.3	0.7
BGR	96.6	100	100	94	67.5	30.2	98.2	33.3	7.5	27.2	100	50	82.6	43.4	19.6	2.5
CYP	98.9	100	100	76	67.8	29.3	96.4	100	24.1	79.1	100	50	0	78.8	85.6	0
DEU	99	100	100	100	91.3	31.4	98.2	70.9	1	2.2	100	33.3	34.2	80.2	93	3.8
DNK	98.7	100	100	100	90.9	32.9	98.4	95.9	11.9	38	100	16.7	87.1	84.4	94.8	9.2
ESP	99	100	100	100	78.4	20	92.4	32.3	18.5	96.5	100	16.7	49.2	80.9	90.4	9.4
FIN	99.2	100	100	100	92.5	38.1	99.7	99.2	24.1	59.4	100	50	94.6	72	92.2	16.3
FRA	99.1	100	100	100	95.2	27.7	98.6	84.7	7.1	70.4	100	33.3	5.5	79	95.1	5.7
GBR	98.9	100	100	100	93.6	29.6	99.2	84.7	28.9	68.7	100	50	64.9	83.2	89.6	1.2
GRC	98.8	100	100	100	73.4	28.4	97.9	91.9	4.1	11.5	100	33.3	85.3	80.9	84.6	4.3
IRL	98.8	100	100	100	91	29.6	99.2	100	3.5	10.7	92.8	33.3	91.4	90.1	90.5	1.9
ITA	98.9	89.4	100	100	83.8	26.7	93	67.7	12.2	62.6	100	33.3	35.7	85.6	91.5	6.8
NLD	98.3	100	100	100	80.8	31	97	55.9	4.3	14.2	100	33.3	68.1	73.5	93.3	1.3
POL	98.4	100	100	93	76.1	31.8	97.6	89.8	2	18.6	100	16.7	48	73.3	49.4	0.7
PRT	98.2	100	100	100	83	17.2	96.6	81.8	11.7	76	99.2	16.7	91.4	83.4	89	16.4
ROU	95.9	22.4	40.4	91	54.6	30.5	72.6	68.5	18.6	25.2	100	50	47.6	67.3	37.2	9.7
SVN	98.2	100	100	100	81.9	30.4	99	100	0	4.3	100	0	11.5	73.9	85	10.8
SWE	99.3	100	100	100	96.2	36.6	99.7	99.4	14.3	72.7	100	50	93	72.5	96.2	28.1

Table A.20 Discretized data matrix EPI/EU, 16 indicators

	I_1	I_2	I_3	I_4	I_5	I_6	I_7	I_8	I_9	I_{10}	I_{11}	I_{12}	I_{13}	I_{14}	I_{15}	I_{16}
BEL	2	2	2	2	2	1	2	0	0	0	2	1	2	1	2	0
BGR	0	2	2	2	0	1	2	0	0	0	2	2	2	0	0	0
CYP	2	2	2	0	0	1	2	2	2	2	2	2	0	2	2	0
DEU	2	2	2	2	2	2	2	2	0	0	2	1	1	2	2	0
DNK	2	2	2	2	2	2	2	2	1	1	2	1	2	2	2	0
ESP	2	2	2	2	1	0	2	0	1	2	2	1	1	2	2	1
FIN	2	2	2	2	2	2	2	2	2	1	2	2	2	1	2	1
FRA	2	2	2	2	2	1	2	2	0	2	2	1	0	2	2	0
GBR	2	2	2	2	2	1	2	2	2	2	2	2	2	2	2	0
GRC	2	2	2	2	1	1	2	2	0	0	2	1	2	2	2	0
IRL	2	2	2	2	2	1	2	2	0	0	0	1	2	2	2	0
ITA	2	2	2	2	2	1	2	1	1	1	2	1	1	2	2	0
NLD	2	2	2	2	1	1	2	1	0	0	2	1	2	1	2	0
POL	2	2	2	2	1	2	2	2	0	0	2	1	1	1	1	0
PRT	2	2	2	2	2	0	2	2	1	2	2	1	2	2	2	1
ROU	0	0	0	1	0	1	0	1	1	0	2	2	1	1	0	1
SVN	2	2	2	2	1	1	2	2	0	0	2	0	0	1	2	1
SWE	2	2	2	2	2	2	2	2	1	2	2	2	2	1	2	2

Table A.21 Data matrix, based on 16 indicators (see Table 18.1): ASEAN

ISO3Cod	I_1	I_2	I_3	I_4	I_5	I_6	I_7	I_8	I_9	I_{10}	I_{11}	I_{12}	I_{13}	I_{14}	I_{15}	I_{16}
MYS	97.1	91	95.1	71	90	69.6	100	98.6	30.2	97.8	100	33.3	100	65.7	69.2	2.6
JPN	98.9	100	100	100	83.5	21.8	99.8	89.7	26.7	100	100	0	0	80.8	95	6.2
KOR	98.4	85.6	100	100	76.8	17.4	99.2	82.3	8.8	39.5	100	16.7	0.4	67.5	83.6	0.7
PHL	94.4	72.9	67.2	15	72	50.8	99.9	94.5	23.9	100	96.1	16.7	95.7	91.8	79.4	22
THA	95	72.9	98.8	28	53	42.1	99.6	84	34.8	77.2	72.4	0	64.5	79.1	72.4	3.2
IDN	88.6	60.3	41.6	37	34.9	15.4	99.9	99.6	16.8	97.1	100	50	89.6	79.8	69.2	4.6
MMR	60.2	63.9	67.2	0	43.6	11.2	99.8	96.5	11.9	43.2	98.3	33.3	100	97.2	96.3	15.1
CHN	94.1	58.5	31.9	70	44.7	0	35	64.3	41.2	84.3	98.7	0	100	77.3	36	6.3
VNM	91.4	51.3	28.3	2	53.7	36.9	99.6	94.5	12	50.1	82	33.3	100	86.5	52.7	21.6
KHM	49.9	0	0	0	58.3	54.8	99.8	100	56.1	100	100	33.3	100	100	97.3	6.8

Index

The manufacturer's authorised representative in the EU is Springer
Nature Customer Service Centre GmbH, Europaplatz 3, 69115 Heidelberg,
Germany. If you have any concerns regarding our products, please
contact ProductSafety@springernature.com

Printed and bound by CPI Group (UK) Ltd, Croydon, CR0 4YY
23/07/2026
02174985-0002